Phonetics

A Contemporary Approach

Arden R. Thorum, PhD, CCC-SP

Communicative Disorders
California State University, Fullerton
Fullerton, California

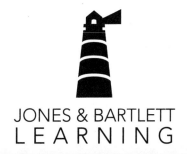

JONES & BARTLETT
LEARNING

World Headquarters
Jones & Bartlett Learning
5 Wall Street
Burlington, MA 01803
978-443-5000
info@jblearning.com
www.jblearning.com

Jones & Bartlett Learning books and products are available through most bookstores and online booksellers. To contact Jones & Bartlett Learning directly, call 800-832-0034, fax 978-443-8000, or visit our website, www.jblearning.com.

Phonetics: A Contemporary Approach is an independent publication and has not been authorized, sponsored, or otherwise approved by the owners of the trademarks or service marks referenced in this product.

Production Credits
Publisher: William Brottmiller
Acquisitions Editor: Katey Birtcher
Managing Editor: Maro Gartside
Editorial Assistant: Teresa Reilly
Production Manager: Julie Champagne Bolduc
Production Editor: Jessica Steele Newfell
Marketing Manager: Grace Richards
Manufacturing and Inventory Control Supervisor: Amy Bacus
Composition: Cenveo Publisher Services
Cover Design: Scott Moden
Photo Researcher: Sarah Cebulski
Cover Image: © dimitris_k/ShutterStock, Inc.
Printing and Binding: Courier Kendallville
Cover Printing: Courier Kendallville

To order this product, use ISBN: 978-1-4496-7889-0

Library of Congress Cataloging-in-Publication Data
Thorum, Arden R., 1935-
  Phonetics : a contemporary approach/Arden R. Thorum.
    p. cm.
  Includes bibliographical references and index.
  ISBN 978-1-4496-3024-9 (pbk. : alk. paper) 1. English language—Phonetics. I. Title.
  PE1135.T56 2012
  421'.5—dc23
                        2011051291

6048
Printed in the United States of America
16 15 14 13 12   10 9 8 7 6 5 4 3 2 1

Dedicated to Jeffrey R. Snelson, a grandson who had everything going for him until cancer took his life at age 23.

He will always be an inspiration to those who knew him.

A percentage of the royalties from this book will be donated to cancer research.

Contents

Contents

Contents

Preface

The study of phonetics encompasses much more than just the ability to recognize the sound/symbols of a language and to develop the skill to transcribe human utterances accurately.

A parallel can be drawn between phonetics and language skills. There are two levels of competency in language usage. One is *performance*, which is the ability of an individual to communicate effectively. The second level is the ability to understand and explain why and how certain language rules apply. This is referred to as *metalinguistics*. These same concepts can be applied to the study of phonetics.

Phonetic performance is the ability to listen to a speaker and accurately transcribe the spoken utterances. *Metaphonetics*, if you will, is the acquired knowledge as to why utterances are spoken the way that they are. This includes an understanding of the historical significance of the origins of words and their pronunciation and spelling (Example: Why do some words contain silent letters?) and the anatomical structures that influence the manner in which the air flow is modified, the placement of the articulators, and whether or not the sound is voiced or unvoiced

In the past, the study of phonetics focused on the development of skills to identify speech sound errors (articulation errors). Recently, it has proven valuable in the identification of phonological processing development and errors. Currently, the study of phonetics has taken on an additional role, that of its relationship to overall literacy, including spelling, reading, and writing.

Phonetics: A Contemporary Approach offers information regarding the historical background of United States English and its dialects. It presents a comprehensive discussion regarding the interrelationship of phonetics and spelling and pronunciation. Dictionary uses and misuses are also discussed.

The organization of the content of the book is based on proven educational learning principles. Because one of the goals of students taking a phonetics course is for them to become competent in sound/symbol recognition, the complete sounds and their phonetic symbols are presented in Chapter 2 rather than throughout the book. This allows the student more time to acquire the skill and reduces the early anxiety that many students have.

The consonant sounds and their phonetic symbols are initially presented in a sequence where those with phonetic symbols that equate to the same alphabet letter come first. For example, the [b] and [p] sound/symbols are presented before the unfamiliar phonetic symbols, such as the *th* sound [Ө]. This allows the student to acquire new information using "familiar" knowledge to assist in the acquisition process.

The sequence of presentation of the vowels and diphthongs follows the same learning principle. They are initially presented in the *traditional* orientation of *front, mid, back,* but the actual study of the vowels and diphthongs is based on attaching to the student's past knowledge of vowel sounds from a *long* and *short vowel* orientation. Thus, the presentation of the vowels is grouped as long vowels, short vowels, and other vowels.

Another educational learning principle is the application of *similarities* and *differences* to gain knowledge and understanding of new information. This principle is applied in the introduction of the *three R sounds*. Rather than presenting these three different sounds with the same alphabet letter in the traditional manner in the vowel and consonant sections of a book, these three sounds are presented in a separate chapter with the intentional purpose of demonstrating their *similarities* and *differences*.

An exciting inclusion in *Phonetics: A Contemporary Approach* is the skill-building activities, which adapt familiar card and board games to the learning of phonetics. In addition, phonetic symbol riddles, word searches, dice, and other game techniques make learning the sounds and their phonetic symbols fun.

STANDARD ENGLISH

Webster's Seventh New Collegiate Dictionary defines *Standard English* as "the English that with respect to spelling, grammar, pronunciation, and vocabulary is substantially uniform though not devoid of regional differences, that is well established by usage in the formal and informal speech and writing of the educated and that is widely recognized as acceptable wherever English is spoken and understood."

During the 1950s and 1960s, there was the *attitude* that if one did not speak Standard English, he or she used substandard speech, with the connotation that something was wrong—not "different" but substandard. As recently as 1996, W. Bryce Evans (Phonics-Phonetics) published a list of words to indicate their "Incorrect and Correct" pronunciation in various dialects in the United States. Give it a try. Which do you say?

women	=	womin	women
winter	=	winder	winter
months	=	mons	months

Years ago when I took a phonetics course, it was drilled into me that the *wh* sound in *when, where, why* had a distinct aspiration of airflow. We would place a thin piece of paper in front of our mouths to visually see the air move the paper. Now, that sound has almost become extinct. There has also been a shift in the use of the [ɑ] sound, such as the first sound in *above* [ɑ-bove]. Instead of saying [opɛn], the more common pronunciation is [opɑn].

And, then there is the ongoing battle I have with my colleagues, who, in my estimation, violate the cardinal rule of phonetics: "Transcribe the sounds as they are spoken." They were taught, as was I, that the last sound in such words as *city* is the same sound as the first sound in *it* regardless of how the word is spoken by the speaker. It was an arbitrary rule! The long *ee* sound has almost entirely replaced the first sound in *it* in the pronunciation of such words as *city*. I hope we can delete that archaic (and erroneous) rule.

I think it was Charles VanRiper, an early pioneer in our field, who defined a speech defect thusly, "A speech defect occurs when it calls attention to itself." In the strictest application of this definition, does that mean that we all have a speech defect when we are speaking to a listener who is not from the same dialect region as we are and he or she is focused more upon *how* we are speaking rather than upon *what* we are saying?

It is somewhat amusing to me when I observe students beginning a class in phonetics. They learn from their peers that not everyone speaks the same way, and it is an eye-opener. Such a situation promotes a discussion on *differences*. It is not wrong when one says *Chicago*, pronouncing the first sound like the first sound in *chair* or the first sound in *shoe*. Students learn that there may be several different ways to pronounce a word and they are all correct by using regional dialects as a standard.

People make subconscious judgments about an individual as soon as they hear the person's spoken words. As listeners, we judge a speaker's character just by how that person pronounces words; any variation from Standard English diminishes that person in our opinion. May we not be found making erroneous judgments and instead focus on *what* is said rather than *how* it is said, and transcribe it accordingly.

Enjoy your adventures in PHONETICS!

Acknowledgments

To my wife, JoAnn, for her assistance in the preparation of the manuscript. To our daughter, Julie Ann Roskelley; without her support and expertise, this publication would not have come to fruition.

I appreciate the encouragement and professional relationship with David D. Cella, publisher, and Katey Birtcher, acquisitions editor, and the high standards and assistance provided through the entire publication process by Maro A. Gartside, managing editor, Teresa Reilly, editorial assistant, and Jessica Newfell, production editor. To Grace A. Richards, marketing manager, for her creativity in marketing this book. To Anupriya Tyagi, project manager, Cenveo Publisher Services, whose attention to the editing of the manuscript was invaluable. To Patti White for her contribution of the original sketches throughout the book. Her artistic abilities are appreciated.

Reviewers

Kelly Scannell Brewer, MS, CCC-SLP
Rehab Manager
Speech-Language Pathologist
Providence Extended Care Center
Anchorage, Alaska

Vannesa Mueller, PhD, CCC-SLP
Assistant Professor and Graduate Advisor
Speech-Language Pathology Program
University of Texas at El Paso
El Paso, Texas

Irene Vogel, PhD
Professor
Department of Linguistics and Cognitive Science
University of Delaware
Newark, Delaware

About the Author

Arden R. Thorum, PhD, is Emeriti Professor of Communicative Disorders, Department of Human Communication, California State University, Fullerton. Dr. Thorum received his doctor of philosophy in speech-language pathology from the University of Utah, his master of arts degree in speech pathology and audiology from California State University, Fullerton, and his bachelor of arts degree in speech pathology and audiology from California State University, Los Angeles.

He began his professional career as a speech and language specialist in the public schools in southern California. He is the author of the Fullerton Language Test for Adolescents and the author and co-author of several books, including *Your Child's Intellect*, which was translated into French. Dr. Thorum is a recognized authority on child language and has appeared on national television. The U.S. Department of Education selected Dr. Thorum as one of a hundred outstanding researchers in special education. He was also awarded a Visiting Distinguished Professor Grant by Rotary International and spent three months in India teaching at various universities, performing clinical demonstrations, and speaking at conferences and seminars.

Dr. Thorum has been recognized several times for his outstanding teaching and has a reputation for his innovative teaching methods. Since his official retirement, he has been invited to continue teaching part-time and is currently in his 41st year.

Chapter 1

What Is Phonetics?

PURPOSE

To describe the science of phonetics and some of its applications.

OBJECTIVES

This chapter will provide you with information regarding:

1. The definition of phonetics
2. Some of the basic requirements needed to study phonetics
3. Background of the International Phonetic Association
4. Symbols used to indicate United States English sounds
5. Phonetic science today and in the future

INTRODUCTION

There are several different approaches to the study of **phonetics**. One is the approach used in this book that focuses on the articulation aspects such as the anatomy of the speech mechanism and the manner in which the airflow is modified, placement of the articulators, and whether or not **sounds** are **voiced** or unvoiced. This approach is referred to as articulation phonetics or **articulatory phonetics** (Stockwell & Minkova, 2001). Another approach

that has gained popularity because of the advancement of available instrumentation is referred to as **acoustic phonetics** (Kent & Read, 2002; Johnson, 1997).

As a beginning student in the study of phonetics, you may be asking yourself, "What exactly is phonetics?" The usual response is, "It is the study of the transcription of *spoken* human sounds into *written* symbols that are designated to each different sound." For example, there are actually two different sounds for the *th* letter combination: the *voiced* /th/ [ð] in the word *the* and the *unvoiced* /th/ [Θ] in the word *thin*. Say these two words while pressing your fingers against your larynx (voice box) and you can feel the difference in vibration.

Granted, that is part of the answer, but it is too simplified to justify the magnitude of the broad scope and impact that the "transcription of sounds to symbols and symbols to sound" has on the modern world. As you will learn, there are many uses for the application of this process.

Phonetic science includes an examination of the following items:

a. Acoustical properties (sound waves) of the sounds—spectrograms
b. Anatomic structures involved in speech sound production (e.g., tongue, teeth)
c. Perception (hearing acuity and discrimination) of the speech sounds; accuracy in hearing the exact sound that is spoken

Aspects of phonetic science are integral parts of many disciplines that often include both subjective (judgment by the human ear) and/or objective (analysis through instrumentation) analysis. Phonetic science has an interdisciplinary orientation, and phoneticians engage in scientific research investigations and clinical applications in the fields of ancient and modern languages, computer science, business and industry, physics, medicine, education, psychology, speech-language pathology, telecommunications, forensic science, entertainment, and for government agencies.

Phonetics is interrelated to other methods of sound analysis such as **phonology** and **phonics**. Phonology includes the analysis of the sound system as it relates to grammatical forms. For example, the "s" sound is a plural marker. If an individual omits the "s" of a plural word, it may indicate that there is not an understanding of the concept of plural rather than it being an articulation error of omission. In phonics, diacritic marks indicate long and short vowels and the pronunciation of other sounds, similar to the markings used in dictionaries.

It is hoped that the information presented here provides you with a broader perspective on the usefulness of phonetic science and motivates you to contribute your knowledge in different disciplines associated with sound-to-symbol and symbol-to-sound transcription.

BROAD NATURE OF PHONETIC SCIENCE

The following information is provided to give you a sense of the usefulness of the discipline of phonetic science. The broad nature of phonetic science can be demonstrated through a series of practical questions:

- What is the relationship between speaking, reading, and writing and each activity's associated auditory and visual disabilities? With the current emphasis on literacy, the sound/spelling/pronunciation relationship of phonetics to speaking, reading, and writing is very significant.

- What characterizes regional varieties of a sound system of a language? The phonetic sound/symbol notation system provides a means whereby specific sounds can be identified and recorded for analyses.

- What is involved in **accent** reduction or acquisition? Elements of phonetic science are involved in the identification of the accent characteristics of speakers. It provides a system to record and analyze the characteristics of accented sounds and words and to modify them when desirable, either to reduce or increase the accent such as in the case of actors. *My Fair Lady*, the musical based on the book *Pygmalion* about how a flower girl in London takes speech lessons from a phonetics professor to pass in high society, is a classic example of this!

- How can voice qualities (**spectrograms**) be objectified and systematically analyzed for voice identification for forensics purposes? This is a relatively new area of development. As technology becomes more valid and reliable in its ability to discriminate speech sounds, application of some of the principles of phonetic science will prove useful.

- How can speech sound disorders be corrected through application of phonetic theory? Phonetic science includes how speech sounds are made correctly. This information provides the framework to assist in the correction of speech sound errors.

- What is the relationship between speech production and speech perception, and how do they affect the deaf and hard-of-hearing populations? Speech sounds have acoustic features that distinguish them from one another. Some sounds are voiced such as the [v] sound. Others, such as the [p] sound, are voiceless (no vibration of the vocal folds). Such phonetic knowledge assists the deaf and hard-of-hearing populations in the development of their sound system.

- What effect does the way one speaks have on interpersonal communication? Aspects of phonetic science include the identification and analyses of different styles of speaking known as the sociolinguistic or pragmatic use of language. For example, you may speak in a more formal manner of precise **articulation** in one setting: "I got you," and in a less formal manner in a different setting: "I gat cha." Or, if you moved away from your hometown and adapted to a new dialect, on arriving back home you discover that you begin to automatically use the mannerisms and dialect of your roots. (And that pleases Grandma!)

- What are the implications for the use of computerized (digital) voices and speech production in business, commerce, government, entertainment, education, medicine, and other fields? The physics of sounds and how to replicate them through digital processing involve phonetic science. Knowledge and application of the uses of "artificial" voice are becoming more and more popular. Most of us have experienced talking on the phone to a "nonhuman." For example, I was walking through a parking structure in a shopping mall and noticed a group of people hovering around an expensive Italian sports car. As I approached them, I heard the following emitted from the car, "You are violating my space. My alarm will go off in 10 seconds if you do not back away!" That is an example of how creative the application of phonetic science is becoming.

Phoneticians throughout the world are engaged in research and development of phonetic science data to answer these questions and other inquiries regarding the usefulness of knowledge in the transmission of sound to symbol and symbol to sound.

CHARACTERISTICS OF SPEECH SOUNDS

Following are some of the characteristics of a speech sound:

1. Each sound has *no meaning* in and of itself. A [t] or [p] sound has no meaning until combined into a recognizable series, such as t-o-p.

2. A speech sound is *maneuverable*. It can occur in different positions within a word such as the [p] in *pie, pepper*, and *stop*.

3. Each sound can be identified by its *physical anatomy*. You will learn how the involvement of the tongue, lips, hard and soft palates, teeth, and alveolar ridge (gum ridge) are used in the production of speech sounds. For example, the upper and lower lips are used to produce the bilabial [p] and [b] sounds. The lower lip and the upper teeth are "articulated" to produce the [f] and [v] sounds.

4. Each sound can be identified by its *acoustic sound waves* that produce a "voice" print displayed on a spectrogram. Such sound properties as frequency, duration, and amplitude can be analyzed. This information is particularly valuable in a **clinical setting** for accent reduction of the vowel sounds.

5. Each speech sound can be *discriminated* in such words as *pet* and *set* for the listener to understand the auditory message. And at a higher cognitive level,

listeners can process homonyms that sound alike but have different meanings, such as *blue-blew*.

6. A speech sound can have a slight **allophonic variation** and still be recognized as the same sound. These similar sounds are referred to as allophones. Notice how the stop and release action of air pressure is slightly different in the production of the two [p] sounds in the word *pop*. The beginning [p] has a greater release of air pressure than does the final [p] sound. However, they are both recognized as the [p] sound and therefore are considered allophones.

WRITTEN VERSUS SPOKEN LANGUAGE

Written language (**orthography**) such as that used in writing and reading consists of printed symbols that represent various combinations of alphabet letters that are sequenced into words. Spoken language consists of the sounds used to speak different words and verbal utterances.

Ball and Lowry (2001) indicate that there are two important problems with English orthography: (1) a symbol does not always represent the same pronunciation: the *c* in *city* and *come*; and (2) a pronunciation can be represented by a range of different symbols, for example, the /f/ sound in *fine* and *phone*.

Both written and spoken language forms convey meaning and serve similar purposes in human communication, but there is a major difference in how each is recorded. Let's use the word *through*, for example. We have learned to spell the word t-h-r-o-u-g-h using seven alphabet letters. However, the number of sounds spoken are only three, th-r-u. These speech sounds are recorded in phonetic symbols: [Өru]. Notice that the /th/ in the word *through* represents only *one* sound and the letters *o, g, h* are silent.

You will discover that there are many exceptions to the rules when it comes to consistency in written language versus the uniform rule that there is a distinct phonetic symbol to represent each of the spoken sounds of words. Take a minute and think of all of the different sounds for the alphabet letter *a*.

Let's analyze just one other difference. For example, consider the words *cat* and *city*. Both begin with the letter *c*, but does that letter have the same sound in each word? You are going to learn a lot about the discrepancies of the English spelling system as you become aware of the phonetic sound/symbol method used to identify the spoken words of United States English. You will discover that there is very little similarity between the written forms of words versus the recorded form of spoken words.

Written language (orthography) consists of groups of alphabet letters arranged in a certain order whereas spoken English consists of a succession of constantly varying noises or speech sounds organized into words. They both convey meaning: One consists of written shapes and the other speech sounds.

These speech sounds are transcribed as phonetic symbols. The symbols for a speech sound might have a different shape from the letter/sound it represents or it might be omitted from the written English alphabet. For example, sh-o-p includes four alphabet letters, *s* and *h, o, p*, but the word has only three sounds: [ʃɑp].

The alphabet letter *c* is used in words like *city* and *car* and represents two different sounds. You will learn that the *c* letter is omitted from the phonetic inventory and is replaced with the [s] and the [k] symbols.

Sound/Symbol Identification

Although some of the *phonetic* symbols for the consonant sounds are the same as the *alphabet* letters such as [p] and [v], several are not. Also, most of the vowel sounds require a different symbol that is not an alphabet letter. For example, the alphabet letter *a*, as you discovered earlier, represents several different sounds as in *sofa* [sofə], *any* [ɛni], *ask* [æsk], and *take* [tek]. Consequently, a different phonetic symbol needs to be written (transcribed) to represent the differences in the sounds.

INTERNATIONAL PHONETIC ASSOCIATION

There was a need to develop a system assigning a different symbol to represent each of the sounds of human speech. What method was used to develop a "phonetic alphabet" and who was responsible for it?

The origin of the International Phonetic Association dates back to 1886. This association promotes the study of the science of phonetics and the application of that science. The membership is worldwide and consists of phoneticians who collaborate on research and issues related to the identification of the human sounds used throughout the world.

The most widely known aspect of its work has been the development and revision of the **International Phonetic Alphabet (IPA)**. The IPA consists of unique symbols assigned to each of the sounds identified by the association. It even includes a different symbol for the *clicking* and *lip smacking* sounds made in some African and Asian languages that convey meaning. Ball and Lowry (2001) note that speech sounds not only include vowels and consonants but also other aspects such as intonation, rhythm, loudness, and tempo.

As it pertains to United States English, the IPA contains a different symbol for each of the vowels and consonants. Although some of the phonetic symbols for the consonant sounds are the same as the alphabet letters, such as the [p] and [f], several are not. Also, most of the vowels and diphthongs (combinations of two sounds) require a different symbol that is not an alphabet letter.

ANALYSIS OF SPEECH SOUNDS

Some of the methods used to analyze speech sounds include the following:

1. *Acoustic properties:* Duration, frequency, and amplitudes of speech sound waves are analyzed and imprinted on spectrograms. This is particularly useful when working with individuals and their accents. It also produces voice prints that can be individualized.

2. *Structures of articulation:* Structures involved in the production of sounds are evaluated for normal structure, absence of structure, deformity of structure, nerve damage such as in dysarthria, and other articulation disorders such as dyspraxia.

3. *Perceptual interpretation:* The listener's ability is accessed in **perceptual phonetics**. Analysis of the listener's acuity (how well he or she hears) and discrimination (the ability to discriminate one sound from another, such as *fin* and *thin*) are analyzed.

BROAD AND NARROW TRANSCRIPTION

Diacritic markings are used for more finite descriptions of speech sound production. For example, the [n] and [d] sounds that are normally *voiced* (the vocal folds vibrate) may be produced with more of a voiceless quality and would thus be transcribed with a small circle under the sound symbol, [n̥] and [d̥]. Transcription using such diacritic markings is referred to as **narrow transcription**. Transcription without these markings is referred to as **broad transcription**.

BASIC COMPETENCY REQUIREMENTS

To become competent in the science of phonetics, you need to acquire knowledge and skills in the following basic areas:

1. *Speech production:* The neuroanatomy and physiology (nerves, bones, muscles) of the articulation process of speech sounds and the interdependency of the speech organs (e.g., lungs, vocal folds, lips, jaws).

2. *Speech acoustics:* The "noises" and human or artificial sounds that produce the acoustic energy that results in the translation of the articulatory (human or mechanical) processes into acoustic vibrations and transmissions.

3. *Speech perception:* The perception and processing of the speech/sound signals by the ear and the brain: listening skills.

4. *Transcription:* The identification of the sound/symbol representation (phonetic symbols) and the accurate transcription of what is spoken into the phonetic symbols that represent the spoken utterance.

The application of this information through study and drill work can result in your becoming proficient in these requirements.

PSYCHOLOGICAL AND SOCIOLOGICAL IMPLICATIONS OF PHONETICS

Although phonetics is defined as the study of the sound system of human speech including its anatomic structures, acoustic energy, and listener's perception, it encompasses much more. In communication, phonetics interfaces with the psychological and sociological aspects of humankind, such as the following:

1. The dialect and speaking style differences of different speakers perceived by different listeners. These styles are determined by the *wh-* factors of who is speaking and listening, what is being said, where it is being said, when, and why it is said in the communication setting. In conjunction with this, you should realize that not all parents desire their children to "speak like everyone else." Speech affects personal identity.

2. The social context and relationships of speaker/listener exhibited in the use of formal, informal, casual, intimate, and threatening relationships. All elements of speech production may change:

"Do you want bread and butter?"

"Day a wan brea 'n budder?"

"Do **you** want bread and butter?"

"Do you want **bread** and butter?"

You can appreciate the role that listening skills play in the perception of the spoken sounds and words that may vary depending on the aspects listed previously.

TECHNOLOGICAL IMPLICATIONS OF PHONETICS

These are exciting times for you as a beginning phonetician for several reasons. Three of these reasons follow:

1. Enhancement of instructional materials

2. Increased level of sophistication in research

3. Prescriptive clinical applications

You should make it a goal to become familiar with the basics associated with these three reasons, and then develop knowledge and skills in the areas of technology and phonetics to be used in your future professional settings.

Also, phoneticians have opportunities to be employed as consultants or employees in the research and development of new products that have aspects related to phonetic science.

Instructional Materials

First, as a benefit to you as a beginning student in phonetics, there is a variety of new electronic teaching aids available at the self-tutoring level. Presently, an abundance of computer programs are user friendly and effective. Some of these programs are instructor produced while others are commercially available. Many include an interactive component with both printed and synthesized voice exercises. You simply need to enter the key word *phonetics* in a search engine on the Web and several options will appear. You are encouraged to search these websites and benefit from such resources.

Hoffman and Buckingham (2000) recognize the need for and value of a computerized laboratory for students. They developed a set of digital videos that allows more flexibility for students to select transcription exercises to practice. They indicate that the advanced technological equipment provides students with improved clinical performances during their beginning clinical practicum experiences.

Research and Technology

Computers have become available for research in voice production related to speech perception, reception, and expression. Because computers are used for research, you should learn their applications in phonetic science so as to assist in future academic and clinical needs.

The computerized methods used to analyze the characteristics of human speech have greatly enhanced the quality and quantity of data acquired in phonetic science. Research results from computerized analyses have increased validity and reliability.

Clinical Application

To reach the level of competency required in clinical interventions, you must become proficient in the use of available electronic equipment. The widespread availability and use of computers continue to affect the manner in which clinicians analyze phonetic production.

Phonetic science has a *subjective* aspect that is determined in a speaker–listener relationship. But as significant and valuable is the *objective* aspect that can be measured by instrumentation. Both the subjective and objective aspects are needed in clinical evaluation and treatment. You will learn more about the relationship between the clinical application of phonetics and the diagnosis and treatment of articulation disorders in your studies.

A Word of Caution

In this age of technology where the tendency may be to shift attention to more objective analyses, you need to keep things in balance. True, aspects of phonetic science lend themselves to instrumentation and you should vigorously pursue competency in these areas. However, there are also essential skills that are subjective in nature. You should be sure to engage in human interaction.

Nothing can replace the experiences of group participation where speakers and listeners gain insight from their dialogue regarding the *spoken sounds* and the *transcription* recorded from listening to one another's speech. You are encouraged to form small study groups and to participate both as the speaker and the listener/transcriber as you practice the drill work.

Always keep in mind that the *sound system* (*dialects*) that we use may be different but still meet the definition of a *correct standard* for any given linguistic geographic region.

SUMMARY

You should not view phonetic science from a narrow perspective of phonetic symbols and sounds but realize that it has great diversity in use both in scientific and nonscientific areas. Basic elements of the characteristics of the sounds and symbols are unique, but once that foundation has been acquired, the application of such knowledge provides many opportunities in a wide variety of settings, including education, industry, medicine, speech-language pathology, linguistics, anthropology, psychology, and more.

Phonetic science includes the study of speech sounds, their acoustic (sound waves) and physical (articulation structures) properties, and the perception of these speech sounds by listeners. Phonetics does not concentrate on the *meaning* of sounds in words but rather on the *features* of the sounds and their influence on one another.

Enhanced listening skills are a requirement to be a successful transcriber of the spoken word. You need to avoid "re-auditorizing" a word spoken by another because there may be a difference between the way the two of you might speak it.

The International Phonetic Association (IPA) developed a set of symbols and other markings to represent the sounds of languages spoken worldwide. Among these sounds/symbols are those used to represent the sounds of United States English. This method of recording is referred to as broad transcription. Narrow transcription is the use of designated marks to indicate variation in pronunciation of sounds within words, primary and secondary syllable stress, and intonation.

Phonetic science has many different disciplines that focus on different aspects of the production and reception of human speech. Two of the more recently involved disciplines include forensic phonetics and synthetic and computerized (digital) phonetics. Other fields of study include phonology and phonics. Each approaches the study of sounds differently and for different purposes; however, much of the theoretical foundation is closely related to phonetics.

The need to incorporate phonetic skills in the teaching of literacy is expanding, and the use of voice-activated technology will continue to increase to meet needs in many consumer and clinical settings.

Good luck to you in your pursuit of competency in transcription of the sounds and symbols of phonetics!

REFERENCES

Ball, M. J., & Lowry, O. (2001). *Methods in clinical phonetics*. London, England: Whurr Publishers.

Hoffman, P. R., & Buckingham, H. W. (2000). Development of a computer-aided phonetic transcription laboratory. *American Journal of Speech-Language Pathology, 9,* 275–281.

International Phonetic Association. (1999). *Handbook of the International Phonetic Alphabet.* Cambridge, England: Cambridge University Press.

Johnson, K. (1997). *Acoustic auditory phonetics*. Oxford, England: Blackwell Publishers.

Kent, R. D., & Read, C. (2002). *Acoustic analysis of speech* (2nd ed.). San Diego, California: Singular Publishers.

Stockwell, R., & Minkova, D. (2001). *English words: History and structure*. Cambridge, England: Cambridge University Press.

What You Will Find in This Text

To help you along the way to proficiency, here is a description of the chapters that follow.

Chapter 2, "Phonetics: Sound/Symbol Recognition," introduces you to the phonetic symbols used to identify the 17 familiar consonant symbols such as [p] and [d], the 8 unfamiliar consonant symbols such as /sh/ [ʃ] and /th/ [θ], the 14 vowels, and 5 diphthongs symbols of United States English. These are presented to you in a step-by-step method that simplifies your acquisition of this information. To further assist you in learning the sound/symbol inventory, games such as card games, word searches, riddles, concentration/memory games, and dice are suggested to make learning fun. Continue playing these games until you are competent in fluently using the symbols and their sounds. The overall purpose of this chapter is to assist you in learning the sounds/symbols used to identify the sounds of United States English.

Chapter 3, "The English Language and United States English Dialects," takes you for a ride on a time machine as you journey from Old English to modern times. You will observe the wide variety of languages that comprise the English vocabulary, sometimes resulting from invasions by other countries or for religious or political reasons. You may be surprised to learn that Queen Victoria's first language was French and that she was later tutored in English. Before the Great Vowel Change toward the end of the period of Middle English, these pairs of words had the same vowel sound: *name/father, wine/mean*. In early Modern English during Shakespeare's time, *reason* had the same vowel sound as *raisin* and *face* as *ask*. After we depart from the Atlantic shore of England and land on the shoreline of the United States, you will learn, among many things, the contributions of the American Indians and the slaves to the sound system and vocabulary of United States English. Also, you may find it interesting that Boston has at least five different accents depending on which side of the river you live on.

Chapter 4, "United States English Spelling and Pronunciation Differences," invites you to explore the historical spelling of words and the changes that have occurred over time, evolving to the current generation of instant messaging and texting. Some learners that speak English as a second language might already appreciate the discrepancies that exist in the pronunciation rules (or lack of rules): *tough-bough-cough-dough*. Some of you may become directly involved in literacy programs and find the information in this chapter most helpful.

Chapter 5, "The Three Ss: Sounds, Syllables, and Suprasegmentals," offers a discussion on sound and how it relates to human listening. You will learn about the three components that interact to produce human speech: (1) energy, (2) sound sources, and (3) the role of resonance. It may surprise you to learn that some spoken languages include *oral clicks* and *glottal stops* to communicate. You will learn about **syllables** and how challenging their identification can be. For example, you will probably readily agree that the word *boundary* has three syllables, but will we agree in the division? Is it *bound-a-ry* or *boun-da-ry* or is the word reduced to two syllables, *boun-dray*? You will learn about the role that prosodic features or suprasegments such as rate, rhythm, intonation, loudness, and stress play in human speech production. Take, for example, the word *present*. Unless you recognize which syllable receives the primary stress, you will not know whether it is used as a noun or a verb: "I will pre**sent** her with a **pre**sent." Suprasegmental features play important roles in accent reduction and correction of monotone speech. At the end of this chapter, you will find some challenging exercises that require you to identify the number of sounds, number of syllables, and which syllable has the primary stress. These exercises are included to assist you in reducing your *alphabet–orthographic* spelling habits and in concentrating on your phonetic transcription skills.

Chapter 6, "Anatomy and Physiology of the Speech and Hearing Mechanisms," provides you with basic information on the parts of the body that are responsible for the production of speech sounds and the reception of these sounds. As mentioned earlier, three distinct features are used to describe the human speech sounds of United States English: plus or minus voicing, the [b] versus the [p] sound; modification of the airflow, [p] stop-release versus [f] constricted/continuous; and placement of the articulators, [b] bilabial (lips) versus [f] lower lip and upper teeth (dental). You will become familiar with these distinctive features and be able to recognize/describe each sound by its anatomic and physiologic features. For example, a voiceless, lingua (tongue), dental, plosive sound is [t].

Chapter 7, "Vowels and Diphthongs," provides an overview of the characteristics of American English vowels and **diphthongs**. Using the oral cavity (mouth) as a reference, the placement of the tongue within the oral cavity is indicated by perimeters of high-, mid-, low- and front, central, and back. Other characteristics include tongue tenseness (eeeee) or laxness (aaaaa) and if the lips are round (ooooo) or unround (eeeee).

Chapters 8, 9, and 10 each present a comprehensive discussion of the vowels and diphthongs. In addition to

a description of how each sound is produced, information regarding the following is provided:

1. Different spelling of the sound: [e] *gate, they*.
2. Different sounds for the same letter: *a* in *father, ask*.
3. Rules for spelling and pronunciation of the sound. For example, some consonants that follow the [e] sound are silent, as in *weigh, day*.
4. Drill work of words that contain each vowel or diphthong.
5. Auditory discrimination exercises.
6. Allophonic and dialect variations.
7. Nonnative speaker pronunciation.
8. Common speech sound deviations.
9. Competency quizzes.

Chapter 11, "The Three Rs: A Consonant and Two Vowels," clusters together the different sounds/symbols for the *r* alphabet letter. For example, the traditional letter *r* is the phonetic [r] symbol for words such as *ring, train*; the *r* becomes an intervocalic stressed vowel sound in such words as *bird, fur*; and it becomes the unstressed counterpart in *mother, father*. The same subtopics are discussed as those that appear in the previous chapters on vowels and diphthongs, and there are ample opportunities to engage in transcription exercises. The chapter concludes with a skill-building exercise that challenges your knowledge of the three basic characteristics of each of the /r/ sounds.

Chapter 12, "United States English Consonants," introduces you to the characteristics of the 25 consonants as determined by placement of the articulation, manner in which the airflow is modified, and plus or minus voicing. The content of this chapter provides you with the foundation to build on as you learn more specifics about each consonant sound in the following chapters.

Chapter 13, "Familiar Phonetic Symbols: Stop Consonants Analysis and Transcription," provides you with comprehensive information regarding the six stop consonants, [p], [b], [t], [d], [k], and [g]. You will learn about the following:

1. Identification and description of how the consonant sounds are produced
2. Different spellings for each sound and different sounds for each of the corresponding orthographic letters
3. Rules for spelling and pronunciation of each sound

4. Various "sound contexts" in which each sound occurs

5. Examples of cognates and other minimal pairs for auditory discrimination

6. Examples of allophonic variations, dialect differences, and nonnative speaker difficulties

7. Normal development and disordered production of each sound

8. Phonetic transcription exercises throughout the chapter and competency quiz

These eight items are presented in each of the following four chapters.

Chapters 14 and 15 present the fricative sounds and familiar symbols [f], [v], [s], [z], and [h]. Unfamiliar symbols include the voiced [ð] and unvoiced [Ө] /th/, the /sh/ [ʃ], [ʒ], as in *azure*, and the [ʍ], as in *when*.

Chapter 16, "Affricative Consonants: Two Sounds Combine to Make One," provides a comprehensive discussion of one set of affricative consonants [ʤ],

jam [ʤæm] and [ʧ] *chin* [ʧɪn]. The main difference in these two cognate pairs is that the [ʤ] is voiced and the [ʧ] is unvoiced. Placement of the articulators and manner of airflow are the same.

Chapter 17, "Nasal and Oral Resonance Consonants Analysis and Transcription," offers a discussion of the three nasal resonance consonants [m], [n], and [ŋ] and the four oral resonance consonants [w], [j], [l], and [r].

Chapter 18, "Clinical Application: 'Make Your Own Articulation Test,'" is the chapter you have been waiting for . . . the *application* of the sound/symbol system in clinical settings. You use your creativity in the development of an articulation test. Yes, your original test!

Post Script

Appendix A, "fʌn wɪӨ fənɛtɪks," includes phonetic activities using game techniques such as phonetic dice, matching, anagrams, word riddles, word searches, various card games, and skill-building activities.

Appendix B includes instructions for "Phonetic Dice" game.

Chapter 2

Phonetics: Sound/Symbol Recognition

PURPOSE

To introduce you to the phonetic symbols that represent the United States English sounds.

OBJECTIVES

This chapter will provide you with information regarding:

1. Some cardinal rules for you to consider
2. Familiar orthographic (alphabet) letters that represent consonant phonetic symbols
3. Unfamiliar phonetic symbols that represent other consonant sounds
4. The symbol used for syllabic consonants
5. The phonetic symbols of vowels, diphthongs, glottal stop, and flap
6. Examples of activities to increase sound/symbol identification
7. Sound/symbol exercises and transcription

INTRODUCTION

Traditionally, the phonetic symbols that represent United States English sounds have been presented in conjunction with a comprehensive discussion of each sound.

For example, the *plosive* sounds of [p], [b], [t], [d], [k], and [g] would be presented in one chapter. Each chapter that followed would continue to introduce sounds/symbols that had some common phonetic features. Generally, transcription exercises would be included as part of the chapter content.

The approach used here is different. It is different for the following reasons:

1. As you realize that there is not an overwhelming number of sounds/symbols to learn, the less apprehensiveness you will experience in acquiring these phonetic symbols.
2. The major prerequisite to mastery in transcription is the acquisition of the *identification of each phonetic symbol* to be used. The introduction of these symbols at the beginning of the book allows more time to acquire and use these symbols.
3. It has been demonstrated that students can learn the sounds/symbols of the International Phonetic Alphabet as a unit and gain information by acquiring this skill early in the course of instruction.

The style of the content of this chapter also is different because its content dictates a different format. The informal presentation of the section on the 41 steps to learn the consonant sounds provides a basic approach to the acquisition of the sound/symbol combinations. This informal approach should also add an element of "fun" to help you realize that it is not a difficult task to acquire the sounds/symbols of the International Phonetic Alphabet.

Many beginning students are apprehensive when they realize they need to learn unfamiliar symbols and apply them to phonetic transcription. For some, this apprehension creates a barrier to learning because the students perceive the acquisition skill of sound/symbol recognition as a difficult task. Students need to invest time and effort because there is an element of exactness required, that is, a different symbol represents each different sound and some of these symbols are unfamiliar. However, the use of a systematic step-by-step approach such as that suggested in this chapter simplifies the task.

The first part of the chapter presents each sound/symbol used in United States English. Key Words accompany each of the sounds/symbols. These Key Words contain an example of the sound in the initial, medial, and final positions. A reference chart can assist you with the transcription exercises until you become independently proficient.

The second part of the chapter provides suggested activities that may be useful in the acquisition of the United States English sounds and their phonetic symbols. The intention of many of these activities is to promote a feeling of "entertainment" rather than the traditional "drill work," thereby reducing the level of concern associated with the introduction of the phonetic symbols and their sounds. It is recommended that you incorporate these activities in study groups that promote group interaction and learning. The last part of the chapter consists of exercises in sound/symbol recognition and phonetic transcription of the sounds of United States English.

Keep in mind that the goal of this chapter is not for you to reach any degree of proficiency in phonetic *transcription*. The goal is to present information that is helpful to you in your quest to obtain a proficient *recognition level* of the United States English sounds and their phonetic symbols. Obtaining such a level at the onset provides the skills you need to perform the transcription exercises throughout the book that lead to transcription proficiency. Before the sound/symbol activities are presented, consider some basic cardinal rules associated with the use of United States English sounds and their symbols.

CARDINAL RULES

One of the first and foremost cardinal rules of transcription is that the sound or words are transcribed the way they are *spoken by the speaker* not by how you think they should be transcribed or how the transcriber speaks the same sound or word only differently. For example, the first sound in the word *train* may be pronounced as the same first sound in *ch*in "chrain" or as the first sound in *time* "train." Similarly, the first sound in *Chicago* may be the first sound in *ch*in or *sh*ip depending on speaker preference. One speaker may say "shore" for the word *sure* whereas another speaker, "ser." In rapid speaking, sounds may be omitted such as in "bread 'n butter" and "Wha cha doin'?" Each different speaker may be surprised that these words are not pronounced the same as he or she pronounces them! Again, the challenge is to *transcribe sounds and words exactly how they are spoken*.

The second cardinal rule is not to be too judgmental. There are other "correct" and acceptable ways that the sounds of a word may be pronounced than just your own. So, for the most part, you need to exclude some words from your "phonetic" phraseology such as "That's wrong." "That's not the way it's supposed to be said," and so forth. Begin to use more often the statement, "Oh, I understand now. You are saying **lemin** (lemon) and I say **lemun** and we're both okay!" And who knows, someone may even say "**lemen**"!

Cardinal rule number 3: There is a different symbol for each sound in United States English or any other spoken sound system of any language. What is the implication of this rule? You find out in the exercise that follows, so keep this rule in mind.

Cardinal rule number 4: All of the phonetic symbols are written in lowercase manuscript form such as [b] not B, [m] not M, and [t] not T. The use of brackets [ ] is preferred to signify a phonetic symbol [p].

When symbols of the alphabet are intended specifically to represent language sounds (Stockwell & Minkova, 2001), they are enclosed in square brackets [tɪk]. Once a symbol is enclosed in square brackets, it no longer refers to the spelling, only to the sound.

LET'S GET STARTED: 41 STEPS TO COMPETENCY!

To some of you, the following guided tour may appear oversimplified and even nonsensical in style. This is exactly the goal of the author who has yet to find a beginning student who did not appreciate and learn from such an approach to acquire a level of competency in phonetic transcription.

Follow each step of the directions in sequence and complete each step before going on to the other steps. We may as well have fun while doing this!

- Step 1: Take a sheet of paper and draw two vertical lines from top to bottom to form three columns.

- Step 2: Above the left column write *Alphabet Letter*. Above the center column write *Phonetic Symbols*, and above the right-side column write *Key Words*.

- Step 3 (**Table 2-1**): Make a list of the alphabet *a* to *z* on the left side of a sheet of paper, top to bottom.

- Step 4: Cross out the five vowel letters.

- Step 5: Just in case you have forgotten, that is *a, e, i, o, u*.

- Step 6: Because you have crossed out the letter *a*, go to the next letter *b* and in the Phonetic Symbol column, write the letter *b* and put brackets on each side like this: [b]. You have just written your first phonetic symbol!

- Step 7 (**Table 2-2**): In the right column, write Key Words that have a [b] sound such as *bed*

(initial position), *obey* (medial position), and *rib* (final position). You should now have this recorded.

Comment: Now as you will read in the chapter on United States English, there are several exceptions to the rules. So, before you get too comfortable thinking that transcription is going to be easy and straightforward, let's go to the letter *c*.

- Step 8: In the right column, write a word that begins with *c*. Now in that *same* column, write another word that begins with *c* but that has a *different* sound. Hmm. Are we in trouble now? What did you discover? The letter *c* represents two *different sounds*. What are these two different sounds?

- Step 9: You probably discovered an [s] sound as in *city* and *sit* and the [k] sound as in *come* and *kite*.

- Step 10: How are we going to resolve the dilemma with the letter *c*? Remember cardinal rule 3: "Only one symbol for each sound!"

- Step 11 (**Table 2-3**): Simple enough! Just cross out the letter *c*, same as you did the *a* letter. It is not a valid phonetic symbol.

Comment: Be forewarned that you may resort to old habits on phonetic quizzes and use the letter *c* for the [k] sound. Hopefully, you won't do it too often!

TABLE 2-1 | **United States English Phonetic Consonants Step 3**

Alphabet Letter	Phonetic Symbols	Key Words
a		
b		
c		

Continue to list through the letter z

TABLE 2-2 | **United States English Phonetic Consonants Step 7**

Alphabet Letter	Phonetic Symbols	Key Words
a	Cross out the letter *a*.	
b	[b]	bed, obey, rib
c		

■ Step 12: Looks like the next letter is *d*. Follow the same procedure that you did for *b*: phonetic symbol [d]. Key Words: *dye, idea, need*.

■ Step 13: Do the same for *f*, *g*, and *h*. Note that the [h] sound does not occur in the final position in words.

■ Step 14: Now count the different symbols in the Phonetic Symbols column. How many did you get?

■ Step 15: My count is 5: [b], [d], [f], [g], and [h]. Notice how the [g] symbol is made.
   Comment: Wow! This is almost effortless. You have only been at it a short time and already you know five phonetic symbols. Give yourself a pat on the back!

■ Step 16: Now let's examine the letter *j*. Historically, and even today, there are languages in which the *j* <u>letter</u> represents the *y* <u>sound</u>. So, why not transcribe the word *yellow* with a *j* symbol? That is okay [jɛlo], but what about the word *jello*? It's spelled with a *j* letter but is not pronounced as the *y* sound.

■ Step 17: Resolution. The *j* letter represents two *different* sounds. The [j] phonetic symbol is used in such words as *yellow* (initial) [jɛloʊ], *kayak* (medial) [kaɪjæk], and dialectual *hay* (final) [haɪj] when the [j] sound is added. Go to the bottom of the page and locate the *y* letter and cross it out. There is no *y* phonetic symbol in United States English pronunciation.

■ Step 18 (**Table 2-4**): The other phonetic symbol [dʒ] as in *jello* [dʒɛloʊ] for the *j* letter is presented later.

■ Step 19: The letter *k* we've already addressed somewhat. Put it in the Phonetic Symbol column [k] and write the Key Words *kite, catch, accord, took*. Remember: no *c* phonetic symbol.

■ Step 20: Follow the same procedure for the letters *l*, *m*, *n*, and *p*. Remember, you have already crossed out the *o* vowel.

■ Step 21: Count the phonetic symbols in the middle column. What is your total?

■ Step 22: How about that, 11. Is this something to write home about or what? And you thought that phonetic transcription was going to be frustrating and difficult.

■ Step 23: Now let's examine the *q* letter. What exactly is the sound of the *q* letter? Say some words that begin with the letter *q*.

■ Step 24: Aha! Another exception or deception in the United States English sound system. Where can you place such words as *quit* and *quiet* as Key Words for a sound you have already identified?

■ Step 25: I had all the confidence in the world in you. I knew you would write *quit* as a Key Word for the [k] sound.

■ Step 26: Cross out the *q* letter like you did the *c*. The [q] is gaining recognition as a

TABLE 2-3	United States English Phonetic Consonants Step 11	
Alphabet Letter	**Phonetic Symbols**	**Key Words**
a	Cross out the letter *a*.	
b	[b]	bed, obey, rib
c	See *k* and *s*.	

TABLE 2-4	United States English Phonetic Consonants Step 18	
Alphabet Letter	**Phonetic Symbols**	**Key Words**
j	[j]	yellow, kayak, hay (Also see [dʒ] listed with the unfamiliar consonant symbols.)

United States English sound (**voiced, velar, plosive**) but is not considered in this edition.

■ Step 27: The alphabet letter *r* requires some discussion. It can represent either a consonant sound such as in the words *red, target,* and *car* or a vowel sound such as in *bird*. Notice that when you say the *r* in *car* that it sounds different from the *r* in *bird*. The "ir" is one example of the r-vowel sound and it is discussed later. For now, use the Key Words *red, target,* and *car* for the consonant [r].

   Comment: Now aren't you impressed with yourself? Look at all of the phonetic symbols you can use.

■ Step 28: The selection of Key Words for the [s] and [t] sounds requires some thought. Avoid words that combine "sh" *ship* and "th" *the*. These are not the [s] or [t] sounds. Also notice that the final *s* letter in *has* [z] is not the same sound as the *s* in *maps* [s]. You will learn the reason later. The [w] sound is silent in the final position of words. Delete any words that end with the *w* letter. Enter initial *was* and medial *award* for examples.

   Comment: Now aren't you impressed with yourself? Look at all of the phonetic symbols you can use. And in such a short period of time.

■ Step 29: The [v] is a valid phonetic symbol as in *vase, have, envelope*. So, add the [v] to your inventory.

■ Step 30: Hmm. What about this alphabet letter *x*? Let's investigate it further. It will take some finger counting. Say the word *extra* one sound at a time. *Hint:* The first sound is a vowel. How many *total* sounds did you get?

■ Step 31: How many "sounds" does the letter *x* represent in the word *extra*? Did you come up with a series of six sounds like this: vowel (letter *e*), consonant [k], consonant [s], consonant [t], consonant [r], vowel (letter *a*)? So, cross out the letter *x* alphabet letter because it represents several different sounds in word combinations. And consider the confused *x* in the word *Xerox*. What different sounds does the letter *x* represent in the *same* word? Hint: [z-ɪr-ɑ-k-s].

■ Step 32: Remember cardinal rule 3: A different phonetic symbol for each sound in United States English. Fill in the *consonant* phonetic symbols for the word *exist*: Vowel (*e*) Consonant _____ Consonant _____ Vowel (*i*) Consonant _____ Consonant _____.

■ Step 33: You are getting so good! Vowel + Consonant _____ _____ Vowel + Consonant _____ _____. Transcription: Vowel + [ks] Vowel [st]. Now some of you may say the [g] sound instead of the [k] sound and that's okay. We discuss that later. On to the *z* letter.

■ Step 34: Enter the [z] phonetic symbol and your Key Words such as *zoo, ozone, amaze*.

■ Step 35: Now let's count all of the phonetic symbols you know that you didn't think you knew.

■ Step 36: How many consonant phonetic symbols did you count? 13, 15, 17, or 19?

■ Step 37: If your count wasn't 17, you need to review and count again.

■ Step 38: What *percentage* of the *total* number of consonant phonetic symbols do you think 17 represents? 68%, 46%, 87%, or 30%?

■ Step 39: Okay, so it wasn't a fair question because you don't know the total number of consonant phonetic symbols. How does 46% sound to you? You would probably be satisfied with the 46%, particularly because you want to become competent with the sound/symbol transcription task.

■ Step 40: Does 68% sound even better? That only leaves about 30% for the nonalphabet letters to represent 8 consonant sounds. So, you have only 8 other phonetic symbols to learn and you will have *all* of the consonant sounds.

■ Step 41: Let's do an inventory of your consonant phonetic symbol knowledge: [b], [d], [f], [g], [h], [j], [k], [l], [m], [n], [p], [r], [s], [t], [v], [w], and [z]. Your competency level just shot above the learning curve considering that you probably spent less than 30 minutes following these 41 steps.

UNFAMILIAR PHONETIC CONSONANT SYMBOLS

Let's examine the eight unfamiliar phonetic symbols that represent the other consonant sounds. They are listed in the right column of **Table 2-5**.

You have identified the 25 phonetic symbols used with the United States English **consonant** sounds. The 14 *vowel* sounds and their symbols and the 5 **diphthongs** that are a combination of two vowel sounds that represent *one* sound will now be identified. Remember, a diphthong begins as one sound and glides

TABLE 2-5 **Familiar and Unfamiliar Consonant Phonetic Symbols: Reference Sheet**

	Familiar Consonant Symbols			Unfamiliar Consonant Symbols	
	Phonetic Symbol	**Key Words**		**Phonetic Symbol**	**Key Words**
1.	[b]	by table tub	18.	[Ɵ]	*th*in au*th*or bo*th* (voiceless "th")
2.	[d]	day fiddle tide	19.	[ð]	*th*e bro*th*er smoo*th* (voiced "th")
3.	[f]	fine differ if	20.	[ʃ]	*sh*ip wa*sh*er wi*sh*
4.	[g]	girl wiggle log	21.	[ʒ]	(no initial) ca*s*ual massa*g*e
5.	[h]	happy perhaps (no final)	22.	[ʧ]	*ch*in tea*ch*er pea*ch*
6.	[j]	yellow kayak hay (dialect)	23.	[ʤ]	*j*am ca*g*es ed*g*e
					Notice that the only difference in the pairs above [Ɵ] [ð] [ʃ] [ʒ] [ʧ] [ʤ] is that the first sound is voiceless and the second sound is voiced (the vocal folds vibrate).
7.	[k]	kite tickle cake	24.	[ʍ]	"wh" *wh*en *wh*at Only in the initial position. The [ʍ] sound is almost nonexistent in American English pronunciation. Most speakers do not differentiate between the *wh* in *why* and the *w* in *was*. The [ʍ] sound is discussed more fully later.
8.	[l]	like totally tell	25.	[ŋ]	si*ng* (final position only)
9.	[m]	moth hamster Tom			
10.	[n]	note Tony ton			
11.	[p]	path pepper top			
12.	[r]	rob arrow car			
13.	[s]	sit sister picks			
14.	[t]	to title not			
15.	[v]	vote haven gave			
16.	[w]	was tower (no final)			
17.	[z]	zero hazard was			

into another sound. For example, in the word *cake*, the long ā vowel is spoken, and then the sound shifts into the long ē sound [i] [keik] or [ɪ] [keɪk].

UNITED STATES ENGLISH VOWEL AND DIPHTHONG SOUNDS/SYMBOLS

The vowels and diphthongs that are presented here are organized in the following manner: (1) vowels and diphthongs that are not influenced by other factors, and (2) vowels and diphthongs that are influenced by other factors.

1. Vowels and diphthongs that are not influenced by other factors include the ones listed in **Table 2-6**.

2. Some vowels and diphthongs are influenced by the amount of stress given to their sounds (see **Table 2-7**). Amount of **stress** is determined by (1) the length of time and (2) the amount of **loudness** given to a sound. Often, these features are rather subtle to the human ear and can be finitely determined only by instrumentation.

This completes the entire set of United States English consonant, vowel, and diphthong symbols.

In addition, you need to note other information that will influence the symbolization of the United States English sounds.

ADDITIONAL SYMBOLIZATION

A few other symbols complete the inventory of phonetic symbols used in United States English. These include the **flap or tap**, the **glottal stop**, and the syllabic consonants.

The Flap or Tap

When you produce the two words *latter* and *ladder* in their usual "informal" manner, you are probably not able to distinguish between the two of them. There is a general rule that when [t] occurs after a stressed vowel and before an unstressed syllable other than [n], it is changed into a voiced sound. This sound is referred to as a flap or tap [ɾ]. Another example is *butter*. Say this word in your natural pronunciation and chances are that you are not saying a *voiceless* [t] sound but rather something that sounds more like a [d]. Using this pronunciation, the flap or tap [ɾ] symbol rather than a [t] or [d] symbol [bʌɾɚ] would be used. When, indeed,

TABLE 2-6		Vowels and Diphthongs Not Influenced by Other Factors
	Symbol	**Key Words**
1.	[i]	eat beet—same as long vowel ē
2.	[ɪ]	it bit—same as short vowel ī
3.	[ɛ]	edge bet—same as short vowel ĕ
4.	[æ]	at mat—same as short vowel ă
5.	[u]	ooze loose—same as long vowel ū
6.	[ʊ]	book took
7.	[ɔ]	ought caught
8.	[ɑ]	far father part—same as short vowel ŏ
9.	[ɔɪ]	oil coil boil—[ɔɪ] is the traditional pronunciation, but the [ɔi] may be pronounced instead
10.	[aʊ]	how mouse
11.	[aɪ]	ice nice price [ai]—same as long vowel ī

TABLE 2-7 Vowels and Diphthongs Influenced by Stress and Position

	Symbol	Key Words	Factor
12.	[e] or	rotate	Long vowel ā. The [e] symbol is used in the unstressed syllable.
13.	[eɪ] or [ei]	rotation cake day	The diphthong [eɪ] or [ei] is used depending on dialect in the (1) stressed syllable, (2) single syllable, and (3) word ending positions.
14.	[o] or	opinion	Long vowel ō.
15.	[oʊ]	emotion note no	The [o] symbol is used in the unstressed syllable and the diphthong [oʊ] is used in the (1) stressed syllable, (2) single-syllable word, and (3) word ending positions.

It is important to note that these general rules have been traditionally applied. The cardinal rule is that the sound is recorded as it is spoken. Some speakers do not "diphthongize" the [e] and [o].

	Symbol	Key Words	Factor
16.	[ɚ] or	sugar	The [ɚ] symbol is used in the unstressed syllable and the [ɝ] is
17.	[ɝ]	circus word	used in the (1) stressed syllable and (2) single-syllable words.
18.	[ə] or	about	Short vowel ŭ. The [ə] *schwa* symbol is used in the unstressed
19.	[ʌ]	enough up	syllable and the [ʌ] symbol is used in the (1) stressed syllable and (2) single-syllable words.

such words are pronounced more precisely and there is an apparent [t] sound, then it is appropriate to use the [t] rather than the [ɾ]. Add to your phonetic sound/symbol reference sheet: flap [ɾ].

The Glottal Stop

A glottal stop occurs, particularly in some dialects, when there is an interruption of the airflow at the point of the vocal folds (glottis). Such an interruption produces a brief stop and then release of the airflow as in the word *bottle* and *cotton* where the "t" sound is replaced with a glottal stop [ʔ] and transcribed as [bɑʔl̩] and [kɑʔn̩]. This is particularly used in British English. Produce the words *bottle* and *cotton* in that manner to become accustomed to how it is produced and how it sounds.

Add to your list of phonetic sound/symbols reference sheet: glottal stop [ʔ].

Syllabic Consonants

The last phonetic symbol to include in your sound/symbol inventory is a small dot under certain consonant sounds. You may have noticed in the transcription of the words *bottle* and *cotton* in the preceding section on glottal stop that there is a dot under the *l* and *n*. This dot symbolizes that the consonant is functioning

as a vowel. Why is it functioning as a vowel? Let's examine the word *bottle* and find out. How many syllables are there in the word *bott-le*? That's right. There are two syllables. The rules of syllabication dictate that each syllable needs to have a vowel. Where is the vowel in the second syllable of *bott-le*? There is not a vowel, only the consonant *l* sound. To indicate the omission of an actual vowel and to show that a consonant is functioning in the vowel "slot," a dot is placed under the consonant phonetic symbol [l̩].

Examine the following words. Say each one aloud using a normal pronunciation style. Be particularly aware of the sound in the last syllable in each word: *sudden, fountain, ribbon, happen, table*. Notice that the last syllable *can* be said without a vowel sound "*sudn*," "*tabl*." When this occurs, a small dot is placed under the consonant to indicate a "syllabic consonant" or one that functions as a vowel. The dot symbol is used in such words as *tab-le* [teɪbl̩], *happ-en* [hæpn̩], and *sudd-en* [sʌdn̩]. Add the examples of these words to your sound/symbol reference sheet to indicate the use of the dot with syllabic consonants. Keep in mind that these words may also be pronounced with a *vowel* such as "sud-den" [sʌddɛn]. The [m] and [ŋ] may also function as syllabic consonants but with less frequency.

This completes all of the phonetic sounds/symbols that you will need to use in the transcription of the United States English consonants, vowels, diphthongs, and other symbols.

HOW TO SURVIVE PHONETIC TRANSCRIPTION

Most of the consonants are rather straightforward in their sound/symbol correspondence and are rather void of dialectical influences. The vowels and diphthongs are not as consistent, and the transcription presented in this book may be different from what you would use. This condition is not unique to this chapter alone but exists within any book on phonetics. To survive the phonetic transcription presented in any of these books, you need to develop an attitude that what is *printed* as an example of the pronunciation of a word may be only *one* way that such a word may be transcribed and that there are other viable options. Notice that the word *printed* is italicized to emphasize the printed form. When transcribing the *spoken* word, it should be transcribed as the speaker *speaks* it, not as you would say it or as it may be suggested in a dictionary or phonetics book. Simply stated, as you refer to the transcribed words in this book you may say, "But that isn't the way I say it." That statement is okay, but realize that there are others who speak the same United States English who will undoubtedly pronounce the words differently. Some of the sounds that may be pronounced differently are listed in **Table 2-8**.

Many of the vowel and diphthong sounds are relative in their placement in the oral cavity in contrast to the consonants that usually have a rather fixed position with at least two articulators making contact, such as the [b] (lips) or [t] (tongue and upper teeth) sounds. Some judgment as to which vowel sound to use is determined by answering the question, "Which of the two sounds does it sound the most like?" It becomes a judgment of *degree* rather than precision. Often, in fact, the actual spoken sound may be located somewhere between two other sounds that are approximate in their location with one another. For example, the [ɔ] "*odd*" and [ɑ] "*odd*" (same word but with dialectual different pronunciations) are adjacent to each other in the oral cavity and in their production.

For you to become successful, you must understand that there is more than one way to pronounce some sounds in words. The difference may be a result of dialect differences or pathologic defect such as a speech disorder. To survive a course in phonetics, this insight and attitude need to be developed and applied.

Another survival technique is to increase your listening skills. These skills involve two basic principles of **audition**. One is hearing *acuity* that determines how well an individual hears (quiet volume or loudness vs. increased loudness) and the second is hearing *discrimination*. A listener can pass a hearing screening test that assesses the ability to hear pure tones (humming sounds), but that ability is not necessarily correspondent with the ability to discriminate sounds or words that are similar. For example, the ability to discriminate whether the words *pin* and *pen* are the same may be influenced by either cultural learning or a decrease in auditory discrimination ability. You need to acquire the ability to listen discriminately to transcribe the spoken sounds accurately.

Be careful when repeating a word to yourself. One of the difficulties encountered occurs when the listener repeats the word as he or she pronounces it rather than how the speaker says it, thereby resulting in a change. For example, the speaker may say *lemon* as [lɛmən] and the listener may repeat the word as [lɛmɪn], and then transcribe it incorrectly as [lɛmɪn].

TABLE 2-8	**Examples of Sounds That Are Pronounced Differently**	
Phonetic Symbol	**Key Words**	**Pronunciation Options**
[ɪ] or [i]	pretty	The last sound may be either [ɪ] as in the word *it* or [i] as in the last sound in *me*.
[ɔ] or [ɑ]	ought	The vowel may be either [ɔ] or [ɑ] depending on the dialect of the speaker.
[æ] or [aʊ]	alphabet	The first sound may be the [æ] as in *ask* or it may be a sound more closely related to the diphthong [aʊ], the first sound in *ouch*.

Listening skills need to be sharpened and habitual listening perception examined. In other words, a person may be so accustomed to perceiving a sound or word in such a manner that it is not heard differently when spoken differently by other speakers. This is true for both native and nonnative listeners.

As listeners, we have a tendency to rely on the *semantic content* for meaning rather than the actual sounds in words. For example, a subtle acoustical sound change occurs within the word *uses*. The person *uses* [juzəz] the phone. The computer has many different *uses* [jusəz]. Some listeners have difficulty in their ability to discriminate between such subtle differences.

Also, take caution about using the spelling of a word as a source of transcription. Remember that there is a group of words that are spelled the same but change meaning depending on which syllable has the primary stress. These words include the following:

Noun:	*Verb:*
present [prɛzənt]	pre**sent** [prisɛnt]
convert [kɑnvɚt]	con**vert** [kənvɚt]

SUMMARY

It is hoped that after this rather step-by-step approach to the introduction of the phonetic symbols to be used in the transcription of United States English sounds that you do not feel too overwhelmed. The inventory of sounds/symbols is shown in **Table 2-9**.

The inventory of sounds and symbols is listed in the Sound/Symbol Reference Guide on the inside front cover of the book. You have developed your own

reference sheet to assist you in identifying the inventory of sounds and symbols. It is highly recommended that you spend considerable time and effort now in learning this information because it is one of the skills required for transcription.

The goal of this chapter was to present information that assists in the identification of the sounds/symbols of United States English. Examples of the 48 different sounds and symbols were presented and suggestions provided to assist in the acquisition of these symbols. The remainder of the book provides other information related to phonetic science, including the characteristics of each of the sounds. The development of the skill of sound/symbol identification is emphasized as a prerequisite for the remaining transcription throughout the book. Your goal should be to acquire this skill as quickly as possible.

To further assist you in the acquisition of this skill, the following section offers some activities to develop sound/symbol identification. Throughout the remainder of this text are many opportunities to increase your skills in sound/symbol recognition and transcription. It is suggested that you refer to the Phonetic Transcription Reference Chart located on the inside front cover of the book. This chart can assist you in the acquisition of the knowledge that is required to become proficient as a beginning student of the phonetic symbols.

Competency Quiz

Identify the phonetic symbol that corresponds with the sound that is in **bold** print.

TABLE 2-9	Inventory of Sounds/Symbols

Number	Different Sounds/Symbols
17	Familiar consonant symbols
18	Unfamiliar consonant symbols
19	Vowels and diphthongs The flap The glottal stop The syllabic consonants

Consonants

1. **th**at ____
2. si**ng** ____
3. **sh**oe ____
4. **ch**in ____
5. a**z**ure ____
6. **j**am ____
7. **th**in ____

Vowels/Diphthongs

1. **a**bout ____
2. abou**t** ____
3. b**u**t ____
4. b**ir**d ____
5. moth**er** ____
6. **a**sk ____
7. b**oo**k ____
8. b**i**t ____

9. **i**ce ____
10. b**e**d ____
11. **oi**l ____
12. **u**se ____
13. **ea**t ____
14. **ough**t ____
15. c**a**ke ____

Remember: There may be some dialect differences.

FUN WITH PHONETICS:
[fʌn wɪθ fənɛtɪks]

The following activities provide you with opportunities to acquire competency in sound/symbol recognition.

Matching or Concentration: [mætʃɪŋ or kansɛntreɪʃən]

This game can be developed at two different levels of difficulty and can be played as an individual or in small groups. Remember, the goal of this game is to assist you in gaining *sound/symbol recognition*.

1. Use card-stock paper and make 124 small squares, approximately 2 inches by 2 inches in size.

2. You will use a total of 62 cards each for Level 1 and Level 2 as shown here.

[θ] [ð] [ʃ] [ʒ] [ʧ] [ʤ] [ʍ] [ŋ]

[i] [ɪ] [ɛ] [æ] [u] [ʊ] [ɔ] [ɑ] [ɔɪ]

[aʊ] [aɪ] [e] [eɪ] [o] [oʊ]

[ɚ] [ɜ] [ʌ] [ʔ] [ɾ] [l̩] [n̩]

Notice: Only the unfamiliar symbols are included.

3. Level 1. Make two sets of the phonetic symbols and include a Key Word. Refer to your Key Words listing.

[æ]	[æ]
ask	ask

4. Level 2. Make two sets of phonetic symbols without a Key Word.

[æ]	[æ]

5. Use the Level 1 set until you become fairly competent, and then use the Level 2 set. You may want to use only half of the sets at one time. There is a total of 62 cards.

6. Position the cards (either Level 1 or Level 2) upside down in a random pattern. As you turn two cards over, say the *sound* that each symbol represents. If the two sounds don't match, turn them upside down again. If they do match, remove them from the set. The game is over when all of the sounds have been matched. The winner is the one with the most matches. Remember to have fun!

Sound Awareness

Matching Sounds

Exercise 1

Match the *first sound* in the words in the numbered columns with the *first* sound in the words of the columns without numbers. For example: the [z] in item 14 *zoom* matches the "z" sound in *zest*. Put a line through the word once it is used.

1. thick	12. cat	<u>14</u> zest	____ holy
2. young	13. weight	____ vote	____ chef
3. bag	14. zoom	____ loose	____ tomato
4. dude	15. ptomaine	____ kite	____ wild
5. gem	16. gas	____ theory	____ rhyme
6. nail	17. whole	____ Czech	____ dare
7. room	18. fan	____ phone	____ yacht
8. pain	19. leap	____ send	____ kneel
9. vest	20. then	____ pest	____ there
10. check	21. cent	____ jest	____ guess
11. shave	22. meek	____ main	____ boom

Exercise 2

Match the *ending sound* of the words in the numbered columns with the *ending* sound of the words in the columns without numbers. For example: item 12 *soap* ends with a /p/ sound as does the word *hope*.

1. tongue	12. soap	____ picked	____ sane
2. rug	13. lace	____ smooth	____ toll
3. pole	14. save	____ lock	____ youth
4. clothe	15. globe	____ gruff	____ love
5. graph	16. rage	____ licorice	____ loss
6. phrase	17. car	____ grub	____ lung
7. sign	18. odd	____ fade	____ rogue
8. both	19. rouge	____ witch	____ care
9. rich	20. dumb	____ beige	____ ridge
10. look	21. fate	____ dome	____ daze
11. wash		<u>12</u> hope	

Exercise 3

Match the *final sound* in the words in the numbered columns with the *initial* sound in the words in the columns without numbers. For example: item 1 *meat* (final sound [t]) and initial [t] in *team*. Circle the words in *either* of the columns if there is no match. Why do you think there is no match for these sounds in these positions?

1. meat	12. Ruth	___ bad	___ vain
2. coach	13. face	___ zone	___ pitch
3. lane	14. maid	___ choke	___ think
4. sail	15. lick	___ shift	___ rake
5. robe	16. comb	_1_ team	___ gel
6. beige	17. rung	___ name	___ safe
7. nose	18. chip	___ head	___ kill
8. rush	19. nave	___ they	___ yell
9. ledge	20. cough	___ goal	___ lace
10. rogue	21. door	___ dame	___ wet
11. breathe		___ mode	___ fun

Word Chains: [wɝd ʧaɪnz]

This activity requires two or more players. Each player prepares a list of 10 word chains that are written with phonetic symbols. The symbols are placed next to one another with *no* spacing between the words. Each word is unrelated to the others. The challenge is to identify the words that have been transcribed by someone else. If a group is participating, compete to see who can decipher the words the fastest. For example: (Cover the Key below until the words have been deciphered.)

[rolwɛstæktɪveɪtʃoʊnkɑrdzhæpn̩itʃɛkskludmɑɵəbʌv]

Key: request activate shown cards happen each exclude moth above

Double Meanings!

Instructions: Transcribe the following phonetic symbols into a short phrase or statement. Use the Phonetic Sound/Symbol Reference Chart located on the inside front cover of the book to assist you in the sounds of the unfamiliar symbols. Cover the answers at the bottom of the box and refer to them on completion.

1. [ə-n-aɪ-s-h-aʊ-s] _____

2. [ə-n-eɪ-ʃ-ə-n] _____

3. [ʤ-ɔ-ɪ-s-l-i-p-s] _____

4. [ə-g-r-i-k-s-p-aɪ] _____

5. [aɪ-s-k-r-i-m] _____

6. [h-aɪ-ʤ-i-n] _____

If you have not already discovered, there are two ways to divide the sounds to make two different answers to the preceding six phonetic phrases. Now write the other answers.

1. _____

2. _____

3. _____

4. _____

5. _____

6. _____

Answers:

1. A nice house. An ice house.
2. A nation. An Asian.
3. Joy sleeps. Joyce leaps.
4. A Greek spy. A Greek's pie.
5. Ice cream. I scream.
6. Hi, Jean. Hygiene.

Phonetic Scrabble: [fənɛtɪk skræbl̩]

Design a game board similar to that used in Scrabble. Cut white card-stock paper into small squares that will fit on the squares on the game board. Print the number of squares indicated at the bottom of the board. Enter a point value next to each symbol: [i] 1. Each player is given seven squares. The first word must cover the "free" square in the center of the board. Follow the same rules that are used for Scrabble. The game ends when all of the sound/symbol squares are gone. The player with the highest points is the winner. (See **Figure 2-1**.)

- 2 squares—[b], [f], [h], [m], [p], [v], [w], [z]

- 3 squares—[g], [k], [r], [ð], [ʒ], [ʧ], [ʤ], [ŋ], [ʍ]

- 3 squares—[d], [l], [s], [t], [ɵ], [ʃ], [j], [r], [i], [ɪ], [ɛ], [æ], [u], [ʊ], [ɔ], [ɑ], [ɔɪ], [aʊ], [aɪ], [ʌ], [ɝ], [ɚ], [o], [oʊ]

- 4 squares—[eɪ], [e], [n], [ə], [l̩], [n̩], blank

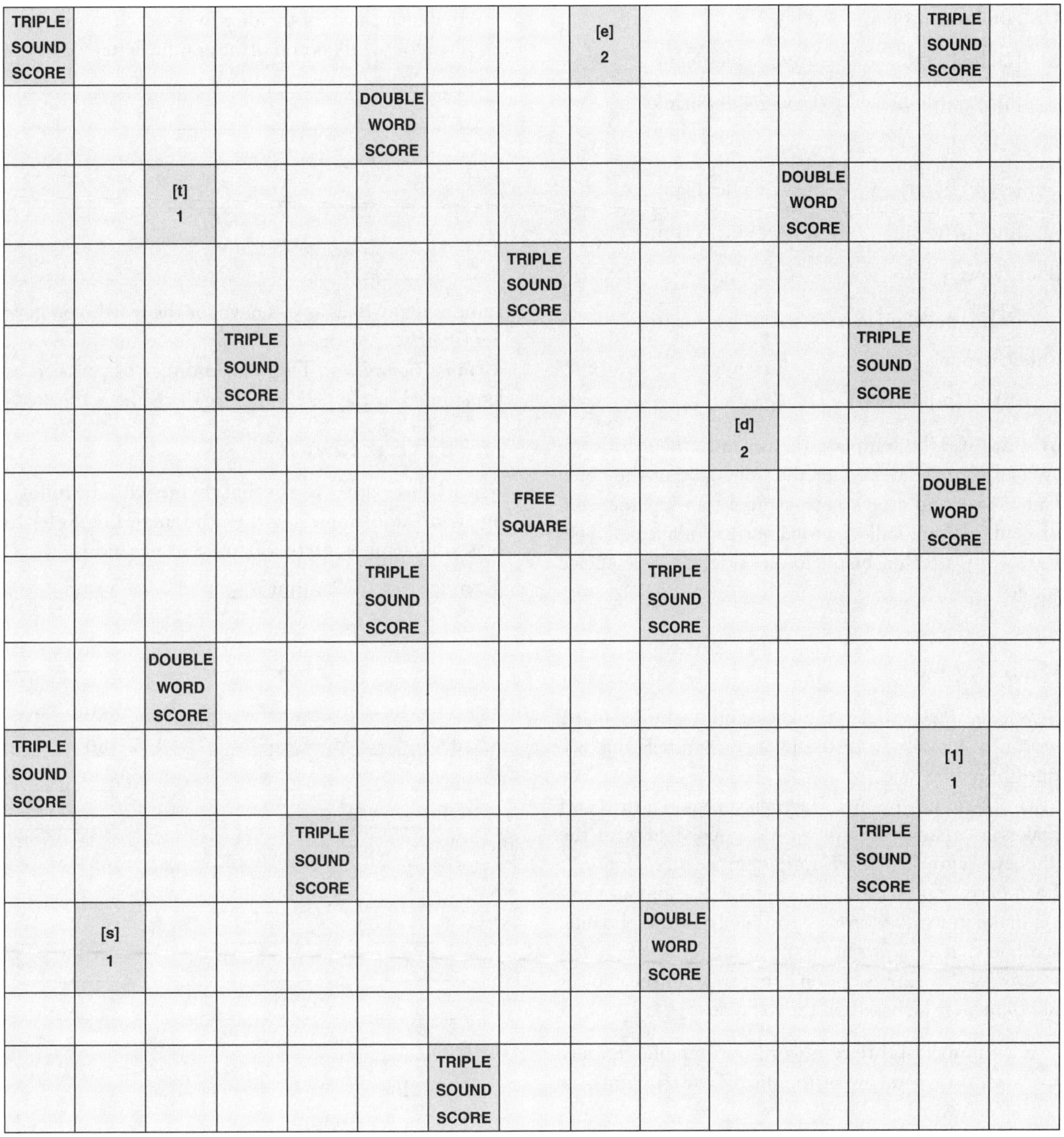

Phonetic Scrabble board contents:

TRIPLE SOUND SCORE							[e] 2					TRIPLE SOUND SCORE		
			DOUBLE WORD SCORE											
	[t] 1									DOUBLE WORD SCORE				
					TRIPLE SOUND SCORE									
		TRIPLE SOUND SCORE									TRIPLE SOUND SCORE			
								[d] 2						
					FREE SQUARE						DOUBLE WORD SCORE			
			TRIPLE SOUND SCORE			TRIPLE SOUND SCORE								
	DOUBLE WORD SCORE													
TRIPLE SOUND SCORE												[1] 1		
		TRIPLE SOUND SCORE									TRIPLE SOUND SCORE			
[s] 1							DOUBLE WORD SCORE							
		TRIPLE SOUND SCORE												

Figure 2-1 Phonetic Scrabble.

Shake Those Dice! Sound/Symbol Dice, That Is

This activity is for individual and/or group skill building and review of the consonants, vowels, and diphthongs. *Materials needed:* Colored marking pens, nine dice-size cubes, and self-adhesive peel-off paper. The wooden cubes are available at most major craft stores, or you can use regular dice.

Instructions:

Familiar consonant symbols

   [b] [d] [f] [g] [h] [j]

   [k] [l] [m] [n] [p]   (leave one side blank)

   [r] [s] [t] [v] [w] [z]

Unfamiliar consonant symbols

[Θ] [ð] [ʃ] [ʒ]   (leave 2 sides blank)

[ʧ] [ʤ] [ŋ] [ʍ]   (leave 2 sides blank)

Long vowels

[eɪ] [e] [i] [aɪ]   (leave 2 sides blank)

[ou] [o] [u] [ju]   (leave 2 sides blank)

Short vowels

[ɪ] [ɛ] [æ] [ɑ] [ʌ] [ə]

Other symbols

[ʊ] [ɔ] [ɔɪ] [l̩] [n̩] [ɾ]

You can use the template in Appendix B. Print each symbol somewhat smaller than one side of the cube. Cut to size and attach each symbol to a separate side of a cube. There will be a total of six symbols per cube. Randomly attach a blank to one side as a free choice sound.

How to Play

Individual Play: Shake the dice and make as many words as possible from the phonetic symbols that are upright on the dice.

Group Play: Option 1: Each player takes a turn and makes as many different words as possible with the phonetic symbols that are upright on the dice. Option 2: Each player takes a turn shaking the dice and all players make as many words as possible from the phonetic symbols that are upright on the dice.

Scoring: Scoring is optional, but some of the choices of points may be based on the following:

1. Number of different words written phonetically with each throw of the dice. Two (2) points for each word.

2. Different points given for the number of sounds (length) of the word. One (1) point for each "sound" used.

Timing: Optional. To be determined by the players.

Sample Score Sheet: (See also Appendix B)

Player's Name: _____ Total Points: _____

Description of point value: To be determined by the players.

_____

_____

After each shake of the dice, write each word(s) using phonetic symbols and orthographic letters.

1. _____/_____   _____/_____

    _____/_____   _____/_____

    _____/_____   _____/_____

2. _____/_____   _____/_____

    _____/_____   _____/_____

    _____/_____   _____/_____

Enter as many lines as you have for the words you have identified.

Game Completed: The total number of turns to be determined by the players before the game is finished.

Words That Rhyme

Identify three other words that rhyme with the following words and transcribe them phonetically. Refer to the sound/symbol reference guide, as needed.

1. much _____   2. thin _____   3. wood _____

   _____   _____   _____

   _____   _____   _____

   _____   _____   _____

4. sneeze _____ 5. base _____   6. did _____

   _____   _____   _____

   _____   _____   _____

   _____   _____   _____

7. witch _____   8. get _____   9. bath _____

   _____   _____   _____

   _____   _____   _____

   _____   _____   _____

10. fix _____

    _____

    _____

    _____

Half and Half: Symbol Recognition
Capital Cities

1-freɪŋk	2-fɹid	3-læns	4-lɪŋ
5-nɪks	6-tən	7-fɚd	8-lənd
9-den	10-kən	11-ɪŋ	12-vɪl
13-sprɪŋ	14-pɔrt	15-næʃ	16-fɚt
17-hɑrt	18-fi	19-trɛn	20-vɚ

1. _____   6. _____

2. _____   7. _____

3. _____   8. _____

4. _____   9. _____

5. _____   10. _____

b	d	f	g	h	j	k	l	m
1	2	3	4	5	6	7	8	9
n	ŋ	p	r	s	t	v	w	ʍ
10	11	12	13	14	15	16	17	18
θ	ð	ʃ	ʒ	tʃ	dʒ	i	ɪ	ɛ
19	20	21	22	23	24	25	26	27
e	æ	ɑ	ɔ	o	ʊ	u	eɪ	ɔɪ
28	29	30	31	32	33	34	35	36
aɪ	ʌ	ə	ɚ	ɝ				
37	38	39	40	41				

Key:

1. 14–8   6. 1–16
2. 18–5   7. 3–11
3. 17–7   8. 4–10
4. 9–20   9. 19–6
5. 13–2   10. 15–12

Cities:

1. Portland   6. Frankfort
2. Phoenix   7. Lansing
3. Hartford   8. Lincoln
4. Denver   9. Trenton
5. Springfield   10. Nashville

Secret Message: Symbol/Sound Identification

Instructions: Write a coded message by using the corresponding phonetic symbols and numbers to create the words of your message.

Example: 7 29 10 = can

— — — — — — — — — — — — —

— — — — — — — — — — — — —

— — — — — — — — — — — — —

— — — — — — — — — — — — —

— — — — — — — — — — — — —

— — — — — — — — — — — — —

— — — — — — — — — — — — —

— — — — — — — — — — — — —

Message:

_____

_____

_____

Scattered Symbols: Sound/Symbol Identification

Instructions: Identify and transcribe the following words. The first sound is in the circle. The other sounds are in clockwise positions, starting at 12 noon.

Example: finger

```
         ɪ
    ɚ  ( f )  ŋ
         g
```

```
   æ              æ              t
 i (t) k      t (dʒ) k       t (s) ɑ
   s              ɪ              p
```

1. _____

2. _____

3. _____

27

[r]
[eɪ] (f) [aɪ]
[d]

[i]
[z] [t] [tʃ]
[ə˞]

[ɑ]
[z] (s) [ð]
[ə˞]

4. _____

5. _____

6. _____

[ɪ]
[o] (w) [n]
[d]

[t]
[t] (s) [r]
[i]

[ɑ]
[t] (r) [k]
[ə]

7. _____

8. _____

9. _____

Key:

1. taxi	4. Friday	7. window
2. jacket	5. teachers	8. street
3. stopped	6. fathers	9. rocket

Transcription Exercises

Enhancing Your Listening Skills

Thus far, the emphasis in this chapter has been on sound/symbol recognition. Another important skill that is required in transcription is to have accurate *listening* abilities. The following exercise may be used to enhance your listening skills. It can be developed at three different levels of difficulty as you progress in your sound/symbol recognition competency.

Level 1

Compile a list of 40 one-syllable *nonsense* words that contain only the 17 familiar consonant sounds. Transcribe the familiar phonetic consonant symbols. The reason for the choice of nonsense words is to eliminate any "sound" contextual clues. For example:

Nonsense Words	Transcription Key
1. gov (like go)	[g __ v]
2. dif	[d __ f]
3. cab (like cake)	[k __ b]
4–40 (continue)	

Presentation:

A. Say the words out loud to another person or small group and have them each transcribe the familiar consonant sound/symbols.

B. Record the 40 words and have another person or small group listen to the recording and transcribe the words.

C. Interchange A and B with others to gain a wider variety of nonsense words and vocal qualities to enhance your listening and transcription skills.

Level 2

Follow the same instructions as in Level 1 and add the *unfamiliar* phonetic consonant sounds.

Level 3

Follow the same instructions as in Level 2 but add five of the vowel sounds.

Level 4

Continue to add nonsense words until all of the consonants, vowels, diphthongs, syllabic consonants, and flap are included.

Recommendation: There are many self-tutorial programs available at different websites. To access these sites, enter the Key Word *phonetics* and scroll through the programs and become familiar with them.

Refer to Appendix A, fʌn wɪθ fənɛtɪks (Fun with Phonetics), for additional activities and exercises.

Spelling Challenge

Using blank card-stock paper, cut to the size of regular playing cards, print each of the phonetic symbols that are used for the Scrabble game. Include the flap [ɾ] and the syllabic [l̩] and [n̩].

For example:

Instructions:

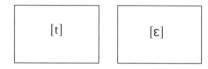

1. Each player is dealt four cards.
2. The remaining cards are placed face down in a pile.
3. The first player draws the top card from the pile.
4. If the player can make a combination of a 1-letter and one 3-letter word, or two 2-letter words, or one 4-letter word (having the fifth card as a discard), that player can lay those cards face up on the table and discard. If the player cannot make

any of these combinations or a 4-letter word, the player must discard a card, and the player to the left takes a turn.

[aɪ] and [t][ʊ][k] plus discard

[r][ə] and [n][z] plus discard

5. That player can either take the discarded card or draw from the pile.

6. When a player can lay down all four cards to spell a word or words, the hand is over. The first player to play must lay down *all* cards, play a discard, and go out.

7. Each player has one turn left. Each player lays down as many words as possible and is allowed to discard one card. Any remaining cards are counted as 1 point each against the player.

8. Continue to add an additional card to each play. The game ends after a hand of 12 cards is played.

9. The player with the lowest score wins. It may be a minus score.

10. If the draw pile runs out, shuffle the discard cards and turn them over face down and resume the game.

11. Bonus points: The players with the (1) longest word or (2) the most single words add a bonus 5 to their score. It may be the same player.

REFERENCE

Stockwell, R., & Minkova, D. (2001). *English words: History and structure*. Cambridge, England: Cambridge University Press.

Chapter 3

The English Language and United States English Dialects

From One Shoreline of the Atlantic to the Other

PURPOSE

To provide an overview of the history of the English language from its origins to its worldwide usage, including in the United States.

OBJECTIVES

This chapter will provide you with information regarding:

1. An overview of the origins and evolution of the English language
2. The development of United States English
3. What constitutes a dialect of United States English
4. Skill-building activities to increase your awareness of the characteristics of United States English

RATIONALE

Generally speaking, books at the introductory level of phonetics provide a brief overview of the history of the English language. Such an overview is perhaps adequate, but there are reasons to include a somewhat more comprehensive discussion on the subject.

This decision is based on several needs that you may have. You need to know:

1. Why there are discrepancies between the spelling and the pronunciation of United States English words
2. What factors influence the sounds of a word from a dialect perspective
3. Why some of the sounds of a language may change from generation to generation
4. How the same issues that confront the choice of speech sounds and language usage today have been debated probably since the time of recorded history

With this knowledge, you will gain a greater understanding and appreciation of the usefulness of the International Phonetic Alphabet (IPA) and its correlation to the sounds/symbols of United States English.

INTRODUCTION

Although the widespread use of the English language is impressive, you must realize that its dialect variations may make it difficult for one English speaker to understand another English speaker. This is particularly true in areas that are isolated from the mainstream of society. These variations are present both in the pronunciation of the sounds, mainly vowels and diphthongs, and in the prosodic features of intonation and inflection. For example, a native Spanish speaker may speak English that has the inflectional patterns typical of the Spanish pronunciation, and the Pennsylvania Dutch can be observed speaking a "Dutchified" version of English.

Understanding the English language and its origins with its variations and idiosyncrasies is essential. There is a need to know how the sound system operates in the following areas:

1. *Pronunciation:* An *ed* ending in such words as *mapped* changes from a [d] sound to a [t] sound.

2. *Spelling: Threw* and *through* have the same number of sounds.

3. *Phonemic or grammatical aspects:* The vowel sound in *man* and *men* changes the grammatical element.

4. *Meaning:* The meaning of the word *conduct* changes from a noun to a verb depending on the vowel used in the first syllable and which syllable is stressed. For example, "She will con**duct**" and "His **con**duct was impressive."

A historical review of any language can help you understand how sounds came into existence in that language, were maintained, and in some cases became extinct or modified in some manner. Such an insight provides the basis for an understanding that sound systems and languages are fluid, continually in a changing state.

While you read about the evolution and development of the English language, think about possible contemporary parallels that are happening throughout the world and within the borders of the United States. What political, commercial, educational, and technological changes are occurring that will affect any language, and specifically the use of United States English?

You can learn about the English language by traveling through the centuries in a time machine. Are you ready? All aboard!

ALL ABOARD THE TIME MACHINE!

We begin our journey around 449 in the current era (C.E.) and we observe the Anglo-Saxons and the Celts using Old English. As we advance to 597 C.E., we see Augustine and the Roman missionaries beginning to arrive on the island of England and ushering in the literary age.

As we stop and examine the first text, we note that it is written in Old English translated from Latin. We now advance to the time period beginning around 866 and watch as the Norsemen arrive from Denmark and the Scandinavian peninsula. They are speaking new words to the people in the villages that include *egg, take, ugly, give*, and others such as *their, they*, and *them*.

As we travel through these villages, we realize that, although Old English is the foundation language, almost every village has its own dialect, some of which still exist in modern time in some isolated areas.

As we pass by a small schoolhouse, we notice on the classroom wall the current alphabet letters of Old English. Omitted from the list are the letters *j, q, w, x*, and *z*. Did I hear you say, "It's amazing that the letters have been in existence for so long"?

As we travel along our route, we pass a sign that says, "Entering the Middle English Period: 1000 C.E." The defining event that separated Old and Middle English was the Norman Conquest. The Normans had established themselves in northern France in the early tenth century, and later we observe them coming across the English Channel and beginning to rule England.

As we flash by the next few centuries, we notice that the kings who rule England, ironically, speak French and that English is their second language! We also notice that the wealthy landowners speak French while the villagers maintain their English dialects.

We also see an example of how powerful the use of a language can be and is through all ages. Those who desired to have a position of influence were required to become proficient in French. Even Queen Victoria, the monarch of England, spoke French and had to be tutored in English.

As our time machine enters the twelfth century, we observe that things are beginning to change. Children of nobility are learning English first, and the status of the French language is diminishing. Wow! What was that we just passed through? It was the Barons' War of 1264–1265, and as we disembark the time machine and attend Parliament, we are somewhat amazed that for the first time it is conducted in English.

The transition from French to English is somewhat confusing because the French listened to the English *spoken* words but imposed their spelling on them. Consequently, we inherited such words as *cueen*, which became *queen*, and *niht*, which became *night*.

As we walk the streets of England during the thirteenth century, we hear many more French words being incorporated into the English vocabulary, and most people that we listen to speak more French than English. By now, the English language has even inherited the word *alkali* from the Arabs.

We notice Dante, who is finishing *Paradiso*. We ask him where he thinks the English language is going. He replies:

> It is a natural thing that man should speak;
> But whether this or that way, Nature leaves
> To your election, as it pleases you.
> For mortal usages are like leaves on trees;
> They fall and others grow.

—Dante's *Paradiso*

As we continue our stroll, we notice a street vendor selling something like a notebook that contains bilingual word lists to assist in the comprehension of French and English. That would be an interesting list to have and to compare with today's vocabulary listings.

We get back in the time machine and begin our travels through the fourteenth and fifteenth centuries and observe an interesting phenomenon taking place. The percentage of English words is diminishing and the percentage of foreign words is increasing. Many Latin words related to medicine, politics, law, religion, and literature are incorporated into the English language. The names of precious stones, such as *ruby, turquoise*, and *pearl*, French words, are included. We also notice that the Scandinavian influence continues adding such words as *get, both, outlaw, birth, trust, knife, window, neck*, and *same*.

As we pass through the time zone of 1400 to 1600, we don't want to appear rude and to laugh, but it does sound humorous to us to hear people using two syllables in the pronunciation of such words as *seemed, stored*, and *laughed*. During Chaucer's time, such words as *stone, wine, name*, and *dance* were two-syllable words. It wasn't until Shakespeare's time that such words were spoken as one-syllable words. As you can imagine, this was a significant change because it affected thousands of words.

We want to get more of a feel for English pronunciation during the Middle English period, so we again disembark the time machine and begin to converse with the people on the streets. We soon discover to our frustration that the usage of some vowel sounds interferes with our conversations. For example, we hear that the word *name* has the same vowel sound as *father, he* is pronounced more like *hey, moon* sounds like *moan, wine* has the same vowel sound as *mean*, and *mouse* is really confusing because it sounds like *moose*!

We get back in the time machine and travel toward the end of the Middle English period. Something is really happening linguistically: Seven of the vowel sounds changed their vowel quality and we enter what is to become known as the Great Vowel Shift.

As we continue to travel to the end of the Middle English period, we discuss how influential the act of invasion is on determining vocabulary and language development, specifically on the English language.

Since the Norman Conquest, England has never been invaded or conquered by others who speak a foreign language; neither has it had to compete with a new invading language. Our time machine has passed through several centuries and now enters the Modern English period, beginning around the fifteenth century.

As our machine silently glides by, we notice a funeral procession. The death of Chaucer marks the end of the Middle English period. English emerges as a national language and increases in variety, versatility, and vocabulary. It also begins to be spread around the world.

Oh, this is a great time to be aboard a time machine. We enter the Renaissance and Reformation periods of the sixteenth century. We, again, want to be out among the people and are intrigued by all of the new words. Most of the new words are taken from Greek, French, Italian, Spanish, and Portuguese. From the Latin and Greek come the following words: *habitual, criterion, drama, comedy, bonus, alumnus*, and *enthusiasm*. French words include *bayonet, anatomy, entrance*, and *tomato*. Some of the Latin words are *carnival, rocket, design*, and *giraffe*. Words from Spanish and Portuguese include *alligator, guitar, tank, tobacco, canoe*, and *banana*.

Shakespeare was the greatest writer of the Early Modern English period. As we attend one of his plays, we noticed that some of the words are pronounced differently from how they are said today. For example, *reason* sounds like *raisin*. The vowel in *face* is the same sound as in *ask* and in words like *palm, could*, and *would*, and the /l/ is pronounced.

Shakespeare makes a prediction about language in *Julius Caesar*:

> How many ages hence
> Shall this our lofty scene be acted o'er
> In states unborn and accents yet unknown

The English language has changed quite a bit from what it was in the 1600s.

As we continue to travel through the next few centuries, we notice that the English language is becoming more like it is today. We stop at a library and find a copy of John Walker's *Pronouncing Dictionary of English* published in 1774. There is also a copy of

Samuel Johnson's *English Dictionary* published in 1755. Earlier in 1603, the first dictionary was published and had 2,500 words briefly defined. Just think of the thousands of words that are in our modern dictionary!

While traveling in our time machine, we saw that English started out as a minor language spoken by people who inhabited a small island and evolved into the most popular language of the world, spoken as a second language by millions of people.

Just for fun, let's take a trip in our time machine around the world and see English being spoken in Australia, New Zealand, the South Pacific, East and South Asia, many parts of Africa, the Caribbean, Canada, and the United States. Naturally, each dialect of English spoken in these various areas is slightly different from the other. I spent several months in India as a visiting professor, and some of my students had difficulty understanding my American dialect.

Our time machine is now ready to cross the Atlantic Ocean and explore the English language in the United States. We notice that the population of the United States has changed dramatically. Diversity in ethnicity, culture, and language has become a hallmark of large U.S. cities and is growing in small communities throughout the country. For example, the student body of a large school district in California speaks more than 50 languages. Such demographics should alert you that it is important to be well informed regarding the ramifications of such diversity, particularly for clinical and nonclinical interventions.

This discussion on the origins of the English language presents information regarding how the language and its sound system have evolved through the centuries. English consists of many borrowed words, some of which lead to confusion in pronunciation and spelling as they have been adapted to English. Some of the issues and conditions related to dialect usage today were discussed and debated during the different periods of development of the English language. It appears that history is repeating itself and that language is fluid and adapts continually to meet the needs of its speakers and listeners. Those who study and apply the rules of the *sound* system of a language need to realize and appreciate this.

UNITED STATES ENGLISH: A COMPOSITE OF DIALECTS

As our time machine passes by a university, we stop and listen to the voice of a professor lecturing on dialects. He has asked, "What determines a dialect?"

He mentions that current research indicates that there are different and often conflicting assumptions about the data we can use to establish a dialect area.

He mentions that dialects are neither static over time nor manifested in precisely the same way in different places. Dialects exhibit inherent variability, which means that they differ from one another. Speakers can move in and out of dialects, changing their language variety according to the topic, to whom they are speaking, and so forth. As mentioned earlier, speakers often shift to their original dialect upon returning to the place of their roots. Some people may not want their children to learn a second dialect because such change may signify a departure from their family ties.

With an estimated 329 different languages spoken in the United States, we can forecast great shifts to come in the sounds of United States English.

SUMMARY

Indeed, it is the multicultural character of this country that is its great strength. As the population becomes increasingly diverse in cultural and linguistic preferences, speech-language-hearing professionals will increasingly be called on to provide services to persons from a wide variety of cultures, each with their own normative behavior, learning styles, social beliefs, and views of the world. It is important that these professionals understand the persons whom they will serve and that they have an understanding of the different approaches necessary to address linguistic differences, accent reduction, and articulation disorders.

Later chapters include sections on allophonic and dialect variations and on nonnative speaker pronunciation. These sections provide more detailed information as it relates to each individual sound.

Skill-Building Activities

1. Compile a list of 20 words and write your pronunciation of the words in a column next to the written words. (See **Table 3-1** for an example.) Then, make three or more other columns and have others pronounce the same words and note any differences in the sounds. You could include such words as *egg, roof, lettuce, lemon, Mary, direction, precious, houses*. Listen for the differences in the vowel and consonant sounds. For example, *lemon* may be pronounced as lem*in*, lem*on*, or lem*en*. The word *lettuce*: lett*us* or lett*ɪs*, and the words

TABLE 3-1	Sound/Pronunciation Samples			
Words	**Me**	**Person A**	**Person B**	**Person C**
Train	chrain	train	train	chrain
Robert	Robert	Wobert	Robert	Robert
Creek	creek	crik	crik	creek

horses and *houses* could have any combinations of [s] and [z] for the two *s* letters in each word.

Important: Do not say the word to others; rather, provide them with a definition such as "What do you call the top of the house that has shingles on it?" Encourage them to pronounce the words in their natural way. You may want to seek out those with different accents to make it more interesting. Attempt to select a group of subjects that includes both native and nonnative speakers and those of different generations and geographic locations. Other words to consider: *roof, athlete* (ath*a*lete), *realtor* (real*a*tor), *horses* and *houses* ([s]s or [z]s or a combination of both), *leg* and *elf* (long *a* or like *e* in *peg*), *settler* (sett*a*ler).

2. Study the sections titled "Introduction," "Guide to Pronunciation," and "Language Changes Especially Common in American Folk Speech,"

in the *Dictionary of American Regional English*, Frederic G. Cassidy, chief editor, 1985.

3. Review some of the definitions and pronunciations of words listed in the *Dictionary of American Regional English* and compare them with your own.

4. In the front pages of most major dictionaries, there is a brief history of the English language. Select two different dictionaries and read these sections.

5. Enter the key words *United States English dialects* or similar descriptors in a search engine and review some of the information available on different websites.

6. Interview people of various ages, nationalities, and social classes, and ask them questions about dialects such as, "Who do you think speaks a dialect of English?" "What do you think a person should do who speaks a dialect?" "What are the pluses and minuses about speaking a dialect?"

Chapter 4

United States English Spelling and Pronunciation Differences

PURPOSE

To provide a historical review of the spelling rules of United States English and a discourse on the use of dictionaries.

OBJECTIVES

This chapter will provide you with information regarding:

1. Background information on spelling reform
2. Discrepancies between written symbols and pronunciation
3. Purpose of dictionaries and their relationship to phonetic symbols
4. Implications for you to consider regarding sound/symbol representation and use of the dictionary
5. Skill-building activities

One of the best ways for you to appreciate the discrepancies between the written form and the verbal form of communication is to read the following poem that I composed for you:

Eye can think of know better weigh to introduce
    you to United States spelling and pronunciation
    than to right a poem four you. Sew hear it is.

Whether you learned United States spelling and
    pronunciation as a native or learned it as a sec-
    ond language
I'm sure it was confusing for you to do.
You may have learned the word *few*
And then discovered it didn't rhyme with *sew*.
And then you didn't know what to do,
When *both, brother*, and *moth*, you did pursue!
At first, you learned such simple words as *do*
    and *so*
And thought you were on the right path to go.
But almost met your limit with *card* and *ward*
    and *sword* and *word*.
When on a spelling test, you spelled the thing
    that has feathers and flies as *bord*!
You learned the sounds in the word *heard* and
    pronounced them right.
But when the word *beard* came along, it blew
    your mind out of sight.
You began to think that you couldn't pronounce
    anything true.
When you tried to pronounce *treat, great*, and
    threat and rhyme they didn't do!
You thought you had it made when you pro-
    nounced *paid*.
But then you tried to rhyme it with *said*.
You learned that *sew* and *low* rhyme but then
    came along *cow*.

I'm sure you thought you'd never learn all of the differences now.

You knew it was totally impossible when you came to the *gh* ending.

To get *through, hiccough, though,* and *laugh* to rhyme, many a rule you would be bending.

You had it made with *dear* and *fear* and then a *bear* came rambling along.

You don't think you'll ever get the lyrics to rhyme in a song

Because so many of the words are not spelled nor pronounced as they belong!

But one thing you have learned to appreciate and to endure,

If you spell the words *phonetically,* you can pronounce them correctly, for sure.

RATIONALE

The need to know more about the relationship between spelling and phonetics has taken on new meaning with the current increased emphasis on literacy. In the past, examples of spelling and pronunciation differences were listed for general information and, perhaps, for novelty. There is a need now to have a more thorough understanding of the significant role that the principles of phonetics play as part of the sound/symbol foundation in the development of reading, spelling, and writing skills.

Through their coursework and clinical practice, speech-language pathologists acquire information that provides them with an understanding of the basics of reading, writing, and spelling. Such items are secondary to many of the speech and language goals associated with speech and language development.

The American Speech-Language-Hearing Association (ASHA, 2000) established guidelines: *Roles and Responsibilities of Speech-Language Pathologists with Respect to Reading and Writing in Children and Adolescents.*

The guidelines set forth the following:
The rationale for SLPs to play a crucial and direct role in the development of literacy with children and adolescents is based on established connections between the spoken and written language, including that (a) spoken language provides the foundation for the development of reading and writing, (b) spoken and written language have a reciprocal relationship, such that each builds on the other to result in general languages and literacy competence starting early and continuing through childhood into adulthood, (c) children with spoken language problems frequently have difficulty learning to read and write, and children with reading and writing problems frequently have difficulty with spoken language, and (d) instruction in spoken language can result in growth in written language, and instruction in written language can result in growth in spoken language. (pp. 1–2)

This chapter provides you with basic information regarding the important role that the phonetic sound system plays in the development of sound- and word-level awareness for grasping the alphabetic principle and alphabet-letter knowledge. In addition, as each consonant, vowel, and diphthong is described later in this text, sections are included that list the different alphabet letters for each sound: [t] = t-*top*, tt-*butter*, bt-*debt*, ed-*picked*, th-*Thomas*, ght-*thought*, cht-*yacht*, ct-*precinct*, and z-*pizza*. Also included are the different sounds for the same letters, th = voiced th *the*, voiceless th *with*, and silent t *listen*. You will find these listings particularly enlightening and gain further insight into the many discrepancies between the written and spoken word.

INTRODUCTION

Ship, ocean, machine, fuchsia, special, sugar, conscience, nauseous, tissue, mission.

As you become more aware of the relationship between the number of symbols (orthographic alphabet letters) in a word and the actual number of sounds within a word, such as *thought* (seven letters and three sounds), you will begin to realize the discrepancies that exist in the pronunciation rules of United States English. A review of the history of spelling reform in the United States provides insight into how some of these discrepancies came into existence. There will, no doubt, continue to be scholarly discussions regarding the spelling and pronunciation of United States English words. Although the rules of pronunciation may now be more stable than in the past, you need only to examine the spelling used during earlier centuries in this country to note that some dramatic changes have occurred over time. In modern times, the spelling used in **text messaging**, incidentally, more closely resembles the spelling rules of the past century!

This chapter includes a discussion on dictionaries because both native and nonnative speakers of United States English rely on the dictionary to assist them in determining the number of sounds in words and how these words are pronounced. When you use the pronunciation guides in dictionaries, you must employ certain safeguards. If you rely only on the *transcription* of a word as presented in the dictionary, you will develop a very narrow perspective or maybe an erroneous one on the actual pronunciation of the word by others. Dialect differences are not accounted for in the standard dictionary and neither are examples of misarticulations. Dictionaries may be used as a guide, but the ultimate *sound/symbol* transcription is determined by the spoken word of the individual speaker and the accuracy of the transcriber.

SPELLING REFORM

food, blood, good / low, cow / beard, heard / comb, bomb, tomb / cord, word

Some unique contemporary spellings reflect earlier spelling practices used before spelling revision occurred.

Such spellings as *Nite Klub* and *Wile U Wate* catch the eye of the reader and are easily understood (as is modern texting). British and American spelling rules are still not in agreement as you can note in such word pairs as *programme–program; defence–defense; centre–center; catalogue–catalog; doughnut–donut;* and *mould–mold.*

In the early twentieth century, notables such as Andrew Carnegie and Samuel Clemens advocated changes such as omission of silent letters in words like *dumb* and *wrong* and changing the spelling of the [u] sound in words like *do* [du] so that the vowel sound would not be confused with the vowel in *so* [soʊ].

Complete the following exercise (**Table 4-1**). *Instructions:* Identify words that have the same last *letters*

TABLE 4-1	Letters That Are the Same But Have Different Sounds			
1. oe	_____	_____		
2. eard	_____	_____		
3. ome	_____	_____		
4. ow	_____	_____		
5. oll	_____	_____		
6. ose	_____	_____		
7. ead	_____	_____		
8. ere	_____	_____		
9. ear	_____	_____		
10. orse	_____	_____		
11. eak	_____	_____		
12. ont	_____	_____		
13. ord	_____	_____		
14. ear	_____	_____		
15. aughter	_____	_____		
16. outh	_____	_____		
17. omb	_____	_____		
18. eat	_____	_____	_____	
19. ood	_____	_____	_____	
20. ough	_____	_____	_____	_____

Key: There are several choices of words. Here are a few of the options: *beard, heard, some, dome, cow, bow, doll, poll, close, lose, read, read, here, there, house, worse, beak, break, front, font, cord, word, bear, dear, daughter, laughter, mouth, youth, tomb, comb, bomb, tomb, beat, great, sweat, hood, food, flood, trough, rough, bough, through.*

but different *sounds*. Upon completion, refer to the key at the bottom of the listing.

And then there are words that *rhyme* but that have *different letters*. For example: *sweet, seat, suite; debt* and *threat*, but not *threat* and *treat*!

Eliminating Spelling Irregularities

A concern to eliminate spelling irregularities has been a focus from at least the sixteenth century (Crystal, 1995). Hundreds of reform proposals continue to be devised. The fact that reform bodies continue to be active testifies to a genuine and widespread concern. Crystal (1995) observes that the history of the spelling reform movement indicates that the disadvantages have generally always outweighed the advantages. He states that we know too little about:

1. The way children actually learn and use spelling systems.

2. The kind of errors adults make with traditional spelling.

3. The nature of compatibility of old and new systems.

Crystal (1995) states that the strongest argument of the reformers is that English spelling should be allowed to evolve naturally and that there is nothing sacrosanct about print. He concludes that their biggest problem remains the question of management. How can any such evolution be organized and implemented. (Author's note: Who knows, perhaps the "evolution" has begun with the popularity of the current *phonetic spelling* being used universally in text and instant messaging.) In orthography,

- Different letters may represent the same sound.

- The same letter represents different sounds.

- Combinations of letters may represent a sound.

- Letters may represent no sound.

SPELLING PRACTICES AND PRONUNCIATION

In written English, a number of spelling practices deviate from the phonetic principle of one sound per symbol (Dew & Jensen, 1974):

1. A single letter is used to represent one sound in some words and a distinctly different sound in other words, such as the hard *c* [k] *come* and the soft *c* [s] *city*.

2. In spelling, a single sound is sometimes represented by one letter and at other times by another letter, such as the [z] in *buzz* and *was*.

3. A single sound is represented by a pair of different letters despite the use of each letter individually to represent other sounds, such as the diagraphs [ph] *phone* and [th] *thin*.

4. A pair of letters *tt* and *mm*, as in *butter* and *summer*, represent only one sound.

5. Some letters are silent, as in *doubt* and *dumb*.

The [b], [m], and [n] have only one sound unless they are silent. The range of pronunciation of consonant letters is somewhat more predictable than the pronunciation of there are vowel letters (Avery & Ehrlich, 1992). This is because there are many more vowel sounds in English than there are vowel letters in the Roman alphabet and because historical changes in the pronunciation of English well-to-do speakers affected vowel sounds much more than they did consonant sounds.

Pronunciation of Vowels

There are at least twice as many vowel sounds in United States English as there are in many other languages. For example, in Japanese and Spanish, there are only five vowels and these vowels are rather distinct and easier to produce than United States English vowels, which may be produced in closer proximity to one another. Avery and Ehrlich (1992) indicate that the comparison of the English vowel system to a typical five-vowel system reveals several potential problem areas:

1. The tense/lax tongue tension contrasts such as [i] (tense) in <u>ea</u>sy versus [ɑ] (lax) in <u>au</u>tumn does not exist in a five-vowel system. This may result in confusion in the distinction between sounds such as *beat-bit, bait-bet, book-boot*.

2. Auditory discrimination may be difficult for some listeners and hinder their ability to discriminate between [ɛ] b<u>e</u>d, [æ] <u>a</u>sk, [ʌ] b<u>u</u>t, and [ɑ] <u>a</u>ll. Also, some speakers and listeners have difficulty discerning the [ɑ] and [ɔ] sound differences, which may be more influenced by dialect.

For the most part, vowels have been divided into two categories, long vowels and short vowels. Certain rules apply:

1. When a-e-i-o-u occur in words ending in the silent *e* letter, the letters have the same <u>long vowel</u> sound as their name: *gate, Pete, guide, vote, cute*.

2. When there is no *e* at the end of the word, the vowels are pronounced as short vowels: *sat, met, bid, not, hut.*

3. *Words* related to meaning also have this correspondence of <u>long vowels</u> *same, serene, divine* and <u>short vowels</u> *sanity, serenely, divinity.*

The sound–spelling correspondence of vowels occurs with some regularity, although there are always exceptions to the rule. The particular vowel used in combination with a consonant also can predict the sound of the consonant in a word. For example:

1. The letter *c* is pronounced [s] when followed by *i, e,* or *y: city, receipt, cycle.*

2. The letter *c* is pronounced [k] when followed by *a, o,* or *u: cake, coke, cute.*

In comparison with vowels, the pronunciation of the consonant letters is somewhat more predictable than the pronunciation of vowel letters.

Other Features of Pronunciation

Other aspects of speech production that affect pronunciation are stress, rhythm, and intonation, also known as suprasegmentals or the prosodic features of speech. These elements are more fully discussed in Chapter 5 and in the sections on allophonic and dialect variations on native speaker pronunciation in later chapters.

The key elements of United States English pronunciation include appropriate stress, rhythm, and intonation. Problems can occur with each of these that can lead to some degree of unintelligibility on the part of the speaker or distraction on the part of the listener who finds the differences interfering with the comprehension of the spoken utterance.

Spelling in Other Languages

The Roman alphabet is used in many languages, including English. However, differences in the sound–spelling correspondences of other languages may result in mispronunciation in English. Take, for example, the letter *s* in *sky, shoe,* and *has.* The spelling system of some languages is more straightforward than the English spelling system in representing sounds. There is usually a one-to-one correspondence between sounds and spelling in such languages as Spanish, Hungarian, and Polish. There may be a tendency for these speakers to pronounce every letter of the English word, assuming incorrectly that the English spelling system is like the spelling system of their native language.

Some speakers may assign the sound values of their own spelling system to the letters used in English words. This often results in a process referred to as *spelling pronunciation* (Avery & Ehrlich, 1992). These authors suggest that pronouncing words on the basis of one's native language spelling system does not necessarily constitute a pronunciation problem. It may merely reflect a lack of knowledge regarding the complex sound–spelling correspondence of the English language.

Avery and Ehrlich (1992) recommend that it is beneficial to be familiar with the sound–spelling correspondences of other languages so as to understand where they differ from English.

UNITED STATES ENGLISH PRONUNCIATION AND THE DICTIONARY

Both native and nonnative English speakers sometimes rely on the dictionary as a reference when they enroll in a class on phonetics. Students have a tendency both to use and misuse the dictionary pronunciation key and information on standard usage. Although the dictionary is perceived and used as a guide—and it should be—its use by phonetics students requires some precautions.

This section presents an overview of the historical and contemporary research and issues that have confronted lexicographers (editors of dictionaries) through the years. It concludes with a word of caution regarding the use of dictionaries as a pronunciation guide. Because dictionaries are widely used in conjunction with literacy programs, it is beneficial to understand the background and philosophy of editors of dictionaries. This information assists you in determining the strengths and weaknesses of dictionaries as it relates to their value as a resource for sound/symbol correlates.

Use of Dictionaries

How are dictionaries useful to you in their current form? For general pronunciation guidance they have some merit, but several safeguards need to be taken. This is particularly true when you are a nonnative speaker of United States English. Here are some points to keep in mind:

1. In phonetics, because the goal is to transcribe speech *as any given person speaks it*, you should not rely on dictionary pronunciation as, necessarily, the way any particular word should be spoken or transcribed.

2. Beginning students tend to want to "grasp onto something" that is concrete such as a dictionary pronunciation. This approach probably is more of a detriment than a help when it comes to total understanding of sound/symbol transcription, particularly in a clinical setting. Such an approach also may give the beginning student the impression that there is only one "correct" way to say a word and not make allowances for dialect differences. Here are some examples: *Chicago* has as its first sound either a *ch* or *sh*; *train* begins with a *ch* or the consonant blend *tr*; and differences occur between formal and informal usage such as syllable reduction in the word *chocolate*, choc-o-late versus choc-late. Do you say *di<u>r</u>ection* or *drection*?

3. Some students have difficulty with syllabication. The division of spoken words into syllables may be different from the syllable divisions used in a dictionary, resulting in total confusion. For example, some dictionaries prefer a morphemic (meaning) division of syllables such as in *skat-er* rather than the phonetic division *ska-ter*. Stockwell and Minkova (2001) present an overview of the different types of dictionaries.

Several dictionary representatives indicate that the International Phonetic Alphabet (IPA) may become more prevalent in use with the English as a Second Language (ESL) population. You may find yourself in settings where expertise with the IPA is valuable. There is a real need for research in the effective utilization of the IPA as an instructional methodology to meet the needs of such a diverse population that is ever increasing in the United States.

SUMMARY

The English alphabet mostly is a product of Roman and Greek influences. The spellings of United States English words contain many discrepancies between alphabet letters and sounds. The basic premise of sound/symbol representation can be very useful in demonstrating sound- and word-level awareness and alphabetic-letter knowledge as they relate to literacy in spelling, writing, and reading. Dictionaries are useful but must be used with some caution because all are not consistent in their presentation of pronunciation rules, syllable separation, and dialect diversity. Listening skills are a prerequisite to the accurate recording of speech sounds. A variety of symbols is used to represent sounds, and diacritic markings identify more subtle aspects such as dentalization and minus aspiration. The International Phonetic Alphabet offers a standardized set of symbols for recording different sounds spoken throughout the world.

Skill-Building Activities

1. Compare the pronunciation symbols listed in four different dictionaries. You can usually find the dictionary's pronunciation key on its inside front cover. Set the dictionaries side by side and compare the symbols used to identify the same sounds. Note the similarities and differences in some of the symbols and even the pronunciation. For example:

Letters Sound	Word	Dictionary			
		1	2	3	4
ch /ʧ/	catch	kat**ch**	ka<u>ch</u>	kaʧ	kach

2. Note the number of syllables you say for each of the following words. Compare your sample with that of several dictionaries. For example, some dictionaries acknowledge syllable deletion as an option for a word like *federal: fed-(ə)-rəl* because the common pronunciation of some people is two syllables *fed-rəl* rather than three syllables. In contrast, someone may add a syllable that is not present in the dictionary spelling.

How Many Syllables?

library ___ arctic ___ athlete ___ realtor ___ nuclear ___ mirror ___ chimney ___ every ___ chocolate ___ vegetable ___ poinsettia ___ federal ___ settler ___ asterisk ___

Say the preceding words as both two- and three-syllable words. Make a riddle out of these words. Present a clue to someone. Say, "What do you call a building that houses a lot of books that you can check out?" Note how many syllables others say in these words.

3. Interview a classroom teacher and inquire about the problems he or she encounters when teaching spelling.

4. Interview several people who have learned English as a second language and have them relate

to you the difficulties they had in learning to spell English words.

5. Randomly select words in a dictionary and say them out loud, noticing whether your pronuniciation of syllables corresponds with the dictionary's syllabilization of the word. Notice, for example, the word *grasshopper*. As you pronounce it to yourself, does the last syllable begin with the [p] sound? According to the dictionary, it would be pronounced *gras-hop-er* with no [p] sound in the last syllable. Do not confuse the *written* with the *spoken*. The purpose of the break in the written form is to indicate where the word can be hyphenated at the end of a line or along the right margin of a page, for example. Such breaks may or may not correspond with the spoken syllable pronunciation. The purpose of this activity is to alert you to the potential difficulties in the number of syllables in a word as indicated in a dictionary versus the numbers of syllables spoken in daily life.

6. Search the Web for topics related to spelling. There are many interesting topics related to the history of spelling, teaching strategies, and other concepts.

7. Search the American Speech-Language-Hearing Association website (http://www.asha.org) on the topic of literacy and become acquainted with the professional educational goals of that organization regarding literacy.

8. Visit your college or university library and become acquainted with the content of the *Dictionary of American Regional English*. Write a two-page commentary on your findings.

REFERENCES

Avery, P. W., & Ehrlich, S. (1992). *Teaching American English pronunciation.* Oxford, England: Oxford University Press.

Crystal, D. (Ed.) (1995). *The Cambridge encyclopedia of the English language.* Cambridge, England: Cambridge University Press.

Dew, D., & Jensen, P. J. (1974). *Phonetic transcription: An audio-tutorial program.* Columbus, OH: Charles E. Merrill.

American Speech-Language-Hearing Association. (2000). *Roles and responsibilities of speech-language pathologists with respect to reading and writing in children and adolescents* (Position Statement). Rockville, MD: Author. Retrieved from http://www.asha.org/docs/html/ps2001-00104.html

Stockwell, R., & Minkova, D. (2001). *English words: History and structure.* Cambridge, England: Cambridge University Press.

Chapter 5

The Three Ss: Sounds, Syllables, and Suprasegmentals

PURPOSE

To provide information concerning the units that influence sound production and their relationship to one another.

OBJECTIVES

This chapter will provide you with information regarding:

1. Basic acoustic elements of human speech sounds
2. Characteristics of syllables
3. The role of suprasegmentals (prosody) in speech production
4. Skill-building activities

INTRODUCTION

When embarking on a study of phonetics, you should understand several terms and concepts. These include **sounds, syllables**, and **suprasegmentals**. An understanding of both the acoustic and physical elements of sounds is essential because sounds represent the basic units of phonetics. Just like the alphabet, which is a set of written symbols necessary for reading and writing, the phonetic symbols enable phonetic transcription.

Knowledge of the characteristics and functions of syllables is needed to understand the rules of pronunciation and meaning. In some instances, the primary stressed syllable is indicated with a different phonetic symbol, although the sounds may be quite similar. For example, in the word *above*, the two vowels *a* and *o* have basically the same sound but are transcribed as [əbʌv]. Another example, there are two "r" sounds in the word *murder* [mɝdɚ]. The sound in the first syllable is the stressed "r" and the sound in the second syllable is the unstressed "r." *Also*, knowledge of the characteristics of a syllable is essential as it relates to suprasegmental features such as **stress, rate**, and **intonation** patterns. For example, the printed word *present* can be either a noun or a verb depending on which syllable has the primary stress, **pre**sent versus pre**sent**. In addition to stress and intonation patterns, suprasegmental features include rate and rhythm. The transcription of formal versus informal speaking such as "Come and get them" versus "Come 'n git 'em" is affected by the rate of speaking. The use of a foreign **accent** while speaking English is an example of the suprasegmental features (prosody) of one language imposed on another, for example, speaking English with a Spanish intonation pattern. Accent reduction focuses on changing these features to "fit" the features of the second language.

SOUND

Kreidler (1989) provides an understandable description of sound as it relates to human listening. He says that when "we hear something" we speak of hearing as if it were something that we do, an action that we perform. In reality, hearing a sound is not so much something that we do as it is something that *happens* to us, a stimulus that we receive and to which we react. When we hear a door slam or an airplane overhead, the air around us is disturbed and that causes particles of air to move. These particles of air contact our eardrums and create a different type of air pressure. The difference in pressure affects the tiny bones behind the eardrum, these bones cause changes of pressure in a liquid stored in the inner ear, and the different pressures in the liquid produce different nerve sensations that are telegraphed to the brain and sound is perceived.

Ordinarily, we not only hear, we recognize (discriminate) what we have heard. We can distinguish the ring of a telephone from the ring of a doorbell. This is possible because we have stored such sounds in our memory and we compare each new auditory experience with those we have previously recorded. Thus, hearing a sound is both passive (acts on us) and active (interpretation of auditory stimuli).

Sound in the context of this text refers to human speech sounds that are spoken by a speaker and perceived by a listener. United States English speech sounds consist of consonants, vowels, and diphthongs (combinations of two vowels: *house* [haʊs]) that can be identified by their distinctive features. The characteristics of a speech sound can also be influenced by the meaning of a word or utterance, such as when specifying *the* apple in contrast to using the same word *the* in conversational speech with *th* [ð] in an unstressed context.

The study of speech production from an acoustic point of view provides the means for looking at a very complex process in a simpler way (Fucci & Lass, 1999). That simpler way is the intent of this book rather than to provide an extensive discourse in speech acoustics. That subject is addressed in more depth in courses related to speech science and acoustics. Acoustic phonetics analyzes the amplitude, **frequency**, and duration of human speech sounds, which are displayed on a spectrogram (Johnson, 1997; Kent & Read, 2002). Johnson (1997) discusses three important topics in acoustic phonetics:

1. The acoustic properties of major classes of speech sounds

2. The acoustic theory of speech production

3. The auditory representation of speech

These topics are included in his book *Acoustic and Auditory Phonetics*, which he recommends as a supplement to a general phonetics or speech science text. Another resource on acoustics is *The Acoustic Analysis of Speech* (2nd edition) by Kent and Read (2002).

Fucci and Lass (1999) designed a straightforward model of speech sound production that includes three major components controlled by the central nervous system. Each component is modified by the one that succeeds it as the communication progresses from speaker to listener. The three components are: (1) energy source, produced by the airflow from the lungs; (2) sound source that is voiced, such as the vowels and **voiced consonants** [d] and [z], or voiceless, such as consonants created by noise-like qualities [t], [k], [p]; and (3) resonance source that consists of the hard and soft surfaces of the speech production tract, which begins above the larynx and exits through the openings of the mouth or nose. Vocal fold vibration is the usual sound source, and the vocal tract is the resonance source and acts as an acoustic filter that modifies the sound made by the vocal folds. One of the best demonstrations of the effect of resonance is in the production of the nasal resonance sounds [n], [m], and [ŋ]. Lightly pinch your nose as you produce these sounds and you will sense the vibration created by the sound waves acting on the inner surfaces of the nasal cavity.

Three basic types of airflow modulation provide the sound sources of vowels, diphthongs, and consonants (Pickett, 1999). These types are: (1) an aperiodic or voiceless sound source for voiceless consonants such as *sh* [ʃ] "ssshhhhhh" that is a turbulent, hissing sound source; (2) a periodic or voiced sound source for vowels, diphthongs, and voiced consonants; and (3) a transient, steplike sound source that is produced by the formation of a momentary complete constriction of the airflow, such as the first step in the production of a stop consonant [t] or [k] to the second step release of the stopped airflow. The steplike sound results in a period of silence followed by noise comparable to that provided by turbulent modulation.

Some languages include oral clicks and glottal stops. One of the most distinctive types of nonpulmonic (not originating in the lungs) sounds is the click (Crystal, 1987). Crystal mentions that it is quite possible to make sounds like *tut-tut* or *tsk-tsk* independent of airflow from the lungs. In other words, you can inhale and exhale and still produce this series of sounds. Crystal indicates that "click languages" include some of the southern Africa languages, including the Khoisan languages, that have the most complex click systems, using many different **places of articulation** in the mouth and involving the simultaneous use of other sounds made in the throat or nose.

Crystal (1987) explains that when the glottis makes the air move inward, the sounds are called *implosives*, and when the air is made to move outward, the sounds are called *ejectives*. Implosives and ejectives are particularly common in certain American Indian and African languages and may be heard in certain accents and styles of English such as in the word *bottle* where the [t] sound may be substituted by a glottal stop.

These types of airflow modulations for vowels, diphthongs, consonants, clicks, and glottal sounds are produced by the speaker and perceived (hearing acuity) and interpreted (hearing discrimination) by the listener. Hearing acuity and hearing discrimination are listening skills. Some consonants such as the voiceless [f] and the th [Θ] in thin are high-frequency sounds and are more difficult to hear than such voiced sounds as [v] and [g]. All vowels and diphthongs are voiced and quite easy to hear. Some words because of their spelling may appear to have a certain number of sounds when in actuality it is difficult for the human ear to perceive whether or not a sound is present. For example, unless the listener knows the context in which the word is spoken (by surrounding words or environmental cues), the words *tents* and *tense* are undistinguishable to the human ear. However, a "voice print" of the production of the two words indicates the influence of the *t* in *tents*. Vowel sounds have more acoustic energy than **voiceless consonants** and are therefore more easily audible to the listener. Although there are variations (**allophones**) in the production of human speech sounds (a [t] may have more or less "explosion" to it), a sound is still perceived as such even though there are acoustic differences.

SYLLABICATION

Another skill to be acquired by the phonetic transcriptionist is the ability to identify (1) the number of syllables in a word and (2) which syllables are given the primary and secondary stresses. At first, you may think that these are simple tasks, but in reality many people have difficulty with both. The discussion that follows is intended to help you understand the concept and function of syllabication.

Shriberg and Kent (1995) state that it is difficult to define exactly what a syllable is. A popular conception is that a syllable is a grouping of speech movements usually linked together with other speech movements in a rhythmic pattern. They prefer to think of syllables as highly adaptive units for the articulatory organization of speech.

Most speakers can identify the number of syllables a word has, but in English, they are not always able to say precisely where syllable boundaries occur for certain words. Ball (1993) adds that although we can identify the number of syllables in a word, we usually cannot say how we reached our answer or produce an adequate description of what a syllable is. One of the problems is that individuals may perceive syllables in slightly different ways. For example, for words that end in *-ism*, is the *-ism* ending one or two syllables? Consider *prism, mechanism*. Also consider *real, wheel, fire, hour* and words with neighboring vowels: *heavier, mediate*.

Traditionally, the minimal requirement for a syllable is the presence of a vowel (as in *a-bout*) or a diphthong, which is a combination of two vowels acting as one sound (as in the gliding combination in the word *ice* [aɪs]). This definition holds fairly true except for some consonants that function as a "nucleus," which are discussed in the following subsection.

For both beginning and experienced students, the "bound-a-ries" or "boun-da-ries" of syllables can be confusing and ambivalent. Sloat, Taylor, and Hoard (1978) and Crystal (1995) offer a comforting commentary on the subject to offset the feelings of frustration when you attempt to determine syllable divisions. They state that it is one thing to be able to count the number of syllables in a word (and most people do not have difficulty with this), but it is quite another to decide where the boundaries between the syllables are. Crystal notes that English is full of cases where alternative analyses are possible. He provides three examples that should get you thinking:

1. In the two-syllable word *extra* [ɛktrə], where does the division occur? It is not likely to be [ɛ-kstrə] because that appears very awkward and there are no syllables in English that begin with the consonant sequence of "kstr."

2. There are two syllable in *standing*, but where is the division to be made, "stand-ing" or "standing"? Crystal indicates that two approaches may be used to make the choice. If you follow a phonetic instinct and go for two evenly balanced consonant-vowel-consonant (CVC) syllables, the

result is "stan-ding." The grammatical instinct is to divide between the base form (*stand*) and the inflection (*ing*). This form of syllable division is discussed in Chapter 4 in the section on using a dictionary as a pronunciation guide with the accompanying caution not to rely entirely on dictionary guidelines for the correct pronunciation.

3. There are three syllables in *boundary* and the same question can be asked, "Where does the division occur?" Is it determined phonetically (*boun-da-ry*) or grammatically (*bound-a-ry*) to preserve a semantic link with *bound*? Is *several* three syllables *se-ve-ral* or two syllables *sev-ral*? Crystal concludes that regional accent, speed of speech, level of formality, and context of use can all influence these decisions. The number of syllables may be determined by whether they are being spoken spontaneously or read aloud, and whether they are being said with emphasis, with emotion, or plainly stated.

It also is worthwhile to discuss the hyphenation used in some dictionaries. You may view such marks as indicators of syllable breaks when, in fact, these marks do not necessarily correspond to syllabic boundaries in speech. Rather, they reflect the editor's general publishing practice to indicate where the *printed* word should be divided in written form.

Syllabic Consonants

Under certain conditions and in some contexts, a number of consonants function as the nucleus of a syllable, performing the function of a vowel in the syllable: the [l̩] in *hum-ble* and *bo-ttle*, the [m] in *bo-ttom*, and the [n] in *bu-tton*. *Pick-le* [pɪkl̩] has two syllables but no vowel sound in the second syllable; therefore, the [l] in the second syllable is considered a syllabic consonant. Other words may be written with a vowel in the second syllable but pronounced without the vowel sound, such as *season* [sizn̩], *lesson* [lɛsn̩], and *risen* [rizn̩].

There are more syllabic consonants in rapid speech than in slow, careful speech (Sloat et al., 1978). Speakers have a tendency to drop segments in rapid speech, and if the segment dropped is a vowel, an adjacent consonant may become syllabic. The [l] and nasal sounds of [m], [n], and [ŋ] may become syllabic consonants depending on the adjacent consonant, as in:

[n] room and board = room 'n board
[n] pots and pans = pots 'n pans
[m] up and back = up 'n back

A common pronunciation of *button* does not include a distinct "ton" (as in weight) at the end and excludes the *o* vowel, and the sounds move from one consonant [t] directly to another [n]. In very slow or precise articulation of such words, the vowels may reappear and the consonants may revert to their normal value as in [bɑtəl], but these pronunciations are highly artificial and are not used in conversational speech except in some dialectual instances (Crystal, 1995). Crystal includes as a syllabic consonant the *r* in *perhaps* when said as "pr-haps," but this *r* actually functions as a central vowel [ɝ]; [pɝhæps] that is explained later in this text.

Cardinal Rule

A syllable consists of one vowel, diphthong, or syllabic consonant. Almost everything else regarding syllabication is open to interpretation!

SUPRASEGMENTALS

Suprasegmentals are prosodic features of **stress, intonation, loudness, rate,** and **rhythm** that are imposed on a single sound (phoneme), a series of sounds (syllables), or longer utterances (words, phrases, sentences). These prosodic features provide added meaning or change the meaning of speech productions. The word *prosody* comes from ancient Greek and means a "song sung with instrumental music" (Nooteboom, 1997). In modern phonetics, the words *prosody* and *prosodic* are most often used to refer to such properties as the controlled modulation of the voice pitch, the stretching and shrinking of segment and syllable durations, and the intentional fluctuations of overall loudness. In contrast, an utterance spoken in a monotone pattern is an example of a complete absence of suprasegmental features. Apart from the consonants and vowels, many other aspects of speech may need to be recorded (especially if you are working with speakers with speech disorders). Ball and Lowry (2001) note that some or all suprasegmental features may be important to a total understanding of the message or to the complete characterization of a speaker's abilities. Tatham and Morton (2006) define the terms *prosody* and *prosodic* as relating to a dimension of speech that goes beyond the individual sounds and how they are strung together.

Three main suprasegmental features need to be determined to understand prosody in speech production and perception: stress, intonation, and rhythm.

Rhythm is the melody of the utterance that includes intonation and inflectional patterns.

Stress is associated with pitch, which is produced by the speaker on a relative scale of low to high and is subjectively perceived by the listener, and it exhibits pattern changes in the duration and loudness of an utterance. It can occur in a single sound, such as "Oh, that is eeeeeasy," and within a word or words within an utterance: "I want you to SIT DOWN NOW!" or "LOOK OUT FOR THAT CAR!" The nature of stress is simple enough (Roach, 1983). Almost everyone can agree that the first syllable of words like *father, open, camera* is stressed; that the middle syllable is stressed in *potato, apartment*; and that the final syllable is stressed in *receive, perhaps*. Roach (1983) indicates that there are two different ways to describe the characteristics of stressed syllables. One is to consider what the speaker does in producing stressed syllables (production), and the other, is to consider what characteristics of sound make a syllable seem to the listener to be stressed (perception). The production of stress requires the speaker to use more muscular energy than is used for unstressed syllables. The muscles used to expel air from the lungs and other muscles of speech are more active.

From a perceptual point of view, Roach (1983) notes that all stressed syllables have one characteristic in common, and that is called prominence. Stressed syllables are recognized as stressed because they are more prominent than unstressed syllables are. There are at least four factors that create prominence: (1) loudness: stressed syllables are louder than unstressed syllables; (2) length; (3) pitch; and (4) vowel quality. Pitch in speech is closely related to the frequency of vibration of the vocal cords and is a perceptual characteristic of speech. When one syllable is said with a pitch that is noticeably different from the others, it makes that syllable prominent. Roach concludes that these factors tend to work together, though syllables may be made prominent by only one or two of these factors.

Word meaning can also be changed depending on the stressed syllable. You need to know the context of the word *conduct* before you can pronounce it correctly. Notice the difference in these two statements: "Your conduct (*noun*) is excellent" and "She will conduct (*verb*) the orchestra." In the noun form, the emphasis is on the first syllable, but the emphasis is on the second syllable in the verb form. Also, did you notice that the vowel sound changed in the first syllable? In some Asian languages, a word spelled the same as another has a different meaning depending on the tonal inflection, as discussed in a moment.

Intonation contours are patterns of pitch variations that are associated with rhythm. An example is the intonation used to produce a declarative statement versus a question. Experiment with this by "humming" the intonation pattern rather than verbalizing. Hum . . . "Where did you go?" Now hum, "I went home." Notice the difference in the inflectional pattern. In the question form, the contour tends to end in an upward pattern. The statement form ends in either a neutral or downward pattern. In United States English, one of the main functions of intonation is to differentiate between sentence types.

As mentioned, some languages are tonal languages, in which the tone used on a particular word or morpheme determines the meaning, and a different word or meaning is produced when a different tone is applied (Roach, 1983). English does not use tone in this way. You can, however, observe from time to time a nonnative English speaker who speaks English with their native intonation patterns imposed on English utterances.

Not often considered as a prosodic feature, but rather one that has a function is the pause. A pause is a silent interval that can occur within a word or a phrase. When intentionally produced, it can add emphasis to a statement, create anticipation in a listener, and influence the meaning of what is said. Situations such as "I wish he would hurry up and say something" signal that the listener desires a reaction on the part of the speaker. Think of a child who is about to be informed of a punishment. The parent may use a "deadly" silence or may mete out the punishment by saying, "For your punishment you will (*pause*). . . ." Also, a phrase is defined as an utterance that is bounded by silent intervals, or pauses.

Pronunciation changes occur in connected or conversational speaking versus saying words in isolation. Repeat the following words in citation form: "We-want-them-to-go-with-us." In connected speech, the same utterance would be something like this, "We wan' 'em to go with us." The contour pattern of the less stressed portion of the utterance contains omitted sounds. The omitted sounds in the words *want* and *them* do not indicate a speech defect; in this context, they are a result of the operations of conversational speaking and are considered normal.

Cardinal Rule

Suprasegmentals are imposed on sounds, syllables, words, phrases, and longer utterances to provide meaning and intent. Words that are spelled the same (present) *can change from a noun to a verb merely by altering the pattern of stress applied. Loudness and intonation patterns can provide emphasis to critical elements of an utterance, and pitch variation adds tonal qualities to the spoken utterance.*

SUMMARY

The production of speech sounds requires an energy source, which is the airflow from the lungs; a sound source created by the opened or closed vocal folds; and a vocal tract wherein the sound waves are shaped by contact with the surfaces of the tract. Human speech sounds are spoken by a speaker and perceived by a listener. United States English speech sounds consist of consonants, vowels, and diphthongs. The characteristics of a speech sound can also be influenced by the meaning of a word or utterance.

Syllabication rules are somewhat controversial. Although most people can identify the total number of syllables in a word, they might find it difficult to select where the break between syllables occurs and which syllables have primary and secondary stresses.

Suprasegmental features include stress, intonation, rhythm, rate, loudness, and pitch. Suprasegmental features add meaning to utterances. Nonnative speakers sometimes superimpose the prosodic features of their native language on their second language. For example, some people might speak English with a Spanish intonation pattern.

Skill-Building Activities

Sounds and Syllables

Instructions: Pronounce each of the following words. Pronounce each again in isolated sounds as naturally as possible.

1. Step 1: Record the number of sounds.
2. Step 2: Record the number of syllables.
3. Step 3: Indicate which syllable has the primary stress.

There should be close agreement between the number of sounds and syllables. The primary stress of the speaker may vary from that indicated in the answer key in the right-hand column. Refer to the key after completing each word for immediate feedback.

Set 1

Example:

Word	Number of Sounds	Number of Syllables	Stressed Syllable	Key
camera	5	3	1	
exclamation	11	4	3	

Word	Number of Sounds	Number of Syllables	Stressed Syllable	Key
1. banana	_____	_____	_____	6-3-2
2. constitution	_____	_____	_____	11-4-3
3. unwanted	_____	_____	_____	8-3-2
4. grandfather	_____	_____	_____	9-3-1
5. Mississippi	_____	_____	_____	8-4-3
6. everything	_____	_____	_____	7-4-3
7. imitation	_____	_____	_____	8-4-3
8. avalanche	_____	_____	_____	7-3-2
9. judicial	_____	_____	_____	7-3-2
10. amphibian	_____	_____	_____	8-4-2
11. Sacramento	_____	_____	_____	10-4-3
12. iodine	_____	_____	_____	5-3-1
13. diagnosis	_____	_____	_____	8-3-3
14. deliver	_____	_____	_____	6-3-2
15. evidence	_____	_____	_____	7-3-2
16. anything	_____	_____	_____	6-3-2
17. whoever	_____	_____	_____	5-3-2
18. generator	_____	_____	_____	7-4-3
19. population	_____	_____	_____	9-4-3
20. November	_____	_____	_____	7-3-2

Set 2

Word	Number of Sounds	Number of Syllables	Stressed Syllable	Key
1. planetarium	_____	_____	_____	11-5-3
2. December	_____	_____	_____	7-3-2
3. condition	_____	_____	_____	8-3-2
4. somebody	_____	_____	_____	7-3-2
5. erosion	_____	_____	_____	6-3-2
6. unusual	_____	_____	_____	8-3-2
7. hippopotamus	_____	_____	_____	11-5-3
8. average	_____	_____	_____	5-3-1
9. navigator	_____	_____	_____	8-4-3
10. providing	_____	_____	_____	8-3-2
11. aptitude	_____	_____	_____	7-3-1
12. agility	_____	_____	_____	7-4-2
13. customer	_____	_____	_____	7-3-2
14. understand	_____	_____	_____	9-3-3
15. cantaloupe	_____	_____	_____	8-3-2
16. endurance	_____	_____	_____	8-3-2
17. uncommon	_____	_____	_____	7-3-2
18. romantic	_____	_____	_____	8-3-2
19. acrobat	_____	_____	_____	7-3-2
20. populate	_____	_____	_____	8-3-2

Set 3

Word	Number of Sounds	Number of Syllables	Stressed Syllable	Key
1. apartment	_____	_____	_____	9-3-2
2. gasoline	_____	_____	_____	7-3-2
3. hamburger	_____	_____	_____	7-3-2
4. regulation	_____	_____	_____	10-4-3
5. comedy	_____	_____	_____	6-3-2
6. department	_____	_____	_____	10-3-2
7. important	_____	_____	_____	9-3-2

Word	Number of Sounds	Number of Syllables	Stressed Syllable	Key
8. improvise	_____	_____	_____	8-3-2
9. election	_____	_____	_____	7-3-2
10. irrigation	_____	_____	_____	8-4-3
11. definition	_____	_____	_____	9-4-3
12. engineer	_____	_____	_____	7-3-1
13. carpenter	_____	_____	_____	8-3-2
14. ignition	_____	_____	_____	7-3-2
15. declaration	_____	_____	_____	9-4-3
16. whenever	_____	_____	_____	6-3-2
17. abilities	_____	_____	_____	8-4-2
18. tomorrow	_____	_____	_____	6-3-2
19. meteorite	_____	_____	_____	7-4-3
20. mechanic	_____	_____	_____	7-3-2

STRESS IN HOMOGRAPHS

Homographs are words that are spelled the same but that can be pronounced differently, primarily to change the part of speech. Insert the diacritic stress mark (′) to indicate the syllable with the primary stress. Notice in many of the noun–verb pairs that the vowel sound changes as an indication of the part of speech.

Example: ′re cord n.   re′cord v.

protest n. _____	protest v. _____
conduct n. _____	conduct v. _____
subject n. _____	subject v. _____
extract n. _____	extract v. _____
permit n. _____	permit v. _____
insert n. _____	insert v. _____
desert n. _____	desert v. _____
rebel n. _____	rebel v. _____
combat n. _____	combat v. _____
conflict n. _____	conflict v. _____
present n. _____	present v. _____
convert n. _____	convert v. _____

SHH! WHERE ARE THE SILENT LETTERS?

Instructions: Indicate which letter or combination of letters in the following words is silent. Refer to the key in the right-hand column to check your answers.

Example: dead   a

Set 1

Word	Silent Letter	Word	Silent Letter	Key
1. doubt	____	11. scene	____	b, c
2. handsome	____	12. come	____	d, e
3. off	____	13. sign	____	f, g
4. honest	____	14. weird	____	h, i
5. knife	____	15. salmon	____	k, l
6. mnemonics	____	16. column	____	m, n
7. famous	____	17. raspberry	____	o, p
8. often	____	18. guess	____	t, u
9. answer	____	19. yacht	____	w, ch
10. bough	____			gh

Set 2

Word	Silent Letter	Word	Silent Letter	Key
1. align	____	23. benign	____	g, g
2. bomb	____	24. comb	____	b, b
3. condemn	____	25. crumb	____	n, b
4. daughter	____	26. dough	____	gh, gh
5. dumb	____	27. eight	____	b, gh
6. fourth	____	28. ghastly	____	u, h
7. ghost	____	29. gnash	____	h, g
8. gnat	____	30. gnaw	____	g, g
9. hymn	____	31. indebted	____	n, b
10. knack	____	32. knave	____	k, k
11. knee	____	33. kneel	____	k, k
12. knit	____	34. knob	____	k, k
13. knock	____	35. knot	____	k, k
14. know	____	36. knuckle	____	k, k
15. plumber	____	37. pneumatic	____	b, p
16. pneumonia	____	38. prompt	____	p, p
17. psalm	____	39. psychology	____	p, p
18. through	____	40. thumb	____	gh, b
19. tomb	____	41. womb	____	b, b
20. wrap	____	42. wreck	____	w, w
21. wrench	____	43. wretch	____	w, w
22. wring	____	44. write	____	w, w

Set 3

Word	Silent Letter	Word	Silent Letter	Key
1. accompaniment	____	16. accuracy	____	i, u
2. aspirin	____	17. bachelor	____	i, e
3. boundary	____	18. casualties	____	a, u
4. considerable	____	19. criminal	____	e, i
5. definite	____	20. different	____	i, e
6. delivery	____	21. family	____	e, i
7. frivolous	____	22. history	____	o, o
8. ignorant	____	23. lengthening	____	o, e
9. liable	____	24. luxury	____	a, u
10. magazine	____	25. memory	____	a, o
11. misery	____	26. Niagara	____	e, a
12. operate	____	27. particular	____	e, u
13. privilege	____	28. regular	____	i, u
14. scenery	____	29. similar	____	e, i
15. temperature	____	30. victory	____	a, o

REFERENCES

Ball, M. J. (1993). *Phonetics for speech pathology*. London, England: Whurr Publishers.

Ball, M. J., & Lowry, O. (2001). *Methods in clinical phonetics*. London, England: Whurr Publishers.

Crystal, D. (1987). *The Cambridge encyclopedia of language*. Cambridge, England: Cambridge University Press.

Crystal, D. (1995). *The Cambridge encyclopedia of the English language*. New York, NY: Cambridge University Press.

Fucci, D. J., & Lass, N. J. (1999). *Fundamentals of speech science*. Boston, MA: Allyn & Bacon.

Johnson, K. (1997). *Acoustic and auditory phonetics*. Cambridge, MA: Blackwell Publishers.

Kent, R. D., & Read, C. (2002). *The acoustic analysis of speech*. Albany, NY: Singular.

Kreidler, C. W. (1989). *The pronunciation of English: A course book in phonology*. Oxford, England: Blackwell.

Nooteboom, S. G. (1997). The prosody of speech: Melody and rhythm. In W. J. Hardcastle & J. Laver (Eds.), *The handbook of phonetic sciences*. Oxford, England: Blackwell Publishers.

Pickett, J. M. (1999). *The acoustics of speech communication*. Boston, MA: Allyn & Bacon.

Roach, P. (1983). *English phonetics and phonology: A practical approach*. Cambridge, England: Cambridge University Press.

Shriberg, L. D., & Kent, R. D. (1995). *Clinical phonetics*. Boston, MA: Allyn & Bacon.

Sloat, C., Taylor, S. H., & Hoard, J. E. (1978). *Introduction to phonology*. Englewood Cliffs, NJ: Prentice Hall.

Tatham, M., & Morton, K. (2006). *Speech production and perception*. New York, NY: Palgrave.

Chapter 6

Anatomy and Physiology of the Speech and Hearing Mechanisms

PURPOSE

To provide a concrete overview of the speech and hearing anatomy and physiology responsible for speech reception and production.

OBJECTIVES

This chapter will provide you with information regarding:

1. The anatomy and physiology of the speech mechanism
2. The anatomy and physiology of the hearing mechanism

SPEECH PRODUCTION FEATURES

The process of speech production involves three basic features: (1) manner in which the airflow is modified; for example, continuous constricted flow for the [f] sound or a tightness of the lips to stop the airflow that is then released for the [p] sound. (2) Placement of the articulators, such as the **bilabial** position of the lips involved in the [p] sound or contact between the lower lip and upper teeth as in the [f] sound. (3) Voicing, or whether a sound is voiced such as the [v] sound (lightly touch your larynx and feel the vibration) or unvoiced (no vibration) such as the [f] sound. The anatomic structures for speech production are discussed from the perspective of these three basic speech production features. **Figure 6-1** shows the anatomic structures involved in speech. **Table 6-1** lists the anatomic structures and their function in speech production.

Basically, the diaphragm, lungs, and ribs are responsible for the amount of air (power source), and the trachea directs the airflow into the larynx. The vocal cords in the larynx remain inactive to produce the voiceless sounds such as [f] and [t] or begin to vibrate to produce voiced sounds such as [v] and [d]. The manner in which the airflow is modified and the placement of the articulators involve the lips, teeth, alveolar ridge, hard palate, soft palate (velum), and tongue. The mandible (jaw) is active in the production of such sounds as [f] and [v] as it lifts the lower lip upward to make contact with the upper teeth. It is also responsible for the degree of openness in the production of vowel sounds such as [ɑ] "ahhh" in contrast to the [i] "eee" sound. The oral cavity provides the resonant quality for other sounds, including the vowels and diphthongs.

The central nervous system functions to integrate and interpret incoming and outgoing stimuli, such as differentiating between homonyms such as *due, do,*

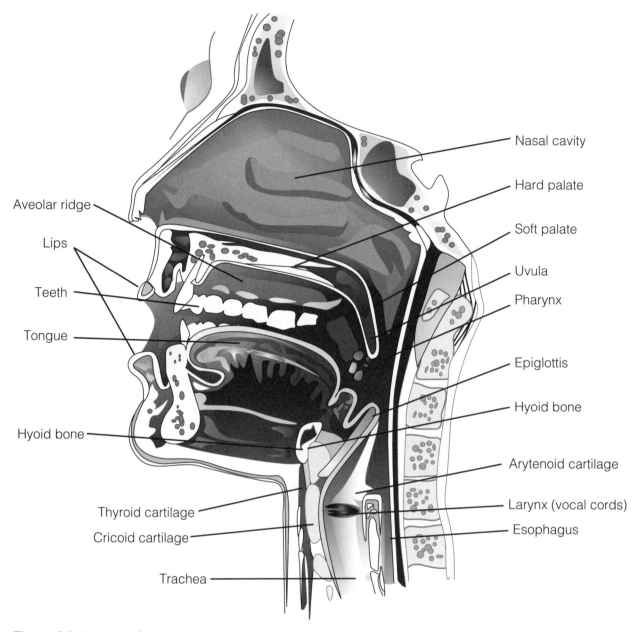

Figure 6-1 Anatomy of the speech mechanism.

TABLE 6-1	Anatomic Structures Involved in Speech Production	
Process	**Function**	**Anatomy**
Respiration	Air supply/direction	Diaphragm, lungs, rib cage, trachea
Phonation	Plus or minus voicing	Larynx (vocal cords)
Articulation	Placement of articulators	Lips, teeth, alveolar ridge, mandible, hard palate, soft palate, tongue
Resonation	Resonance quality	Pharynx, oral and nasal cavities

and *dew*, and organizing the sequence of sounds that are combined into words.

The peripheral nervous system functions to control such operations as the amount of pressure placed on the lips for the production of the [b] sound. The autonomic nervous system affects the emotional state of the individual and is directly related to processes of respiration, phonation, articulation, and resonance. The functioning of any or all of these processes affects speech production and reception.

A discussion of the anatomy begins with respiration: the source of the air supply.

RESPIRATION

The act of respiration for speech production includes both the inhalation and the exhalation of air. Unlike respiration for life support, which follows a rhythmic pattern of rather equal proportions of inhalation and exhalation, the respiratory act involved in speech production includes rather quick intakes of air and metered exhalations. The principal anatomic structures involved in respiration are the diaphragm, ribs, lungs, and trachea. All of these structures are located below the larynx. Respiration supplies the initial energy source and air that is acted on by one of the distinctive features of sound production, including voicing, manner, and placement. (See **Figure 6-2**.)

The location of the bones, muscles, nerves, and tissues involved in respiration include the abdomen where the diaphragm is located and the thorax, which includes the rib cage and lungs. The trachea also plays a vital role in channeling the airflow (inhalation and exhalation) into and out of the lungs.

The Diaphragm

The diaphragm serves a major purpose in respiration. It is a large muscle located between the abdominal cavity and the thoracic (chest) cavity. It is attached laterally to the abdominal wall. In its at-rest position, it forms a dome shape and makes contact with the lower portion of the lungs. As it is activated, it becomes flattened and taut to allow space for the lungs to expand. It is estimated that this process of expansion (exhalation) and flattening (inhalation) takes place about 12 times per minute during normal breathing in an adult.

The Rib Cage

The ribs border the thoracic cavity and consist of a set of 12 matching pairs of bones. They are thin, curved shafts of bone that surround and protect the lungs. They are attached posteriorly to the thoracic vertebrae and anteriorly to the sternum (breastplate). The upper 10 sets of ribs are attached to the sternum by the costal cartilage and the remaining 2 lower sets are referred

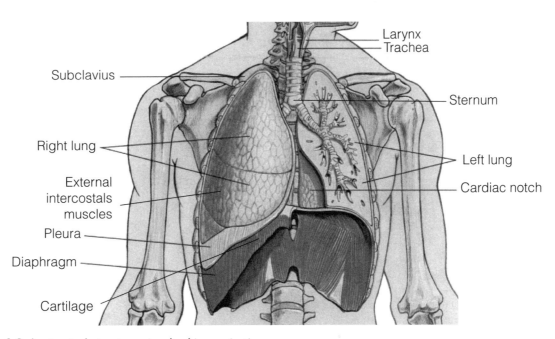

Figure 6-2 Anatomical structures involved in respiration.

to as floating ribs because they attach only in the back. The ribs are flexible to allow them to move upward or downward during respiration.

The ribs are bound together by intercostals muscles (Perkins & Kent, 1986). These muscles are divided into two groups, the external intercostals and internal intercostals. As the diaphragm lowers, the rib cage expands by the action of the external intercostals and the thoracic cavity is enlarged. The enlarged space allows for air to be inhaled into the lungs, which become inflated. The rib cage becomes reduced in size during exhalation through the action of the internal intercostals and abdominal muscles (Fucci & Lass, 1999). See **Figure 6-3**.

The Lungs

The lungs are cone-shaped and consist of millions of tiny air sacs. They adhere to the skeletal walls of the thorax and move in conjunction with them (Perkins & Kent, 1986). Upon inhalation, the air enters the tubular bronchi and then is directed into smaller tubes, the bronchioles, and from there into the air sacs of the lungs. The process is reversed for exhalation. See **Figure 6-4**.

The Trachea

The trachea is a tube of cartilaginous rings embedded in muscle tissue that is attached to the lungs and extends to the lower section of the larynx. The trachea serves as a connection between the lungs and the larynx (McMinn, Hutchings, & Logan, 1994).

The process of respiration varies depending on the situation. For normal vegetative breathing, the ratio of inhalation to exhalation is about 1:1. This relationship changes during speech production when inhalation may take approximately 10–20% of the time and the controlled exhalation is 80–90% of the time. Naturally, a different ratio occurs during physical activities or to blow out a candle.

PHONATION

The structures of the larynx are responsible for the process of phonation. **Phonation** is discussed as either plus or minus voicing. Voicing is one of the three speech production features of a sound. Sound is produced when the airflow that has traveled from the lungs and through the trachea reaches the areas where the vocal folds are located in the larynx. When the vocal folds are lengthened and forced together (**adduction**) by the cartilages, muscles, and nerves of the larynx, the vocal folds vibrate and produce sound waves. Such voiced sounds as [b] and [v] become audible. When the airflow proceeds unobstructed through the opened (abducted) vocal folds, voiceless sounds such as [p] and [f] are produced.

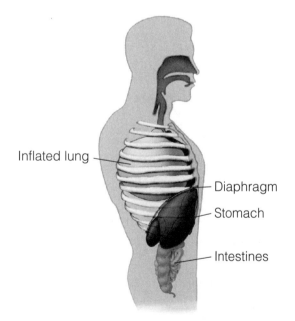

Inhalation: Intake of air supply into the lungs. Rib cage is expanded.

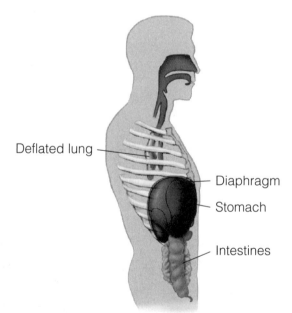

Exhalation: Release of air supply. Rib cage size is decreased.

Figure 6-3 The inhalation and exhalation processes of respiration.

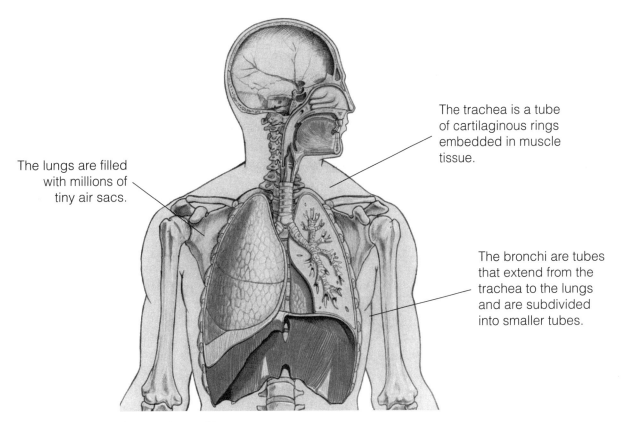

The lungs are filled with millions of tiny air sacs.

The trachea is a tube of cartilaginous rings embedded in muscle tissue.

The bronchi are tubes that extend from the trachea to the lungs and are subdivided into smaller tubes.

Figure 6-4 Anatomy of the trachea and lungs.

The Vocal Folds

To further understand this process, engage in this simple exercise. Place the tips of your fingers firmly against the sides of your larynx and prolong the production of the long vowels: "aaaaaaaaa," "eeeeeeeee," "iiiiiiiii," "ooooooooo," and "uuuuuuuuu." Sense the vibration as you produce these sounds.

Next, alternate the vowel sounds with the [f] sound and notice the lack of the vibration with the [f] sound with **abduction** of the vocal folds. That is because the [f] sound is voiceless and the vowels are all voiced sounds. Then, alternate the [f] and [v] sounds with your articulators "frozen" and notice that the only change is in the distinctive feature of voicing [f] minus voice and [v] plus voice. The manner in which the airflow is modified and the placement of the articulators remain the same.

The Larynx

Cartilages and muscles form the larynx (Palmer, 1984). The lower section of the larynx is attached to the trachea and the top broad curtain-like ligament section is attached to the hyoid bone. This bone has muscular attachments to the tongue and to the mandible.

The vocal folds are attached in front to the thyroid cartilage and to the arytenoids cartilages in back. Each vocal fold is connected to a separate arytenoids cartilage. These cartilages are attached to the superior portion of the cricoids cartilage that encircles the larynx. The cricoids resemble a signet ring with the narrowest portion toward the front and the widest portion toward the back. The thyroid cartilage is attached at the sides to the cricoids.

RESONATION

The vocal quality of resonation occurs when the airflow accompanied by sound waves produced by the vibration of the vocal folds is directed through the cavity of the pharynx and then through the oral (mouth) or nasal passageways and cavities. These three cavities contribute to the resonance quality of human speech sounds. Not all speech sounds are resonated. For example, the [t] and [k] sounds are produced with aspirated noises. Sounds that are resonated include vowels (oral resonance) and [n], [m], and [ŋ] (nasal resonance). The speech sounds that are affected by resonation are discussed later in the sections on oral and nasal cavities.

The primary structures that determine the direction of airflow are located in the oral-nasopharyngeal areas that begin above the larynx and include the pharyngeal area (lower throat) and the velum. Action of these structures determines whether the air flow and sound waves will exit through the mouth or the nares (nostrils). This action is called the velopharyngeal process.

Velopharyngeal Process

Shortly after the airflow exits the laryngeal area (larynx), it enters the pharyngeal area (lower throat) and proceeds upward toward the back of the throat, approaching the oral and nasal cavities, which are separated by the hard and soft palates. The velum (soft palate) acting in unison with the back of the throat determines whether the airflow is directed into the mouth or nose.

When the velum closes against the back of the throat, referred to as **velopharyngeal closure**, the airflow is directed into the oral cavity. If the airflow remains unobstructed as a result of the velum remaining in a relaxed position and in contact with the surface of the back of the tongue, the airflow mainly enters the nasal cavity. See **Figure 6-5**.

Oral Cavity

The oral cavity consists of the hard and soft surfaces of the mouth that are acted on by the sound waves contacting these surfaces. Traditionally, the speech sounds that are classified as oral resonant sounds include all of the vowels and diphthongs (combinations of two vowels) and the following consonants: [w], [j] as in *yellow* [jɛloʊ], [l], and [r].

Nasal Cavity

The nasal cavity consists of the inner hard and soft surfaces of the nose. Sound waves acquire their resonant characteristics on contact with these surfaces. The speech sounds that are classified as nasal resonant include [m], [n], and [ŋ] as in the "ng" in *sing* [sɪŋ]. These sounds may become denasaled or hyponasal resulting in a "muffled" type sound such as when a person has a cold and the inner surfaces of the nose may be swollen and blockage occurs. Other nonnasal sounds such as vowels may become nasal or hypernasal as a result of dialect preference or anatomic insufficiencies, both of which are a result of lack of sufficient velopharyngeal closure.

Nasal resonance is easier to sense than oral resonance. For example, place your fingers against the sides of your nose but do not pinch the nostrils closed. Allow the airflow to continue to exit through the nose. Now prolong the production of the "mmmmmmm" and feel the resonating sensation of vibration against your fingers. Contrast the nasal resonance of "mmmmm" with the nonnasal resonance of the [f] sound by alternating the production of each as in "mm-mmmmm–ffffff." Note the "turning on and off" of the nasal resonating vibration.

ARTICULATION

Articulation includes two of the speech production features mentioned earlier, *manner in which airflow is modified* and *placement of the articulators*. Articulation occurs when two or more of the articulatory structures modify the manner of the airflow. The following anatomic structures are involved in the process of articulation: lips, teeth, alveolar ridge, hard palate, velum (soft palate),

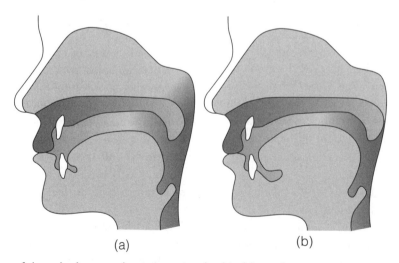

(a)   (b)

Figure 6-5 Illustration of the velopharyngeal processes involved in (a) nasal resonance—passageway open into nasal cavity—and (b) oral resonance—passageway to nasal cavity closed.

TABLE 6-2	Anatomic Structures Involved in Articulation

Movable	Stationary
Lips	Teeth
Tongue	Alveolar ridge
Mandible Velum Pharynx	Hard palate

tongue, mandible, and pharynx. These articulators can be classified as movable or stationary (see **Table 6-2**).

The mandible (lower jaw) moves to assist the lower lip in making contact with the upper teeth [f] and in the openness feature of vowel sounds, such as the [a] "ahhh" versus the [i] "eee" sound. The oral and nasal cavities are stationary and do not articulate with (contact) other structures. However, they do play a role in the characteristics of the voice by adding their distinctive resonation qualities to speech sounds. (See **Figure 6-6**.)

DESCRIPTION OF ANATOMIC STRUCTURES INVOLVED IN ARTICULATION

Examples of a few of the consonant sounds are provided to demonstrate the function of each of the articulators. Not all consonant sounds are presented. Each speech sound is discussed in detail in later chapters. The Latin roots of the terms are also provided.

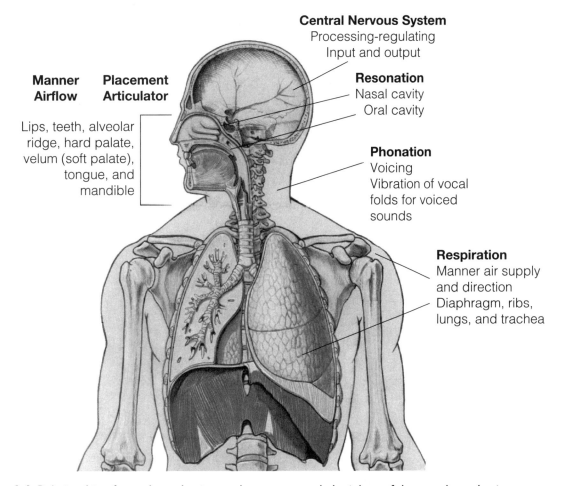

Manner
Airflow

Placement
Articulator

Lips, teeth, alveolar ridge, hard palate, velum (soft palate), tongue, and mandible

Central Nervous System
Processing-regulating
Input and output

Resonation
Nasal cavity
Oral cavity

Phonation
Voicing
Vibration of vocal folds for voiced sounds

Respiration
Manner air supply and direction
Diaphragm, ribs, lungs, and trachea

Figure 6-6 Relationship of speech production to the anatomy and physiology of the speech mechanism.

The Lips

Prefix: *labio*; suffix: *labial*.
Examples:

- Placement: Lips pressed firmly together
- Manner: Temporary interruption (stop) of the airflow
- Results: Production of the [p] or [b] (**bilabial stop**) sound
- Placement: Lower lip pressed lightly against upper teeth (dental)
- Manner: Constriction (friction) of the airflow
- Results: Production of the [f] or [v] (**labio-dental fricative**) sound

The lips can also be described in terms of roundness for vowel production. For example, in [i] "eee," the lips are unrounded, and in [o] "ooo" they are rounded.

The lips are made of muscles and other tissues (McMinn et al., 1994). They have a great capacity for varied movements, and much of their range of motion is used in the production of the bilabial sounds of [p], [b], [m], and the labiodental sounds [f] and [v].

One of the major muscles of the lips, the *orbicularis oris*, with muscle fibers in a circular pattern around the periphery of the mouth, can cause the lips to contract or protrude. From the upper jaw, or maxilla, other muscles are responsible for raising or lowering the upper lip and moving the corners of the mouth up and back. Originating from the lower jaw, or mandible, are the muscles that raise and lower the bottom lip, protrude it, and draw down and back the corners of the mouth. Experiment using these muscles by protruding and retracting your lips. Exaggerate the pronunciation of the words *you* and *he* and you will sense these muscles in operation. You can also feel another speech production feature of the lips, that of rounding: Lips are rounded in *you* and unrounded in *he*.

Closures of the lips vary in firmness, and some are rapid motions of short duration. These actions require active muscular closure by the upper and lower lips moving simultaneously to the center of the mouth.

The Teeth

Prefix: *dento*; suffix: *dental*.
Example:

- Placement: Upper and lower teeth and tongue (lingua) together
- Manner: Constriction (friction) of the airflow
- Results: Production of *th* [Ɵ] [Ɵɪn] (**lingua-dental fricative**) sound

The upper teeth play a passive role in speech production because they are not movable whereas the action of the mandible (jaw) facilitates the movement of the lower teeth for the production of certain speech sounds. Adults have 32 permanent teeth with equal numbers located in the maxilla (upper) and mandible (lower portions of the mouth) (Perkins & Kent, 1986). Beginning at the midline, the teeth are indentified as central incisor, lateral incisor, canine, first bicuspid, second bicuspid, first molar, second molar, and third molar (wisdom tooth). These are arranged symmetrically with sets of eight teeth on either side, top and bottom.

The production of speech sounds that involve the teeth may be imprecise or distorted after the loss of the deciduous teeth (baby teeth) until the permanent teeth are in place. Also, malocclusion resulting from an over-, under-, or cross-bite that causes the teeth to be out of functional alignment may cause distortion or substitution of certain speech sounds, mainly [s] and [z].

Alveolar Ridge (Gum Ridge)

Prefix: *alveolo*; suffix: *alveolar*.
Example:

- Placement: Tongue pressed against the alveolar ridge (**lingua-alveolar**)
- Manner: Temporary blockage (stop) of airflow
- Results: Production of the [t] or [d] (**lingua-alveolar stop**) sounds

The alveolar processes consist of both the maxilla (upper) and the mandible (lower) ridges in which the teeth are embedded. The alveolar ridge behind the maxillary incisors and canine teeth form a pronounced ridge that plays a predominant role in the production of several consonant sounds, such as [t] and [d]. For some speakers, the tip or front portion of the tongue makes contact embedded behind the lower ridge in the production of the [s] or [z] sound. In this position, it is the blade or middle of the tongue that is in contact with the alveolar ridge to create the friction feature. For others, the tongue tip is elevated and positioned lightly against the upper alveolar ridge.

Palate

Prefix: *palato*; suffix: *palatal*.
Example:

- Placement: Lingua (tongue) **palatal** (Palate)
- Manner: Constriction (friction) of the airflow
- Results: Production of the [ʒ] in *azure* and [ʃ] in *she* (**lingua-palatal fricative**) sounds

Located posterior to the upper alveolar ridge is the *palate*, commonly referred to as the hard palate (Palmer, 1984). Its structure serves as both roof of the mouth and floor of the nasal cavity. The palate arches upward to form the palatal vault, which varies greatly with facial structure. The upper (superior) surface of the floor of the nasal cavity contributes to vowel resonance. As the roof of the mouth, the palate assists in directing the airflow toward the front of the mouth for the production of most of the consonant sounds. In contrast, when there is a cleft (opening) in the palate, such as in cleft palate, a portion of the airflow reaches the nasal cavity and escapes through the nose.

Velum

Prefix: *velo*; suffix: *velar*.
Example:

- Placement: Contact of the back of tongue (lingua) to **velum**

- Manner: Temporary blockage (stop) of airflow

- Results: Production of [k] or [g] (**lingua-velar stop**) sound

Attached to the end of the hard palate is the soft palate, or velum (McMinn et al., 1994). It consists of muscle and connective tissue covered with the same mucous membrane of the palate. It is very flexible and mobile, opening to permit the airflow into the nasal cavity as it is funneled through the throat. The velum is responsible for the direction of the airflow into either the nasal cavity or the oral cavity. This is accomplished by the process called velopharyngeal closure. In its relaxed position, the airflow is permitted to enter the nasal cavity to resonate as for the [m], [n], and [ŋ] consonants. When the velum actively presses against the pharyngeal (back of the throat) area, the airflow is directed into the oral cavity and minimal or no air enters the nasal cavity.

The mobility of the velum is controlled by a group of muscles that are located above, below, and behind it.

Tongue

Prefix: *lingua*; suffix: *lingual*.
Example:

- Placement: Tip of tongue (**lingua**) in contact with upper front teeth

- Manner: Constriction (frication) of airflow

- Results: Production of the *th* [Ɵ] (lingua-dental fricative) sound

The tongue is one of the most critical structures in the production of speech sounds. It is highly mobile because of intrinsic and extrinsic muscles that are responsible for its movement in the oral cavity. The anatomic sections of the tongue include its root, or the posterior portion connected with the hyoid bone and epiglottis; apex at the anterior end; dorsum, or superior surface; and septum, or midline structure of connective tissue (McMinn et al., 1994). The lingual frenum is connected to the lower front of the tongue and to the mandible.

In terms of speech production, it is convenient to identify the tongue by section: the back, middle, front, tip, and point (which appears when the tongue is narrowed and pointed such as in the production of the [l] sound—produce this sound and sense how the tip of the tongue approximates a "pointer"). The front and back of the tongue can be elevated or lowered by subtle degrees to produce the vowel sounds. Another characteristic of the tongue is tenseness of the muscles: tense in "eee" and relaxed in "ahhh." Experiment with some of the other vowel sounds and identify the tongue's degree of tenseness. All of the vowel sounds are influenced by the action of the tongue. The consonants [p], [b], [f], [v], and [m] appear to be the only consonants that have little dependence on the tongue.

Mandible (Jaw)

Prefix: *mandibulo*; suffix: *mandibular*.
Example:

- Placement: Lower mandibular changes shape of oral cavity

- Manner: Allows for unobstructed airflow for vowel production

- Results: Vowels such as "ah" [ɑ] and "o" [o]; mandible also moves to assist in the placement of the lip for [f] and [v]

The **mandible**, or lower jaw, functions in both a passive and active manner in articulation. It is the foundation for the large genioglossus muscle of the tongue, and the lower teeth are embedded in it. It can be elevated to close as in the "eee" [i] sound or lowered to open the jaw for the "ah" [ɑ] vowel articulation. These movements are made possible by four major muscles: temporal muscle, masseter, internal pterygoid muscle, and external pterygoid muscle. The temporal muscle originates over a large fan-shaped area of the temporal bone of the skull and converges downward and forward to form a tendon inserted into the mandible. It elevates and retracts the mandible to close the jaw. The masseter also closes the jaw and is connected to the zygomatic arch, or cheek bone. The internal pterygoid muscle assists in closing the jaw and protruding the mandible; and the external pterygoid muscle gives the mandible lateral movement for chewing (Perkins & Kent, 1986).

Pharynx

Prefix: *pharyngo*; suffix: *pharyngeal*.
Example:

- Placement: Contact with velum to produce velopharyngeal closure

- Manner: Directs airflow from the top of the trachea to the back of the throat

- Results: Primarily the oral [r], [l], [w], [j], or nasal sounds [m], [n], [ŋ]; secondarily influences all other sounds

The pharynx (throat), although not as active as some of the other articulators, nonetheless plays a vital role in the production of speech sounds. It is one of the primary structures that determines the direction of the airflow. It is also referred to as the pharyngeal cavity because it adds resonance to some sounds. It extends from the posterior portion of the nasal cavity downward through the back of the oral cavity to the larynx. The pharynx is a vertical tube with three parts: the nasopharynx, a continuation of the nasal cavity; the oropharynx, a continuation of the oral cavity; and the laryngopharynx, the area above the larynx. It is lined with mucous membrane over a number of muscles (Palmer, 1984).

The velopoharyngeal sphincter includes the area from the midline of the velum around the sides of the pharynx and the back of the pharynx. The superior constrictor muscle contracts the pharynx in the nasopharyngeal region to assist with the raising and circular closing action of the velopharyngeal port.

ORAL AND NASAL CAVITIES

Although not considered in the strictest sense as articulators, the oral and nasal cavities, in some functions, meet the same criteria as other articulators. The oral cavity sets the perimeter in which other articulators are contained, such as the tongue and hard and soft palates. It assists in the modification of the airflow. However, its primary role is to add a resonance quality to the speech sounds. The primary role of the nasal cavity is to add resonance, and it also contributes to the modification of the airflow.

Oral Cavity

Prefix: *oro*; suffix: *oral*.
Example:

- Placement: Oral cavity in conjunction with tongue positions

- Manner: Resonation of sound waves in oral cavity

- Results: Production of **oral resonant** consonants [r], [l], [w], [j]

The oral cavity extends from the oral aperture (opening), or mouth, to the front of the posterior wall of the pharynx, from the palate and velum to the base of the tongue, and laterally between the right and left sides of the cheeks (Hedge, 2001). Its surface is composed of different surfaces. The hard surface of the palate tends to deflect sounds, whereas the soft palate and the density of the inner cheeks tend to absorb sounds. The oral cavity is indeed the cavity in which the articulators of the mandible, tongue, palate, velum, alveolar ridge, and lips shape speech sounds. It adds the resonance quality to a voice.

Nasal Cavity

Prefix: *naso*; suffix: *nasal*.
Example:

- Placement: Nasal cavity (fixed structure)

- Manner: Resonation of sound waves in nasal cavity

- Results: Consonants [n], [m], and *ng* [ŋ]

The nasal cavity extends from the nostrils (nares) in the front to the posterior wall of the pharynx and from the base of the skull to the palate and velum (Fucci & Lass, 1999). The active participation of the nasal cavity in speech production is controlled by the opening or closing of the velopharyngeal port, which opens to allow sound waves to enter the nasal cavity and closes to create a barrier and divert the waves into the oral cavity. With the velopharyngeal port closed, the nasal cavity resonates in conjunction with the oral cavity to provide the unique voice sounds of an individual. With the velopharyngeal port open, the nasal cavity can produce the nasal consonants [m], [n], and [ŋ]. With some firmness, press against the sides of your nose while producing the prolonged "mmmmmmmmm" sound and sense the resonation occurring in the nasal cavity.

ANATOMY AND PHYSIOLOGY OF THE HEARING MECHANISM

Traditionally, the hearing mechanism has not been included, but as Studdert-Kennedy and Whalen (1999) indicate, "There is a powerful link between the way we perceive (hear) speech and the way we produce it." (p. 21) These authors state that modern studies of speech perception and speech production have generally followed separate paths at laboratories where only one or the other topic was of interest. They comment that only quite recently have researchers begun to argue that a viable theory of speech perception must be grounded in a viable theory of speech production, and vice versa.

Acuity and Discrimination

You need to understand two concepts regarding **audition** (hearing). Hearing reception includes both acuity and discrimination. Auditory acuity relates to how well a person hears or how loud a sound needs to be in order to be heard by an individual. One test to determine acuity is when the person responds to a humming sound while wearing a headset. Auditory discrimination deals with how well a person can discriminate two sounds that are closely related such as the voiceless *th* in *thin* and the voiceless *f* in *fin* without visual or contextual clues. In extreme conditions, such as in auditory agnosia, a person may perceive that a sound is present but cannot discriminate or recognize whether the sound is a train whistle or a knock on a door.

Anatomic Structures of the Ear

The anatomic structures of the hearing mechanism are divided into three major sections: the outer ear, the middle ear, and the inner ear. (See **Figure 6-7.**) The nature of conveyance of the auditory signals is as follows: **outer ear**—catches airborne sound waves; **middle ear**—mechanical vibrations of the tympanic membrane (ear drum) activate the three bones of the ossicular chain; **inner ear**—hydrodynamic energy in the fluid of the inner ear moves the hair cells, which convert the fluid motions into neural signals (electrochemical energy) whose impulses are transmitted to the brain through cranial nerve VIII.

The Outer Ear

The two main structures of the outer ear are the auricle (or pinna) and the external auditory meatus.

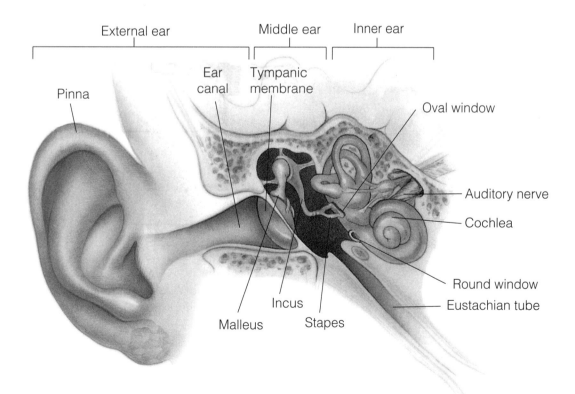

Figure 6-7 Detailed illustration of the anatomy of the ear.

The auricle is the protruding outside section of the ear that is formed in a half-funnel shape that serves to capture auditory signals such as noises and voices. It is constructed of soft tissue and cartilage. The auditory signals advance past the auricle and enter the small tunnel of the external auditory meatus. This ear canal, as it is commonly called, is responsible for channeling the auditory signals to the surface of the tympanic membrane that divides the outer and middle sections of the ear.

Because the tympanic membrane (ear drum) is delicate, the external auditory meatus serves as a protection by filtering foreign matter that may find its way into the ear. This is accomplished by the presence of a lining of small hairs nearest the auricle and by wax called cerumen that is a lubricant that keeps the canal supple and clean. As mentioned, in the outer ear the method of conveyance of the auditory signal is airborne as the sound waves travel from the auricle through the external auditory meatus.

The Middle Ear

The auditory signal becomes a mechanical signal when it contacts the tympanic membrane. The tympanic membrane functions as a partition and creates a seal between the outer ear and middle ear. The airborne auditory signals apply pressure to the tympanic membrane and set in motion a series of vibrations that activate the three smallest bones in humans, the ossicles.

The ossicles form a chain beginning with the malleus, which is directly attached to the tympanic membrane. The malleus is attached to the incus, and the stapes, the third bone, is attached to the incus. (See **Figure 6-8.**) The footplate of the stapes is inserted into the fenestra vestibule (oval window), which separates the middle ear from the inner ear. The names of the small bones derive from the Latin words that describe their resemblance to common objects: malleus for hammer; incus for anvil; and stapes for stirrup, like on a saddle. The small bones of the ossicular chain are bound together by ligaments and two tiny muscles, the tensor tympani and the stapedius. The action of these muscles safeguard the tiny bones against the tightening of the ossicular chain, thereby providing a means to accommodate excessive pressure.

The Inner Ear

The structure of the inner ear serves two functions, balance and transmission of sound. The vestibular apparatus is responsible for sense of balance and spatial orientation.

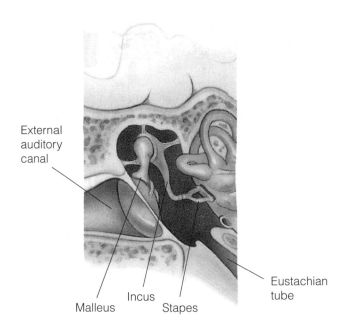

Figure 6-8 Detail of ossicular chain of middle ear.

Contained within the inner ear are three semicircular canals that are located in the superior, lateral, and posterior positions. Each represents a body plane (horizontal or vertical) in space and signals to the person aspects of balance and equilibrium. (See **Figure 6-9.**)

The canals are filled with fluid that moves in conjunction with head and body movements. Spatial balance is maintained as the movement of the fluid sends signals to the brain that, in turn, sends neural signals to the peripheral nervous system. The muscle motor processes adjust to the neural messages to affect equilibrium (balance). Appropriate body posture and stability are maintained in reference to the surrounding spatial environment.

The second function of the inner ear, transmission of sound, occurs in the snail-shell-shaped cochlea. The cochlea communicates with the middle ear through two small windows: the fenestra vestibuli (oval window), which is occupied by the footplate of the stapes, and the fenestra rotunda (round window), located slightly below the oval window. The round window is covered with a thin flexible membrane to allow for expansion when fluid movements occur within the cochlea. Imagine looking into the base opening of an empty snail shell and visualizing three separate channels that extend from the opening surface to the tip (apex). This can give you the concept of the structural interior of the cochlea. Thin, flexible, membranous walls that allow fluid movement from one channel to the others

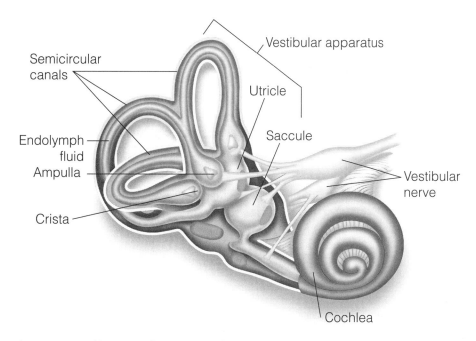

Figure 6-9 Spatial orientation of location of inner ear and major anatomic structures.

separate these channels. The upper channel (scala vestibuli) works in conjunction with the back and forth movements of the stapes footplate within the fenestra vestibule. These movements activate the fluid in the cochlea, creating a wave motion. These wave motions influence the middle channel (scala media), which contains the organ of Corti, the sensory end organ of hearing located on the basilar membrane. The organ of Corti contains tiny hair cells that are situated in one inner and three to four outer rows from the base of the cochlea to its apex. These hair cells function as sensory receptor cells. The cilia, small hairlike projections, occupy the top portion of the inner and outer hair cells and are imbedded in the tectorial membrane above.

COMMENTS

It is important to remember that speech production and hearing rely on specific anatomic structures and that aspects other than simple physiology influence the functioning of these anatomic structures.

These influences have to do with human behavior. One is compensatory or adaptive behavior that compensates for abnormal conditions of these anatomic structures. A deformity in or absence of any part of the speech production anatomy could present major obstacles

to a speaker. However, human beings have great compensatory abilities and can accommodate such conditions and bring about results that are acceptable to both speaker and listener. There is not a reader of this book who is not aware of someone who has demonstrated such abilities. Second, emotions influence the functioning of the anatomic structures of speaking and hearing. All of the physiologic structures may be intact and, indeed, be near perfection and yet may malfunction as a result of the emotional state of the speaker or listener. When emotions are high or low, they take precedence over higher-level communication needs. Breath control can be erratic, speech may be slurred, and voice may be weak or absent. Depending on the situation, auditory vigilance and listening skills may diminish or increase. The pragmatic factors of who, what, where, when, and why come into play to influence the level of sound production competencies and intelligibility. There are different conversational styles of speakers such as casual, informal, and formal production. This may result in omission of sounds or substitutions. "Whatcha got goin'?" versus "What have you got going?" The suprasegmental features of loudness, stress, intonation, and rate can be influenced by pragmatic factors. The urgency of the message may come as a rapid rate versus a more casual production.

SUMMARY

Humans have a set of anatomic structures for speech production and reception of speech sounds. Among individuals, these structures may vary, but there is a wide range of normalcy. For example, all tongues are not the same length and width, lips are not the same shape, and teeth are not all positioned in the same formation. The process of accommodation is constantly operating as a speaker relays the spoken word and the listener receives it.

The emotional state of both the speaker and listener affects speaking and hearing. For example, a frightened person does not have much conscious control over the inhalation and exhalation processes that supply air for speaking, so speech may not be smooth and rhythmic. Likewise, a person who is fatigued may exhibit slurred speech or lack projection of voice. A person's ability to hear and to discriminate sounds can be affected by the listener's state of mind.

The specific anatomic structures responsible for speech production include the diaphragm, lungs, trachea, larynx, pharynx, velum, palate, alveolar ridge, teeth, oral cavity, lips, mandible, and nasal cavity. The processes of speech production include respiration, phonation, resonation, and articulation. The hearing mechanism is divided into the outer, middle, and inner ear and is responsible for the transmission of speech signals to cranial nerve VIII. All of these structures and processes work together in a highly sophisticated and integrated manner.

REFERENCES

Fucci, D. J., & Lass, N. J. (1999). *Fundamentals of speech science*. Boston, MA: Allyn & Bacon.

Hedge, M. N. (2001). *A pocket guide to assessment in speech-language pathology*. San Diego, CA: Singular and Thompson Learning.

McMinn, R. H. M., Hutchings, R. T., & Logan, B. M. (1994). *Color atlas of head and neck anatomy*. St. Louis, MO: Mosby.

Palmer, J. M. (1984). *Anatomy for speech and hearing*. Baltimore, MD: Williams & Wilkins.

Perkins, W. H., & Kent, R. D. (1986). *Textbook of functional anatomy of speech, language and hearing*. London, England: Taylor and Francis.

Studdert-Kennedy, M., & Whalen, D. H. (1999). *A brief history of speech perception in the United States*. In A. Bronstein, J. Ohala, & W. Weigel (Eds.), *A guide to the phonetic sciences in the United States*. Berkeley, CA: University of California Press.

Chapter 7

Vowels and Diphthongs

PURPOSE

To introduce you to the United States English vowels and diphthongs.

OBJECTIVES

This chapter will provide you with information regarding:

1. The identification and description of United States English vowels
2. The identification and description of United States English diphthongs
3. Skill-building exercises

VOWELS

Vowels are more difficult than consonants to describe from the perspective of the articulators (Ball & Rahilly, 1999) because no contact or near contact is made between the articulators during the production of vowels. Vowels require a very wide articulatory channel within the oral cavity where the tongue can take various postures to make vowels. Traditionally, therefore, phoneticians have attempted to describe vowels in part by stating where the tongue is placed within the oral (vowel) area.

The articulation of vowels is described by the following factors:

1. *Height.* Tongue position within the oral cavity: high, mid, low.
2. *Depth.* Tongue position within the oral cavity: front, central, back.
3. *Tension.* Oral-facial muscles, particularly the tongue: tense or lax.
4. *Rounding.* Lip configuration: rounded, with protrusion, or unrounded, more toward a horizontal plane (flat).

The purpose of these descriptors is to provide a convenient quadrilateral matrix to describe and define the similarities and differences among the United States English vowels. These descriptions may be more applicable when a vowel sound is produced in isolation because the characteristics of vowels change during the ballistic movements of contextual speech and when intermingled with consonants and prosodic features of rate, stress, loudness, and dialect variations.

The precise acoustic makeup of vowels, or indeed any sound, varies among speakers and within the speech of the same speaker. Each vowel has a formant structure that indicates vowel height, tongue advancement, and lip shape (Ball & Lowry, 2001).

Shriberg and Kent (1995) ask a simple question, "What is a vowel?" They then proceed to explain how, in reality, it is very difficult to define the characteristics of a vowel that can be universally accepted. They quote several earlier phoneticians who conclude that even their definitions are unsatisfactory and not approved by critics and other writers of phonetics.

The vowel is identified in part by the acoustic quality (Stetson, 1951) and by the physiologic shape defined by the movement of the tongue and the jaw and lips. It is important to note that these movements are reciprocal and that there is a whole range of positions possible for the production of each vowel.

Shriberg and Kent (1995) offer this definition:

"A vowel is a speech sound that is (1) formed without a significant constriction of the oral and pharyngeal cavities from the larynx through the lips and (2) that serves as a syllable nucleus, i. e., only one vowel sound can occur within the boundaries of a syllable unit." (p. 25)

In other words, one of the prerequisites of a syllable is the presence of a vowel.

In addition, Shriberg and Kent (1995) stress three aspects of vowel production: (1) a *spatial* aspect: the position of the articulators is such that there is no constriction of the oral and pharyngeal cavities; (2) a *temporal* aspect: the sound can be sustained indefinitely; and (3) a *functional* aspect: a vowel serves as the nucleus of a syllable.

The consonants such as the /f/ in *fun* can be described rather explicitly as contact made between the lower lip and the upper teeth. The position of the tongue within the oral cavity both in its height (high to low) and in its depth (front to back) distinguishes the formation of the vowel sounds. You should realize that these height and depth parameters are relative features and that many variables are present, such as the sounds before and after the vowel, to determine the actual height and depth.

For example, the [i] in *beet* [bit] is the highest front vowel and the [u] in *ooze* [uz] is the highest back vowel, but that does not necessarily mean that the *height* of the two are exact. Indeed, during conversational speaking, speakers may make a lot of accommodation and adjustments. There is a difference between pronouncing a vowel in isolation, where it remains in a rather *fixed* position, versus pronouncing it during rapid conversational speech, where the posturing of the same vowel may be different during the overall ballistic movements of speaking.

A quadrilateral matrix, as presented in **Figure 7-1**, displays the position of the vowels visually within the oral cavity. Keep in mind that, as Shriberg and Kent (1995) caution, "The features conform to general articulatory properties of vowels and are motivated largely by the requirements of simplicity and convenience." (p. 26)

- Long vowels. ā = [e] *rotate*; ē = [i] *eat*; ī = [aɪ] *ice*; ō = [o] *occur*; u = [u] *ooze*

- Short vowels. ă = [æ] *ask*; ě = [ɛ] *bet*; ĭ = [ɪ] *it*; ŏ = [ɑ] *not*; ŭ = [ə] and [ʌ] *above* [əbʌv]

- *r*-influenced vowels. ur = [ɝ] *fur* [fɝ] and er = [ɚ] *mother* [mʌðɚ]

- Other vowels. â and ô = [ɔ] when followed by *l, ll, w,* or *u,* as in *talk, all, saw, haul;* or ô as in *cot, ought;* oo = [ʊ] *foot, good*

In addition to height and depth, other features used to describe vowels include the rounding of the lips (round or unround) and tenseness (tense or lax) of the oral-facial muscles, including the tongue.

Vowel Height

Vowel height (House, 1998; Shriberg & Kent, 1995) is affected by both the position of the mandible (open or close) and the vertical position of the tongue (low to high). There are four variables to consider:

1. *Open.* The mandible (jaw) is dropped in a rather wide-open posture with the tongue resting on or near the floor of the mouth, as in the "ahhh" sound [ɑ] in f<u>a</u>ther. Because the jaw supports the tongue, it is natural that the tongue follows the direction of the lowered jaw and rests on the floor of the mouth.

2. *Midopen.* The mandible is still below the midline of the facial plane but somewhat elevated from completely opened. The tongue posture is raised from the floor of the mouth and is located approximately halfway between the floor and the alveolar (gum) ridge and palatal (hard and soft palates) areas. These vowels include [ʌ] p<u>u</u>t and [ɔ] <u>au</u>ful (Eastern dialect).

3. *Midclosed.* The mandible is nearly closed, but the upper and lower teeth do not make contact. The tongue posture is basically the same as for midopen and is halfway between the floor of the mouth and the palatal areas. Vowels produced are [e] as the "a" long vowel in d<u>o</u>n<u>ate</u> and the long vowel [o] <u>o</u>bey.

4. *Close.* The mandible is in a near closed or elevated position with the tongue in contact with the sides of the alveolar ridge. Vowels produced include [i] as the long "ee" sound in b<u>ee</u>t and the long vowel [u] in <u>ooze</u>.

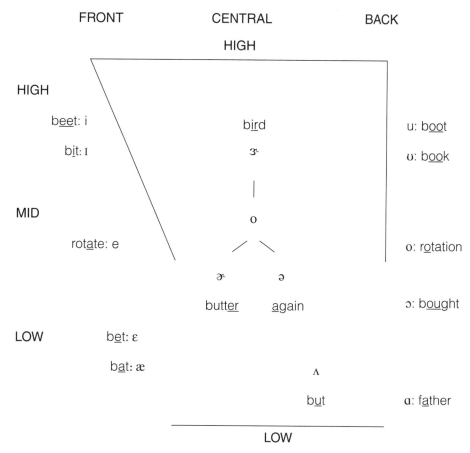

Figure 7-1 Depth (front–central–back) and height (high–mid–low) of vowels in a quadrilateral matrix.

House (1998) indicates that several vowels are not clearly defined using these four positions and that phoneticians use additional terms such as *near open* to describe the vowel [æ] as the "a" sound in _ask_ because its position is between the midopen and open vowels. The [ɪ] as in _it_ and [ʊ] as in _book_ are *near close* vowels and are located between the close and midclose vowels.

Although the tongue and jaw work together in vowel articulation, the more closed the jaw position, the higher the tongue position; the tongue can also move independently of the jaw (Shriberg & Kent, 1995). For example, a [i] high tongue position can be accomplished with jaw positions ranging from closed to more than an inch of opening. Individual speakers vary somewhat in the tongue height feature of vowel articulation.

To demonstrate the concept of height (low, mid, high), repeat the following words and notice the shifting of the tongue posture from the floor of the mouth to a raised position.

Low	*Mid*	*High*
ahhhh [ɑ]	aaaaaaa [e] _ache_	eeeeeee [i] _eat_

Depth: Front to Back

Front to back describes the depth movement of the tongue from front, central, to back (see **Figure 7-2**). A section or division description is all that is needed to explain the depth aspect of vowel production.

1. *Front.* The front one-third of the tongue is positioned in the front one-third section of the oral cavity. The position of the tip of the tongue varies with the particular vowels and ranges from the lower and upper incisors. The front vowels are (from top to bottom in height) [i] *beet;* [ɪ] *it,* [e] *donate,* [ɛ] *bed,* and [æ] *ask.*

2. *Central.* The body of the tongue is in a neutral position, basically in the center of the mouth. The central vowels cannot be described without reference to stress (Shriberg & Kent, 1995). The sounds of the central vowels are determined by stress patterns. For example, the word *murmur* has two r-like sounds. The first syllable is stressed and the r symbol is the [ɝ]. The [ɚ] symbol is used for the r in the secondary stressed syllable at

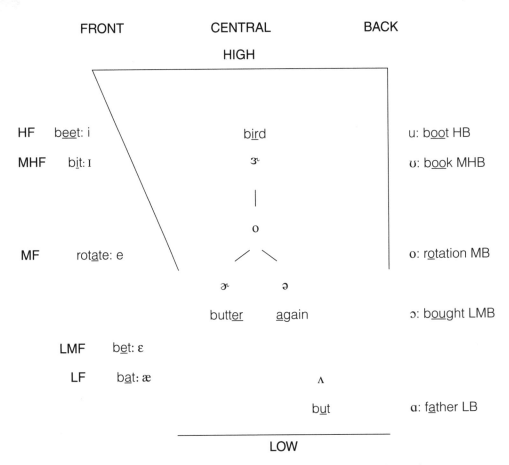

FRONT   CENTRAL   BACK

HIGH

HF	beet: i		bird		u: boot HB
MHF	bit: ɪ		ɝ		ʊ: book MHB
			o		
MF	rotate: e				o: rotation MB
		ɚ	ə		
		butter	again		ɔ: bought LMB
LMF	bet: ɛ				
LF	bat: æ			ʌ	
			but		ɑ: father LB

LOW

Figure 7-2 A visual representation of the depth of United States English vowels in the oral cavity.

Key

HF	High Front	LF	Low Front	MB	Mid-Back
MHF	Mid-High Front	HB	High Back	LMB	Low Mid-Back
MF	Mid-Front	MHB	Mid-High Back	LB	Low Back
LMF	Low Mid-Front				

Central vowels are positioned as indicated on above chart.

the end of the word. Thus, [mɝməɚ] is the correct transcription of this word, primarily based on the stress pattern. The same principle applies to the schwa sound, as in *above*. There are two syllables, "a" and "bove," and the second syllable has the primary stress indicated by the [ʌ] symbol. The first syllable is unstressed, and the symbol is [ə]. The transcription for *above* is [əbʌv]. The four central vowels are [ʌ], [ə] and [ɝ], and [ɚ].

3. *Back.* The tongue is positioned near the back of the mouth. The back vowels are (from top to bottom in height) [u] *ooze*, [ʊ] *book*, [o] *rotation*, [ɔ] *awful*, and [ɑ] *hot*.

You can sense the effect of tongue depth by repeating the contrasting front vowel sound [i] *beet* and the back vowel [u] *ooze*. Continue repeating aloud just the vowel in the following words. The key words are provided to assist in the identification of the sound.

Front		*Back*
[i] beet	⇒	[u] ooze
[ɪ] it	⇒	[ʊ] book
[e] donate	⇒	[o] rotation
[ɛ] bed	⇒	[ɔ] awful
[æ] ask	⇒	[ɑ] ahhhh

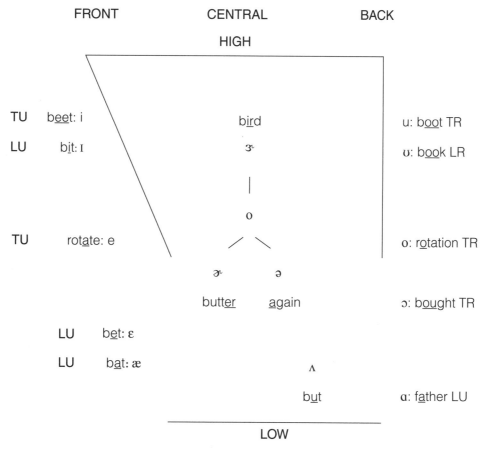

Figure 7-3 Tension and roundness features of United States English vowels in a quadrilateral matrix.

Key

TU	Tense Tongue, Unrounded Lips	TR	Tense Tongue, Rounded Lips
LU	Lax Tongue, Unrounded Lips	LR	Lax Tongue, Rounded Lips

Note: [ʌ] and [ə] are unrounded and lax. [ɝ] and [ɚ] are unrounded and tense.

Tension

The terms *tense* and *lax* represent extremes along a continuum of tenseness (Shriberg & Kent, 1995). These terms are difficult to define as they apply to (1) the degree of muscle activity involved in the articulation of a vowel and (2) the duration of the vowel. Tense vowels have greater muscle activity and longer duration. These vowels include [i] *beet*, [e] *donate*, [ɝ] *bird*, [u] *ooze*, [o] *rotation*, [ɔ] *awful*, and [ɑ] *father*. The lax vowels include [ɪ] *bit*, [ɛ] *bed*, [æ] *ask*, [ʌ] *put*, and [ʊ] *book*. The unstressed *r*-like sound [ɚ] *mother* is variable in its tenseness. **Figure 7-3** presents a quadrilateral matrix of the tension and roundness features of vowels in United States English.

Shriberg and Kent (1995) offer additional insight into the concept of tension by examining the distributional properties of vowels, that is, the different phonetic conditions of their occurrence:

1. A lax vowel cannot occur in stressed open syllables. It cannot be the terminating (last) sound in a stressed syllable. For example, in some dialects the terminating sound in *pretty* is the lax vowel [ɪ]. Note that the last syllable is also unstressed.

2. A lax vowel can occur in stressed closed syllables. For example, in the context of consonant-vowel-consonant (CVC) as in [ɪ] *hit* [hɪt].

3. A tense vowel can occur in either open or closed syllables as in [i] *be* [bi] (open) and *beet* [bit] (closed).

4. Both a tense vowel [ɝ] *herb* [ɝb] and a lax vowel [ɪ] *it* [ɪt] can initiate a syllable.

These authors conclude that because tense and lax vowels are treated differently in the phonology of English, there is sufficient reason to divide vowels into tense and lax groups for phonetic purposes.

Rounding

Rounding refers to the position of the lips during the production of the vowel. The lips are separated (opened) and somewhat protruded for the production of the rounded vowels. The rounded vowels include the central [ɝ] and [ɚ] and the back vowels [u], [ʊ], [o], and [ɔ]. An inventory of the unrounded vowels includes all of the front vowels, [i], [ɪ], [e], [ɛ], and [æ]; the central vowels [ʌ] and [ə]; and the lower back vowel [ɑ].

A sense of rounding can be detected in the prolongation of the following vowel combination: [i] *beet* and [u] *blue*. Prolong the iiiiiii and then move directly to the uuuuuuu sound and notice the difference in the roundness of the lips during the transition from [i] to [u].

DIPHTHONGS

A diphthong is formed when two vowel sounds are combined and emitted as one sound in the same syllable. A diphthong begins by approximating the position of one vowel and then "gliding" into the position of a second vowel. For example, the [e] in *donation* [doʊneʃən] is the beginning (on-glide) sound, and [ɪ] or [i], depending on the dialect, is the ending (off-glide) sound in the word *cake* [keɪk] or [keik]. The two vowel symbols can be considered a digraph similar to the consonants *th* and *ch*, which are two letters that can individually represent two separate sounds—[t] as in *ten* and [h] *here*—but represent only *one* sound, as in *th* in *the* [ðʌ] and *ch* [tʃ] in *chair* [tʃhɛr]. Therefore, the word *cake* has three sounds: [k-ei-k] or [k-eɪ-k].

The five diphthongs that most phoneticians recognize are the following:

[ei] or [eɪ] Primary stressed syllable: *donation* [doneɪʃən]

Word ending: *today* [tudeɪ] or [tudei]

Single syllable: *cake* [keɪk] or [keik]

[aɪ] *ice* [aɪs]

[aʊ] *house* [haʊs]

[ɔɪ] or [ɔi] *oil* [ɔɪl] or [ɔil]

[oʊ] Primary stressed syllable: *donate* [doʊnet]

Word ending: *hello* [hɛloʊ]

Single syllable: *doe* [doʊ]

Most of the diphthongs [ei]–[eɪ], [aɪ]–[ai]–[æ], and [ɔi]–[ɔɪ] are greatly influenced by dialect variations, which are explained later in this text.

The movement from one vowel to another vowel to form the single sound of a diphthong is rapid. From a functional viewpoint, the distinctive feature classification applied to vowels such as high, low, front, back, and so forth is difficult to isolate in the production of diphthongs because their production is so complex. The features of the initiating vowel may differ from the terminal vowel in many aspects. Keep in mind that these features are not exact from one position to another but serve as approximate targets for the diphthong's on-glide and off-glide segments. See **Table 7-1**.

The acoustic characteristics of diphthongs include the movement of the tongue from the position required for one vowel sound to the required position for the second sound. Ball and Lowry (2001) state that this results in a change in the format structure in the course of the spectrogram so that it displays a combination of the characteristic patterns by both components of the diphthong.

Kent and Read (2002) state that diphthongs are like vowels in that they are produced with a relatively open vocal tract and a well-defined formant structure. They indicate that vowels and diphthongs are different in that they cannot be characterized by single vocal tract shape of a single formant structure. Diphthongs are dynamic sounds in which the articulatory shape and the formant slowly change during the sound's production.

Ladefoged (2005) offers a comprehensive discourse on the sounds of vowels including their acoustic structure. The acoustic characteristics of fricatives (Ball & Lowry, 2001) occur when the airflow is forced through a narrow channel between two articulators (for example, the [ff] fricative sound is produced when the lower lip and upper teeth form a narrow channel). They state that this results in noise energy occurring at very high frequencies. Fricatives are located on the spectrogram according to their place of articulation. An examination of the variations in the combined phonetic features of diphthongs demonstrates the complexities of their production. The only variable that appears to be constant is that each diphthong begins at a lower position and ends at a higher position.

The principle of *relativity* applies to the understanding of the operational processes involved in the production of diphthongs. Shriberg and Kent (1995) explain

TABLE 7-1	Diphthongs

Diphthong	Phonetic Feature Variations
[ei]–[eɪ] *cake* [keik] or [keɪk]	Height: mid to high Depth: front to front Tension: tense to tense [i] or lax [ɪ] Roundness: unround to unround
[ai]–[aɪ] *I* [ai] or [aɪ]	Height: low to high Depth: front to front Tension: lax to tense [ɪ] or lax [i] Roundness: unround to unround
[aʊ] *house* [haʊs]	Height: low to mid-high Depth: front to back Tension: lax to lax Roundness: unround to round
[ɔɪ] or [ci] *oil* [ɔɪl] or [ɔil]	Height: mid to high Depth: back to front Tension: tense to lax [ɪ] or tense [i] Roundness: round to unround
[oʊ] *echo* [ɛkoʊ]	Height: mid to mid-high Depth: back to back Tension: tense to lax Roundness: round to round

Noteworthy also is the phonemic characteristics of the diphthongs. Diphthongs that represent two different sounds that can be reduced to one sound, such as the [ei] or [eɪ] reduced to [e], *without changing the meaning*, as in *cake* [keik] or [keɪk], and [oʊ] to [o], as in *oats* [oʊts] to [ots], are considered to be phonemic. The other diphthongs [aɪ], [aʊ], and [ɔɪ] are nonphonemic because the same rule cannot be applied.

Also, the two phonemic diphthongs share another characteristic in common that is mainly determined by their usage in stressed and weaker stressed syllables. The [ei] and [oʊ] occur in stress syllables *donation* [doneɪʃən] and *open* [oʊpən], and the [e] and [o] occur in unstressed syllables *donate* [doun̪et] and *rotation* [roteɪʃən]. Because of this phonemic characteristic, the diphthongs [eɪ] and [oʊ] are discussed in conjunction with the [e] and [o] vowels, and the remaining nonphonemic diphthongs [aʊ], [aɪ], and [ɔɪ] are each discussed individually later.

Skill-Building Activities

1. Construct the vowel quadrilateral matrix and indicate the positions of the vowels according to depth (front-mid-back) and height (high-mid-low).

2. List the vowels and indicate their characteristics of tension and roundness.

3. List each of the vowels and diphthongs and provide a key word that contains each of their sounds.

REFERENCES

Ball, M. J., & Lowry, O. (2001). *Methods in clinical phonetics*. London, England: Whurr Publishers.

Ball, M. J., & Rahilly, J. (1999). *Phonetics: The science of sounds*. London, England: Whurr Publishers.

House, L. I. (1998). *Introductory phonetics and phonology: A workbook approach*. Mahwah, NJ: Lawrence Erlbaum.

Kent, R. D., & Read, C. (2002). *The acoustic analysis of speech*. Albany, NY: Singular.

Ladefoged, P. (2005). *Vowels and consonants: An introduction to the sounds of languages* (2nd ed.). Victoria, Australia: Blackwell Publishing.

Shriberg, L. D., & Kent, R. D. (1995). *Clinical phonetics*. New York, NY: Macmillan.

Stetson, R. (1951). *Motor phonetics* (2nd ed.). Amsterdam, The Netherlands: North Holland.

that there is little agreement among phoneticians as to which vowels should be used to symbolize the English diphthongs. Most agree that two symbols are required, one to represent the on-glide (initiation) and one to represent the off-glide (termination), but phoneticians often hear different vowels for both the on-glide and off-glide segments. For example, consider the word *bye* with the possible transcriptions of *b*+ /aɪ/, /ay/, /ai/, /ɑɪ/, /ɑy/, /ɑi/, /æ/. Shriberg and Kent (1995) offer the explanation that it is not surprising that variable sounds are produced because different speakers may use different on-glide and off-glide segments from one occasion to another, depending on phonetic context, rate of speaking, and the degree of stress.

Chapter 8

Long Vowels and Diphthongs

PURPOSE

To introduce you to the long vowels and diphthongs and their phonetic symbols

OBJECTIVES

This chapter will provide you with information regarding:

1. Characteristics of the five long vowels
2. Different spellings for the long vowels
3. Rules for spelling and pronunciation
4. Allophonic variations and dialect differences
5. Nonnative speaker pronunciation
6. Speech deviations
7. Transcription exercises

INTRODUCTION

The decision to present the vowels and diphthongs in the order of long vowels and diphthongs, short vowels and diphthongs, and other vowels and diphthongs is based on several observations made while teaching over many years. In the past, as the vowels were presented, students would ask for clarification by saying, "Is that the same as the long vowel ā?" and so on. They were seeking a reference point to apply to the new information they were attempting to learn. Also, when the vowels are introduced for the first time in

an elementary school setting and when instruction in English as a second language is presented, the vowels are introduced in a series of long, short, and others. In addition, with the current trend toward promoting literacy, the beginning phonetician needs to become aware of the terminology used with phonics and other approaches to reading as he or she interacts with teachers, reading specialists, and others.

Traditionally, the vowels have been presented from a "position" perspective on a quadrilateral matrix. Whereas this approach continues to be used, other approaches may be as effective or even more so. As mentioned earlier, the organization or sequence of presentation of the vowels and diphthongs begins with the long vowels and related diphthongs, proceeds to the short vowels and then the remaining other vowels and diphthongs. The long vowels are listed in **Table 8-1**.

Some generalizations regarding long vowels include the following. Remember that there are always exceptions to the rules. Long vowels usually have the following characteristics:

1. Two adjacent vowels, as in *seat, coat, greet*
2. Single vowel that ends a word, as in *me, go*
3. Medial vowel with a final *e* ending, as in *hope, cute, tape*
4. How *y* functions at the end of a word, as in *my, day, gray*

TABLE 8-1	The Long Vowels of American English

Vowels	Long Vowels
ā	[eɪ] (stressed syllable, one-syllable word or word ending) *rotation* = /roteɪʃən/, *cake* = /keɪk/, *Kaye* = /keɪ/ [e] (unstressed syllable) *rotate* = /routet/
ē	[i] = *he* = /hi/
ī	[aɪ] = *ice* = /aɪs/
ō	[oʊ] (stressed syllable, one-syllable word or word ending) *rotate* = /routet/, *coat* = /koʊt/, *go* = /goʊ/
ū	[u] = *ooze* = /uz/

PHONETIC SYMBOLS [e] AND [eɪ]

EXHIBIT 8-1	Phonetic Symbols [e] and [eɪ]

Phonetic Symbol	[e] unstressed [eɪ] stressed
Grapheme Symbol	See the section titled "Different Spellings of the [e], [eɪ] Sounds," which follows.
Diacritic Symbol	ā
Phonic Symbol	ā Unstressed, Stressed
Sound Class	Long Vowel or Diphthong Word Ending
Tongue Position	Height: (Upper) Mid Depth: Front Tension: Tense
Lips	Unrounded
Phonetic Features	[eɪ] Progresses from [e] upper-mid, front, tense, unrounded to [ɪ] lower-high, front, unrounded, lax
International Phonetic Alphabet (IPA) (1999)	[e] #302 Close-Midfront, Unrounded

The [e] vowel and the [eɪ] diphthong represent the unstressed and stressed long ā sound and are discussed as they relate to one another rather than in separate sections in this text.

How the Sound Is Produced as a Vowel

The airflow from the lungs activates the vibration of the closed (adducted) vocal folds (voiced), and the sound waves travel through the pharyngeal cavity. The velopharyngeal port is closed, and the sound enters the oral cavity and exits through the mouth. The sides of the tongue are against the upper molars. The middle and front portions of the (tense) tongue are raised somewhat above (upper) the midplane (mid) and shifted forward (front) with the tip of the tongue positioned behind the lower front teeth. The lips are apart in an unrounded position. In the front vowel positions, the [e] is above the [ɛ] and below the [ɪ] vowels.

How the Sound Is Produced as a Diphthong

The [eɪ] diphthong is produced as the sound progresses from the [e] position (upper-mid, front, tense, unrounded) to the [ɪ] position (lower-high, front, unrounded, lax). The [e] segment is the longer nucleus and the [ɪ] is the shorter glide. The movement of the glide process is relative and may result in variable positions between the [ɪ] and [i] depending on context and speaker preference. Refer to the discussion on [ɪ] and [i] later in this chapter for more details concerning these sounds.

Commentary

Edwards (1997) states that in United States English, there is a tendency to diphthongize [e] in stressed syllables, and many phoneticians typically transcribe [e] as a diphthong. Carrell and Tiffany (1960) add that many phoneticians, indeed, would prefer to use such symbols as [eɪ] or [ei] instead of [e] to represent the articulation of this sound. MacKay (1987) offers the example of the English phoneme [e] and indicates that the word *bay* in different dialect areas may be pronounced as [ei], [ɛɪ], [eɪ], and so forth. Small (1999) agrees and states that the stressed form of the vowel [e] becomes a diphthong, written as [eɪ]. The use varies with syllable context and regional pronunciation. He indicates that because the substitution of the articulatory production of [e] for [eɪ] or vice versa would not result in the creation of a different phoneme, these two sounds should be considered as allophones. Calvert (1986) summarizes the viewpoint of the majority of phoneticians by stating that in United States English, the [eɪ] (or [ei]) is substituted for the [e] in the primary accent in words, as in matin*ee* and m*a*king. It also occurs with secondary accent as in polysyllabic words with *–ate* endings, as in lubric*ate* and incorpor*ate*. The [e] is pronounced in the unaccented syllable. This usually occurs when the sound is in the syllable next to the accented syllable. The unaccented [e] may also be pronounced [ə], as in *fatality*: [fe] or [fə]. When [e] loses its stress, it often becomes an [i] or [ɪ] sound, as in *Monday*: [mʌndi] or [mʌndɪ]. The unaccented [e] also occurs in bisyllabic words ending in an unaccented *–ate*, as in don*ate*, reb*ate*, immediately following the accented syllable. The [eɪ] (or [ei]) is usually used when the [e] is the last sound in a word.

Carrell and Tiffany (1960) offer this timely insight: The amount of stress given [e] has a great deal to do with its actual pronunciation in American speech. The diphthongization of the [e] sound varies with length of the sound, which in turn depends on its stress and context. Also, the speaker may have a reason to stress a word such as *cake*, and it may be heard as either [keɪk] or [kek] depending on the amount of stress given to the vowel. Shriberg and Kent (1995) state that the [e] is a monophthongal variant of a more common diphthongized form [eɪ]. The monophthong is shorter than the diphthong and does not have the tongue-raising characteristic. Examples of [e] include *locate, operate, alteration, ballet*. The [e] appears in the stressed accent in *locate* and *alteration* where some other phoneticians would use the [eɪ]. The [eɪ] is essentially an allophone, alternative to [e]. It is more likely to occur when the syllable is strongly stressed or spoken at a slow rate. The actual extent of tongue and jaw movement varies with stress, rate, and phonetic context. Bernthal and Bankson (1998) describe [e] as a front, tense, unrounded vowel and [eɪ] as a variant of the vowel [e] rather than a true phonemic diphthong. The meaning would not change if either sound were used: *bay* [be] or [beɪ].

There appear to be two prominent trends in the usage of the [e] and [eɪ]. One, the [e] is used in unstressed accent syllables and the [eɪ] is used in stressed, accented syllables and word endings; two, the two sounds [e] and [eɪ] are used interchangeably and the sound to be transcribed depends on the contextual production of the speaker and the perception of the listener. Some phoneticians consider [e] and [eɪ] as two separate sounds while others consider them as allophones of the same sound. There appears to be consensus that the meaning of the word will not be misunderstood (nonphonemic) regardless of the usage of the sound [e] or [eɪ].

The rules stated earlier provide some guidance in the appropriate choice of symbol transcription [e] or [ei] or [eɪ], but it still remains rather subjective for both the speaker and the listener to determine which sound is actually spoken and heard.

For the purpose of uniformity, the following will serve as a guideline for the transcription exercises in this book. The [e] vowel symbol is used when the sound occurs in the *unstressed* syllable, and the [eɪ] diphthong symbol is used in the *stressed* syllable, *single-syllable words*, and *word endings*.

From Simple to Complex!

One could also use a parallel statement to this section's heading, "From naïve to informed" or "From unsophisticated to sophisticated." Certainly, for the beginning phonetician, it is more complex. The great pioneer phoneticians John S. Kenyon and Thomas A. Knott who provided *A Pronouncing Dictionary of*

American English in 1944 and revisions through 1953 did not recognize the diphthong [eɪ] and only used the [e] sound such as in *rotate* [rotet] (primary stress, first syllable) and *rotation* [roteʃən] (primary stress, second syllable). How simple it would have been for the beginning phonetician in that time not to have to consider the use of the diphthong [eɪ] and not to have to analyze the sound as to whether it appeared as the only sound in the word, such as *cake*, or as the stressed or word-ending sound to adhere to the "rule." If history repeats itself, as it often does, perhaps sometime in the future there will be a return to Kenyon and Knott's interpretation of the use of the long ā sound. On the other hand, with the ability of the sophisticated technology of today to detect subtle changes in sound production that justifies the use of the diphthong [eɪ], the differentiation between the [e] and [eɪ] will probably remain. For that reason, this author decided to maintain the difference and follow the rule used by the majority of contemporary phoneticians.

Different Spellings of the [e] and [eɪ] Sounds

The following may represent dialectical differences. Transcribe the following words. Refer to the Key at the right upon completion. As you complete the transcription exercises, refer to the key provided in the Sound/Symbol Reference Guide on the inside cover of this book or to your own sound/symbol reference cards.

Different Spellings				*Key*
a	gate ___ taste ___ place ___			geɪt, teɪst, pleɪs
	atrium ___ Abraham ___			etriəm, ebrʌhæm
ai	gain ___ pain ___ tail ___			geɪn, peɪn, teɪl
ay	say ___ delay ___ play ___			seɪ, dɪleɪ/dʌleɪ, pleɪ
ea	steak ___ break ___			steɪk, breɪk
ey	hey ___ obey ___ prey ___ they ___			heɪ, obeɪ, preɪ, ðeɪ
e	mesa ___ debris ___			meɪsə, deɪbri
au	gauge ___			geɪdʒ
uet	bouquet ___			bokeɪ
ae	Gaelic ___			geɪlɪk
et	sachet ___ chalet ___ ballet ___			sæʃeɪ, ʃæleɪ, bæleɪ
ei	neighbor ___ eight ___ freight ___			neɪbɚ, eɪt, freɪt
e	matinee ___ melee ___			mætɪneɪ, mɛleɪ

Different Sounds for the Same Letters for the [e] and [eɪ] Sounds

This listing is not all-inclusive but does represent a major sample. Transcribe the following words. Refer to the Key at the right upon completion.

Alphabet Letters	*Different Sounds*	*Words*		*Key*
a	[e] or [eɪ]	gate	___	geɪt
	[æ]	ask	___	æsk
	[a]	father	___	faðɚ
	[ɑ] or [ɔ]	auto	___	ɔtoʊ
	[ɛ]	fair	___	fɛɪr/fɛɚ
	[ə]	about	___	əbaʊt
ai	[e] or [eɪ]	again	___	əgeɪn
	[ɛ]	again	___	əgɛn
ea	[e] or [eɪ]	steak	___	steɪk
	[i]	each	___	itʃ
ey	[e] or [eɪ]	hey	___	heɪ
	[i]	key	___	ki
au	[e] or [eɪ]	gauge	___	geɪdʒ
	[ɑ] or [ɔ]	autumn	___	ɔtəm
uet	[e] or [eɪ]	bouquet	___	bokeɪ
	[ɛ]	duet	___	duɛt
et	[e] or [eɪ]	chalet	___	ʃæleɪ
	[ɛ]	get	___	gɛt
ee	[e] or [eɪ]	matinee	___	mætɪneɪ

Rules for Spelling and Pronunciation of the [e] and [eɪ] Sounds

1. When [e] is the only vowel in a syllable or word, it usually is pronounced as a long ā sound.

2. Some consonants that follow the [e] sound are silent, as in *weigh, day*, and *Faye*.

Words That Include the Unstressed [e] Sound

Transcribe the following words. Refer to the Key at the right upon completion.

	Medial		*Key*
became _____	rebate _____		bikem, ribet
fatality _____	vibrate _____		fetælɪti, vaɪbret
rotate _____	nativity _____		roʊtet, netɪvɪti
donate _____	vacation _____		doʊnet, vekeɪʃən
vacate _____	orate _____		vekeɪt, ɔret
chaotic _____			keɔtɪk

Words That Include the Stressed [eɪ] Sound

Transcribe the following words. Refer to the Key at the right upon completion.

Initial	*Medial*	*Final*	*Key*
able ___	table ___	bay ___	eɪbl̩, teɪbl̩, beɪ
age ___	spaceship ___	birthday ___	eɪdʒ, speɪsʃɪp, bɝ̩Ѳdeɪ
apron ___	stay ___	baseball ___	eɪprən, steɪ, beɪbɑl
ate ___	player ___	anyway ___	eɪt, pleɪɚ, ɛnɪweɪ
agent ___	away ___	payment ___	eɪdʒɛnt, əweɪ, peɪmənt
Asia ___	rayon ___	pray ___	eɪʒə, reɪjɔn, preɪ

Auditory Discrimination

Contrast Minimal Pairs

Allophonic and dialect differences may occur with the pronunciation of the [eɪ]. The reader should realize that the following [eɪ] columns could also represent the [e] sound depending on the phonetician. Transcribe the following words. Refer to the Key at the right upon completion.

[eɪ]	*[ɪ]*	*Key*
lake _____	lick _____	leɪk, lɪk
break _____	brick _____	breɪk, brɪk
case _____	kiss _____	keɪs, kɪs
pain _____	pin _____	peɪn, pɪn
tape _____	tip _____	teɪp, tɪp
laid _____	lid _____	leɪd, lɪd
ale _____	ill _____	eɪl, ɪl
eight _____	it _____	eɪt, ɪt

[eɪ]	*[i]*	*Key*
male _____	meal _____	meɪl, mil
great _____	greet _____	greɪt, grit
wave _____	weave _____	weɪv, wiv
laid _____	lead _____	leɪd, lid
main _____	mean _____	meɪn, min
wake _____	week _____	weɪk, wik
pace _____	peace _____	peɪs, pis
shape _____	sheep _____	ʃeɪp, ʃip

[eɪ]	*[ɛ]*	*Key*
mate _____	met _____	meɪt, mɛt
gate _____	get _____	geɪt, gɛt
bale _____	bell _____	beɪl, bɛl
laced _____	lest _____	leɪst, lɛst
wait _____	wet _____	weɪt, wɛt
paint _____	pent _____	peɪnt, pɛnt
taste _____	test _____	teɪst, tɛst
fade _____	fed _____	feɪd, fɛd

Allophonic and Dialect Variations

Perhaps the most important aspect of [e] is its prominent diphthongal quality as it shifts from a more lax [ɛ]-like quality toward a more tense [i]-like quality, [eɪ], [ɛɪ], [ej], and [ɛj] (Tiffany & Carrell, 1977). In less-stressed syllables between certain consonants, [e] is relatively monophthongal and short, as in *cake* [kek] or [keɪk].

The diphthong [eɪ] as in *hay* varies considerably in different forms of English (Ladefoged, 1993). Some speakers begin with a vowel much like [ɛ] as in *head* and others start with a sound much closer to [ɪ]. The [ɛ] replaces the [ɪ] in words like *egg* [ɛg] for [eg] or [eɪg], and *make* becomes [mɛk]. Tiffany and Carrell (1977) and Edwards (1997) report that in words that end with "day," the [ɪ] may be substituted as in *Monday* [mʌndɪ], [mʌndi], [mʌnde], or [mʌndj] according to stress and style. Also, the insertion of the [ə] before [l] as in *jail* [dʒeiəl] may occur. As with other vowels, the [e] may assimilate nasality when in the context of nasal consonants [m], [n], and [ŋ].

Nonnative Speaker Pronunciation

The long ā [e] is common among many languages, but one of the conspicuous differences occurs in some

English and Australian dialects that have a variant of the United States English [aɪ], as in "Take if today" sounds like "Tike it to die" [taɪk ət tɔdaɪ].

Speech-Sound Deviations

This sound is relatively stable (Edwards, 1997), even in children with speech impairments. When the diphthongal nature of [e] (e. g., [eɪ]) is maintained, the most frequent substitution is [aɪ]. When the sound is laxed or lowered, the adjacent vowel [ɛ] is substituted.

Summary

The [e] is an (upper) mid, front vowel that is produced with a tense tongue and unrounded lips. This sound occurs in the unstressed, long ā context with the [eɪ] sound pronounced in the stressed and word-ending syllables. Among phoneticians, the interpretation of the [e] varies from a single, nonphonemic sound with [eɪ] as an allophone to two separate sounds, a vowel [e] and diphthong [eɪ]. Many allophonic and dialect variations are possible with this sound, which has at least 12 different spelling possibilities. The sound is present in many sound systems of languages worldwide, and nonnative speakers have minimal difficulty with it. Speech deviations occur as a result of changes in tongue tension (tense vs. lax) and positioning that result in substitutions of adjacent sounds or diphthongs of various combinations.

Competency Quiz

Transcribe the following [eɪ] words. Cover the Key at the right side and refer to it upon completion.

Set 1

		Key
1. aid	_____	eɪd
2. cable	_____	keɪbl̩
3. base	_____	beɪs
4. maybe	_____	meɪbi
5. native	_____	neɪtiv
6. raise	_____	reɪz
7. Mable	_____	meɪbl̩
8. waste	_____	weɪst
9. cape	_____	keɪp

10. face	_____	feɪs
11. ape	_____	eɪp
12. weight	_____	weɪt
13. create	_____	kreɪt
14. stay	_____	steɪ
15. game	_____	geɪm
16. payday	_____	peɪdeɪ
17. safe	_____	seɪf
18. pace	_____	peɪs
19. plain	_____	pleɪn
20. scrape	_____	skreɪp

[eɪ] Transcription Exercises

Remember, the [eɪ] is used in one-syllable words, the stressed syllable, and word endings.

Set 2

				Key
1. ate	_____	11. bait	_____	eɪt, eɪt
2. cave	_____	12. crane	_____	keɪv, kreɪn
3. lace	_____	13. place	_____	leɪs, pleɪs
4. take	_____	14. scale	_____	teɪk, skeɪl
5. rate	_____	15. waste	_____	reɪt, weɪst
6. pay	_____	16. flake	_____	peɪ, fleɪk
7. grade	_____	17. blade	_____	greɪd, bleɪd
8. skate	_____	18. slate	_____	skeɪt, sleɪt
9. state	_____	19. phase	_____	steɪt, feɪz
10. strain	_____	20. quake	_____	streɪn, kweɪk

Set 3

				Key
1. paint	_____	11. freight	_____	peɪnt, freɪt
2. train	_____	12. sleigh	_____	treɪn, sleɪ
3. braid	_____	13. bay	_____	breɪd, beɪ
4. grain	_____	14. may	_____	greɪn, meɪ
5. praise	_____	15. hey	_____	preɪz, heɪ
6. straight	_____	16. play	_____	streɪt, pleɪ
7. fate	_____	17. stay	_____	feɪt, steɪ

8. quaint _____ 18. mate _____ kweɪnt, meɪt

9. steak _____ 19. gray _____ steɪk, greɪ

10. weigh _____ 20. prey _____ weɪ, preɪ

Circle the Words with the [eɪ] Stressed Sound

Set 4

have	fame	rail
stale	dance	male
cage	grade	chance
haste	aisle	reign
prance	shape	neigh
wait	slave	said
ail	pace	plaid

Key: Stale, cage, wait, fame, grade, shape, slave, pace, rail, male, reign, neigh.

Circle the Words with the Unstressed [e] Sound

Set 5

became	matinee	rotate	rotation
baseball	stay	nativity	rebate
player	payment	vibrate	chaotic
age	apron	fatality	spaceship
donate	table	orate	agent
Abraham	ballet	atrium	neighbor

Key (Note that dialect may influence individual stress patterns): Donate, matinee, ballet, rotate, nativity, fatality, orate, chaotic.

This completes the discussion of the long ā [e] vowel and [eɪ] diphthong.

PHONETIC SYMBOL [i]

EXHIBIT 8-2	**Phonetic Symbols [i]**

Phonetic Symbol	[i]	**[i]**
Grapheme Symbol	See the section titled "Different Spellings for the [i] Sound," which follows.	
Diacritic Symbol	ē	
Phonic Symbol	Long ē	
Sound Class	Cardinal, Front, High, Vowel	
Tongue Position	Position: High-Front Depth: Front Tension: Tense	
Lips	Unrounded	
IPA (1999)	[i] #301 Close, Front, Unrounded	

A discussion of the long ē [i] vowel is now presented.

How the Sound Is Produced

The airflow from the lungs activates the vibration of the closed (adducted) vocal folds (voiced), and the sound enters the oral cavity because the velopharyngeal port is closed or nearly closed. The tongue is in a forward position (front), and the blade of the tongue is elevated (high) toward the hard palate. The [i] has the highest tongue position of the front vowels. The sides of the tongue are in contact laterally with the alveolar ridge. The tip of the tongue is positioned behind the lower front teeth and exerts tension (tense) during the production of the [i] sound.

Different Spellings for the [i] Sound

The following examples may represent variations in dialect and usage. For example, *remember* [rimɛmbɚ] and [rəmɛmbɚ]. Transcribe the following words. Refer to the Sound/Symbol Reference Guide as needed. Compare your transcription to the Key at the right upon completion.

Different Spellings				Key
i	machine ___ prestige ___			məʃin, prɛstiʒ
	pizza ___ ski ___ chic ___			pisə, ski, ʃik
e	recipe ___ me ___			rɛsɪpi, mi
	remember___ even ___			rimɛmbɚ, ivən
ee	beet ___ see ___ greet ___ teepee ___			bit, si, ɡrit, tipi
ei	deceive ___ receipt ___ neither ___			disiv, risit, niðɚ
ie	believe ___ relieve ___			biliv, riliv
	chief ___ cookie ___			ʧif, cɔki
ae	Caesar ___ eon ___			cizɚ, iɔn
ea	meager ___ meat ___ eat ___ read ___			miɡɚ, mit, it, rid
eo	people ___			pipl̩
oe	amoeba ___ Phoenix ___			əbibə, finɪks
ey	monkey ___ donkey ___ key ___			mʌnki, dɔnki, ki
y	tidy ___ city ___			taɪdi, sɪti
	worthy ___ dirty ___			wɝði, dɝti

Different Sounds for the Same Letters That Represent [i]

Transcribe the following words. Refer to the Key at the right upon completion.

Alphabet Letters	Different Sounds	Words		Key
i	[i]	ski	___	ski
	[ɪ]	in	___	ɪn
e	[i]	bee	___	bi
	[ɛ]	bet	___	bɛt
	Silent	cake	___	keɪk
oe	[i]	Phoenix	___	finɪks
	[oʊ]	toe	___	toʊ
y (dialect)	[i]	city	___	cɪti
	[ɪ]	city	___	cɪtɪ
	Silent	key	___	ki
	[j]	yes	___	jɛs

Rules for Spelling and Pronunciation of the [i] Sound

1. Because the written symbol e̲ represents the name of the letter *e*, it is considered to be a long vowel, as in *see, key,* and *be*.

2. In the unstressed position, the letter *y* is pronounced either with an [i] or [ɪ].

3. When *e* is the only (vowel) letter in a syllable or word, it is pronounced as either the long vowel ē *mē* or the short vowel ê *gêt*.

4. The [i] before [r] is frequently substituted with the [ɪ], as in when *near* [nir] becomes [nɪr] and *peer* [pir] becomes [pɪr].

5. The [i] sound is very consistent for two adjacent *ee*, as in *see, feet, seed, agree*.

6. The *ea* frequently represents the [i] sound as in *each, tea, leave, please, east*. When two different vowels are adjacent, the second one is silent.

Words That Include the [i] Sound

The pronunciation may vary depending on differences in dialect. Transcribe the following words. Refer to the Key at the right upon completion.

Initial	Medial*	Final	Key
each ___	sweet ___	city ___	iʧ, swit, cɪti
equator ___	beat ___	me ___	ikweɪtɚ, bit, mi
erupt ___	deceive ___	candy ___	irʌpt, disiv, kændi
eel ___	amoeba ___	tea ___	il, əmibə, ti
event ___	seat ___	teepee ___	ivɛnt, sit, tipi
elongate ___	ravine ___	see ___	ilɔnɡet, rivɪn, si
eliminate ___	retrieve ___	ski ___	ilɪmɪnet, ritriv, ski
even ___	meager ___	party ___	ivɔn, miɡɚ, pɑrti
emit ___	piece ___	free ___	imɪt, pis, fri

VanRiper (1979) has a solution, but this author does not recommend it. He states, "Use [ɪ] in unaccented endings of words (*city* [sɪdɪ]), even if it sounds like [i] to you. In the word *candy*, the second syllable is unaccented, and therefore requires the [ɪ] symbol." (p. 57)

---

*In word-final position in words like *city* and *petty*, the choice between [i] and [ɪ] can be difficult and most phoneticians prefer [ɪ] (Shriberg & Kent, 1995). For words such as *warranty-warrantee*, the [ɪ] is suited for the *y* in *warranty* and the [i] for the *ee* in *warrantee*. A review of several dictionaries indicates pronunciation of [i] at the end of both words!

Auditory Discrimination

Contrast Minimal Pairs

The following pronunciation may be influenced by dialect differences. Transcribe the following words. Refer to the Key at the right upon completion.

[i]	[ɪ]	Key
least _____	list _____	list, lɪst
meet _____	mitt _____	mit, mɪt
week _____	wick _____	wik, wɪk
lead _____	lid _____	lid, lɪd
feel _____	fill _____	fil, fɪl
each _____	itch _____	iʧ, ɪʧ
read _____	rid _____	rid, rɪd
meal _____	mill _____	mil, mɪl
green _____	grin _____	grin, grɪn

Other Minimal Pairs

[i]	[ɛ]	Key
heed _____	head _____	hid, hɛd
seal _____	sell _____	sil, sɛl
mean _____	men _____	min, mɛn
teen _____	ten _____	tin, tɛn
keep _____	kept _____	kip, kɛpt
lease _____	less _____	lis, lɛs
seed _____	said _____	sid, sɛd
beast _____	best _____	bist, bɛst
each _____	etch _____	iʧ, ɛʧ

[i]	[eɪ]	Key
feet _____	fate _____	fit, feɪt
free _____	fray _____	fri, freɪ
be _____	bay _____	bi, beɪ
feel _____	fail _____	fil, feɪl
ease _____	as _____	iz, eɪz
we _____	way _____	wi, weɪ
least _____	laced _____	list, leɪst
see _____	say _____	si, seɪ
me _____	may _____	mi, meɪ

Allophonic and Dialect Variations

The possibility of nasalization exists for the production of [i] (Shriberg & Kent, 1995). The velopharynx is normally closed for [i], but it may be open in a nasal context as in *me* and *mean*. Some linguists regard the [i] as being a diphthong [iy] rather than a monophthong. Edwards (1997) provides the example of this occurrence of the [i] becoming diphthongized in open and stressed syllables, as in *flee* [fliɪ]. In many cases, the tongue nearly touches the hard palate, with an approximation so close that a fricative sound is often heard (Tiffany & Carrell, 1977). As with most vowels, [i] becomes "reduced" in unstressed positions, and such words as *revise* [rivaɪz] may be spoken as [rɪvaɪz] or [rəvaɪz]. Also, an insertion of the [ə] may occur before an [l], as in *seal* [siəl]. A final weak, unstressed [i] sound varies markedly, as in *city* and *twenty*, resulting in a somewhat more lax and simple [i] that is spoken somewhere between the range of the [ɪ] and [i]. Tiffany and Carrell (1977) conclude that this is probably more or less the rule in United States English. Calvert (1986) and Ladefoged (1993) state that in United States English dialects, either [i] or [ɪ] is pronounced in such unstressed contexts as those mentioned above: *city, baby,* and so forth.

In some dialects, the [i] is seldom heard as a tense vowel before [r], and words like *beer* and *we're* may be spoken more like [bɪr] and [wɪr] (Tiffany & Carrell, 1977). A common dialect difference in United States English is found in words that end in [k], such as *creek*, pronounced as either [krik] or [krɪk] (Edwards, 1997). Some Eastern American speakers make a distinct diphthong in *heed* and they "glide" through the sound, starting with [ɪ] and ending with [i] (Ladefoged, 1993).

Nonnative Speaker Pronunciation

Nonnative speakers have minimal difficulty with this sound because it appears quite universally (Edwards, 1997), but the [i] may be substituted for the [ɪ]. However, this may be another example of the prominence of the [i] that is shifting in other languages as well as in United States English.

Speech-Sound Deviations

The [i] sound is relatively easy to acquire and children usually develop it without any problems. When a deviancy is encountered, as can be predicted, substitutions of the other vowels, particularly [e], will occur (Edwards, 1997). Shifting from a tense [i] to a more relaxed posture may result in the [ɪ] sound.

Summary

The [i] is a cardinal vowel that marks the high front apex of the vowel quadrilateral. It is the highest in both tongue position and resonance frequency. It is produced with the tongue in the high-front position. The tongue is tense and the lips unrounded. It is classified as a "long" vowel and has more than 11 different spelling combinations whose letters also represent other sounds. The [i] sound occurs in all positions within words—initial, medial, and final. It is in "competition" with the [ɪ] sound in many contexts, particularly in the final sound as in *city, only,* and similar words. There are considerable variations in the allophones and dialects of this sound depending on context, rate, and stress. Diphthongization is also characteristic of this sound, resulting in diphthongs such as [eɪ] and [ai]. Deviations may occur with the substitution of [e] (tense) or [i] (lax).

Competency Quiz

Transcribe the following words. Refer to the Key at the right after completion of each set.

Set 1

				Key
1. be	_____	11. grief	_____	bi, grif
2. beast	_____	12. keen	_____	bist, kin
3. geese	_____	13. grieve	_____	gis, griv
4. beak	_____	14. quay	_____	bik, kwi
5. bean	_____	15. seize	_____	bin, siz
6. bleed	_____	16. glee	_____	blid, gli
7. east	_____	17. bead	_____	ist, bid
8. leave	_____	18. kneel	_____	liv, nil
9. gleam	_____	19. treat	_____	glim, trit
10. key	_____	20. niece	_____	ki, nis

[i] Transcription Exercises

Set 2

				Key
1. bean	_____	11. sneak	_____	bin, snik
2. clean	_____	12. stream	_____	klin, strim
3. eat	_____	13. bead	_____	it, bid
4. seat	_____	14. beast	_____	sit, bist
5. tea	_____	15. cream	_____	ti, krim
6. seem	_____	16. creak	_____	sim, krik
7. dream	_____	17. feast	_____	drim, fist
8. meat	_____	18. heap	_____	mit, hip
9. ream	_____	19. peace	_____	rim, pis
10. scream	_____	20. pea	_____	skrim, pi

Set 3

				Key
1. plead	_____	11. cease	_____	plid, sis
2. squeak	_____	12. feat	_____	skwik, fit
3. steam	_____	13. grease	_____	stim, gris
4. treat	_____	14. plea	_____	trit, pli
5. weave	_____	15. beet	_____	wiv, bit
6. flea	_____	16. feet	_____	fli, fit
7. knead	_____	17. green	_____	nid, grin
8. league	_____	18. squeal	_____	lig, skwil
9. Lee	_____	19. street	_____	li, strit
10. heap	_____	20. teepee	_____	hip, tipi

Set 4

				Key
1. tree	_____	11. heat	_____	tri, hit
2. breeze	_____	12. steep	_____	briz, stip
3. tease	_____	13. week	_____	tiz, wik
4. bleed	_____	14. deep	_____	blid, dip
5. sleek	_____	15. free	_____	slik, fri
6. creek	_____	16. geese	_____	krik, gis
7. creep	_____	17. knee	_____	krip, ni
8. queen	_____	18. greet	_____	kwin, grit
9. seek	_____	19. clean	_____	sik, clin
10. speed	_____	20. seem	_____	spid, sim

Circle the Words with the [i] Sound

Set 5

friend	meal	peel
sleep	break	chief
they	sneeze	pier
steep	edge	keen
great	brief	steak
been	flee	theme
freeze	seize	peep

Key: Sleep, steep, freeze, sneeze, brief, flee, seize, chief, keen, theme, peep.

This completes the discussion of the long ē [i] vowel sound.

PHONETIC SYMBOL [aɪ]

EXHIBIT 8-3	Phonetic Symbols [aɪ]

Phonetic Symbol	[aɪ]	**[aɪ]**
Grapheme Symbol	See the section titled "Different Spellings of the [aɪ] Sound," which follows.	
Diacritic Symbol	ī	
Phonic Symbol	ī	
Sound Class	Diphthong	
Tongue Position	Height: Low [a] to high [ɪ] Depth: Front [a] to front [ɪ] Tension: Lax [a] to tense [ɪ]	
Lips	Unround [a] to unround [ɪ]	
IPA (1999)	Not specified by IPA.	

A discussion of the long ī [aɪ] vowel is now presented.

How the Sound Is Produced

The airflow from the lungs activates the vibration of the closed vocal folds (voiced), and the sound enters the oral cavity because the velopharyngeal port is normally closed except for nasal contexts. The jaw is lowered and the mouth is open in the posture of the [a] sound (nucleus-on-glide), and then it closes somewhat for the off-glide ending. The middle and front sections of the tongue are raised from low, back (on-glide) as the tongue rises in front to a mid-front or high-front [e], [ɪ], or [i] height. The movement is rapid and smooth. The tip of the tongue presses lightly behind the lower front teeth. The overall movement proceeds from a low-back [a] position and glides to a high-front position. During the process, the tongue tension begins rather lax and becomes tense for the sound. The lips begin in an unrounded position and usually move from a slight to a moderate closing during the production process of the diphthong.

Different Spellings of the [aɪ] Sound

Transcribe the following words. Refer to the Key at the right upon completion.

Different Spellings				Key
i	time __ sign __ idea __			taɪm, saɪn, aɪdɪ
	alibi __ wild __ diamond __			ælʌbaɪ, waɪld, daɪmənd
ie	pie __ tie __ tried __ cried __			paɪ, taɪ, traɪd, kraɪd

y	by __ why __ deny __	baɪ, waɪ, dinaɪ
	dry __ psychology __	draɪ, saɪkɔlədʒi
igh	might __ thigh __	maɪt, Өaɪ
	night __ fight __ high __	naɪt, faɪt, haɪ
i-e	nice __ write __ bike __ kite __	naɪs, raɪt, baɪk, kaɪt
uy	buy __ guy __	baɪ, gaɪ
ei	height __	haɪt
ey	eye __ aye __	aɪ, aɪ
ae	maestro __	maɪstroʊ
ai	aisle __	aɪl
oi	choir __	kwaɪr
ui	guide __ disguise __	gaɪd, dɪskaɪz

Different Sounds for the Same Letter(s) for the [aɪ] Sound

The following is a representative sample of the different sounds used for [aɪ]. Dialect variations may also influence pronunciation. Transcribe the following words. Refer to the Key at the right upon completion.

Alphabet Letters	Different Sounds	Words	Key
i	[aɪ]	ice	_____	aɪs
	[ɪ]	city	_____	sɪti
y	[aɪ]	by	_____	baɪ

	[ɪ] or [i]	party	_____	partɪ, parti
ei	[aɪ]	height	_____	haɪt
	[eɪ]	eight	_____	eɪt
ey	[aɪ]	eye	_____	aɪ
	[i]	key	_____	ki
oi	[aɪ]	choir	_____	kwaɪr
	[ɔɪ]	oil	_____	ɔɪl̩
ui	[aɪ]	guide	_____	gaɪd
	[u]	fruit	_____	frut

Words That Include the [aɪ] Sound

The [aɪ] diphthong occurs more frequently in United States English than any other diphthong (Edwards, 1997). It is found in all word positions (initial, medial, and final). Transcribe the following words. Refer to the Key at the right upon completion.

Initial				_Key_
idle	_____	iris	_____	aɪdl̩, aɪrəs
ice	_____	icicle	_____	aɪs, aɪsɪkl̩
item	_____	idea	_____	aɪtəm, aɪdɪə
iron	_____	island	_____	aɪɚn, aɪlənd
ivory	_____	aisle	_____	aɪvɔri, aɪl̩
eyes	_____	ivy	_____	aɪz, aɪvi

Medial				_Key_
pine	_____	light	_____	paɪn, laɪt
shine	_____	child	_____	ʃaɪn, ʧaɪld
myself	_____	rhyme	_____	maɪsɪf, raɪm
style	_____	python	_____	staɪl, paɪθɔn
hide	_____	fright	_____	haɪd, fraɪt
height	_____	wild	_____	haɪt, waɪld

Final				_Key_
sky	_____	lie	_____	skaɪ, laɪ
die	_____	guy	_____	daɪ, gaɪ
fry	_____	apply	_____	fraɪ, əplaɪ
July	_____	deny	_____	ʤulaɪ, dinaɪ/dɪdaɪ
buy	_____	thigh	_____	baɪ, θaɪ
ally	_____	reply	_____	ælaɪ, rɪplaɪ

Auditory Discrimination

Dialect variations may influence how the following words are pronounced, particularly in the use of the [ɔ] and [ɑ] sounds. Transcribe the following words. Refer to the Key at the right upon completion.

Contrast Minimal Pairs

[aɪ]	[ɔɪ]	[aɪ]	[ɑ]	_Key_
sigh ___	soy ___	night ___	not ___	saɪ, sɔɪ, naɪt, nɑt
fire ___	foyer ___	high ___	hah ___	faɪɚ, fɔɪɚ, haɪ, hɑ
imply ___	employ ___	fire ___	far ___	ɪmplaɪ, ɛmplɔɪ, faɪɚ, fɑr
ire ___	oyer ___	mile ___	moll ___	aɪɚ, ɔɪɚ, maɪl, mɔl
try ___	Troy ___	type ___	top ___	traɪ, trɔɪ, taɪp, tɑp
fried ___	Freud ___	side ___	sod ___	fraɪd, frɔɪd, saɪd, sɑd
buy ___	boy ___	like ___	lock ___	baɪ, bɔɪ, laɪk, lɑk
tie ___	toy ___	pipe ___	pop ___	taɪ, tɔɪ, paɪp, pɑp

[aɪ]	[eɪ]	[aɪ]	[ɪ]	_Key_
time ___	tame ___	bite ___	bit ___	taɪm, teɪm, baɪt, bɪt
light ___	late ___	fine ___	fin ___	laɪt, leɪt, faɪn, fɪn
fight ___	fate ___	type ___	tip ___	faɪt, feɪt, taɪp, tɪp
I'll ___	ale ___	sign ___	sin ___	aɪl̩, eɪl̩, saɪn, sɪn
wise ___	ways ___	like ___	lick ___	waɪz, weɪz, laɪk, lɪk
mine ___	mane ___	light ___	lit ___	maɪn, meɪn, laɪt, lɪt
ice ___	ace ___	hide ___	hid ___	aɪs, eɪs, jaɪd, hɪd
ride ___	raid ___	ride ___	rid ___	raɪd, reɪd, raɪd, rɪd

[aɪ]		[aʊ]		_Key_
by	_____	bow	_____	baɪ, baʊ
mice	_____	mouse	_____	maɪs, maʊs
spite	_____	spout	_____	spaɪt, spaʊt
dine	_____	down	_____	daɪn, daʊn
file	_____	fowl	_____	faɪl, faʊl
nine	_____	noun	_____	naən, naʊn
lied	_____	loud	_____	laɪd, laʊd
high	_____	how	_____	haɪ, haʊ

Allophonic and Dialect Variations

Calvert (1986) indicates that for some speakers, the nucleus (beginning) may be closer to the [ɑ] position and the termination of the glide close to the [i] but of short duration. In some dialects, its diphthongal quality may be lengthened [a:] as in *nice* [nas] and *smile* [sma:l], or it may be reduced to the [æ] sound as when *time* becomes [tæm] (Edwards, 1997). It varies in pronunciation depending on adjacent phonemes, dialect variations, and speaking rate (House, 1998; Shriberg & Kent, 1995). The initial [a] phoneme of this diphthong is not commonly used by all speakers in the United States but does occur in the speech patterns of speakers in Boston and other areas of the eastern United States as the vowel in *car* [ka] (Small, 1999). The diphthong is reduced to a monophthong [a] by some speakers in the East and South as in *ice* [as] and *might* [mat]. Although the [a] is considered the best approximation of the initiating resonance (Tiffany & Carrell, 1977), the [ɑɪ] is an acceptable variant, particularly in the South. When words with [aɪ] receive minimal stress, a neutral vowel [ə] may replace it, such as "I'm home" becoming [əm hoʊm].

Nonnative Speaker Pronunciation

The [aɪ] sound is easily perceived by the nonnative speaker and is usually not a problem in pronunciation (Edwards, 1997). The letters used to spell the [aɪ] sound and the intrinsic inconsistencies of these spelling "rules" can cause confusion regarding which sound to use when the same letter(s) that represents different sounds is used, as in *y* for *by* [baɪ] and *y* for [i] or [ɪ] in *city*.

Speech-Sound Deviations

The most frequent error is a result of diphthong reduction, as in [ɑ] (Edwards, 1997). The [aɪ] is the most stable of the distinctive diphthongs that have been studied.

Summary

The [aɪ] diphthong begins its on-glide near the [a] or [ɑ] nucleus depending on dialect variation and other factors such as context and speaking rate. The off-glide ending can vary, with the [e], [ɪ], or [i] termination depending on the height of the front of the tongue. There are at least 11 different alphabet letter combinations that represent the [aɪ] sound, and most of them represent other sounds in United States English. The [aɪ] diphthong occurs more frequently than any of the other diphthongs and it occurs in all positions in words. There are many dialect variations, particularly representative of central, eastern, and southern dialect regions in the United States. The sound does not present pronunciation difficulties to nonnative speakers, other than dialectical variations and some spelling inconsistencies. The substitution of the single vowel [ɑ] may occur as a sound error.

Competency Quiz

Transcribe the following [aɪ] words. Refer to the Key at the right upon completion.

Set 1

				Key
1. night ___	11. grime ___			naɪt, graɪm
2. plight ___	12. line ___			plaɪt, laɪn
3. rice ___	13. kind ___			raɪs, kaɪnd
4. grind ___	14. style ___			graɪnd, staɪl
5. I'm ___	15. ice cream ___			aɪm, aɪs krim
6. aisle ___	16. vice ___			aɪl, vaɪs
7. height ___	17. sky ___			haɪt, skaɪ
8. right ___	18. divide ___			raɪt, divaɪd
9. eye ___	19. sigh ___			aɪ, saɪ
10. fine ___	20. require ___			faɪn, rikwaɪr

[aɪ] Transcription Exercises

Set 2

				Key
1. bike ___	11. mine ___			baɪk, maɪn
2. dime ___	12. pipe ___			daɪm, paɪp
3. hide ___	13. quite ___			haɪd, kwaɪt
4. line ___	14. size ___			laɪn, saɪz
5. nice ___	15. strike ___			naɪs, straɪk
6. time ___	16. vine ___			taɪm, vaɪn
7. dive ___	17. wife ___			daɪv, waɪf
8. drive ___	18. wise ___			draɪv, waɪz
9. ice ___	19. glide ___			aɪs, glaɪd
10. mice ___	20. guide ___			maɪs, gaɪd

Set 3

				Key
1. hike ____	11. crime ____			haɪk, kraɪm
2. knife ____	12. fife ____			naɪf, faɪf
3. pine ____	13. quite ____			paɪn, kwaɪt
4. price ____	14. mite ____			praɪs, maɪt
5. rise ____	15. spike ____			raɪz, spaɪk
6. slice ____	16. stride ____			slaɪs, straɪd
7. spine ____	17. rhyme ____			spaɪn, raɪm
8. tribe ____	18. scribes ____			traɪb, skraɪbz
9. twice ____	19. site ____			twaɪs, saɪt
10. whine ____	20. spice ____			waɪn, spaɪs

Set 4

		Key
1. ride ____	11. right ____	raɪd, raɪt
2. pie ____	12. wild ____	paɪ, waɪld
3. buy ____	13. dry ____	baɪ, draɪ
4. cry ____	14. sigh ____	kraɪ, saɪ

		Key
5. high ____	15. grind ____	haɪ, graɪnd
6. kind ____	16. lye ____	kaɪnd, laɪ
7. my ____	17. tight ____	maɪ, taɪt
8. might ____	18. sign ____	maɪt, saɪn
9. climb ____	19. fright ____	klaɪm, fraɪt
10. try ____	20. bite ____	traɪ, baɪt

Circle the Words with the [aɪ] Sound
Set 5

fine	tide	bridge
prince	live	rye
mind	nine	fight
fringe	hive	since
file	hinge	sly
slide	lime	ridge
give	write	bind

Key: Fine, mind, file, slide, tide, live, nine, hive, lime, write, rye, fight, sly, bind.

This completes the discussion of the long ī [aɪ] vowel sound.

PHONETIC SYMBOLS [o] AND [oʊ]

EXHIBIT 8-4	Phonetic Symbols [o] and [oʊ]

[o] [oʊ]

Phonetic Symbol	[o]
Grapheme Symbol	o
Diacritic Symbol	Long o; ō
Phonic Symbol	ō
Sound Class	Back Vowel Unstressed, Stressed
Tongue Position	Height: Mid Depth: Back Tension: Tense
Lips	Rounded
Diphthong [oʊ]	Progresses from [o] midback, tense, round to [ʊ] midhigh, back, lax, round
IPA (1999)	[o] #307 Close-Mid, Back, Round

A discussion of the long ō [o] vowel or diphthong [oʊ] is now presented.

How the Sound Is Produced as a Vowel

The airflow from the lungs activates the vibration of the closed (adducted) vocal folds (voiced), and the sound waves travel through the pharyngeal cavity. Because the velopharyngeal port is closed or nearly closed, the sound enters the oral cavity and exits through the mouth. The tongue is retracted (back) and positioned in a midplane (mid) posture at the rear of the oral cavity. The tip of the tongue is in contact with the lower front teeth. There is tension (tense) in the muscles of the tongue, and the lips are rounded (rounded) and rather protruded. In the oral cavity, the [o] is positioned below the placement of the [ʊ] sound and above the [ɔ]. The production of the [o] sound is approximately on the same midplane as the midfront [e] vowel.

How the Sound Is Produced as a Diphthong

The [o] has a mid, back, tense tongue position and rounded lips that begin the on-glide aspect of this diphthong. The middle and back portions of the tongue are raised toward the palate (on-glide). The position of the tongue moves from mid to high back, lax, and approximates the [ʊ] sound position (off-glide). The lips remain in a slightly narrow, rounded posture and the tip of the tongue makes light contact with the lower front teeth. The [o] phase is the longer nucleus and the [ʊ] phase is the shorter glide.

Commentary

Phoneticians who distinguish between unstressed [e] and stressed [eɪ] as a diphthong make the same distinction between the [o] and [oʊ]. There will not be a lengthy discourse regarding the use of [o] and [oʊ], but a discussion similar to the pros and cons of [e] and [eɪ] could be presented.

The [o] is one of the complex vowels (Tiffany & Carrell, 1977) and is often diphthongal to the extent that a complex symbol such as [oʊ] is appropriate to indicate the speech movements involved, especially in stressed and final positions. During the production of [o], there is a tendency for the tongue to move to a higher position, near [u] or [ʊ], and for the lips to become more rounded.

Interpretations in the literature can lead to confusion and perhaps frustration when the phonetician attempts to establish how the o̱ and its allophonic variations are to be transcribed. For example, Small (1999), in a comparison of the words *below* (second syllable stressed and ending) and *bellow* (second syllable unstressed and ending), transcribes both with the [oʊ] sound symbol because this sound ends both words and the final phoneme is correspondingly lengthened. His example may be an exception to the rule. However, Calvert (1986) elaborates on this rule and offers some options. He states that as the final unaccented syllable in *window, polo, pillow*, the sound may be transcribed either as [o] or [oʊ] according to listener judgment. He adds that as a last sound of an utterance, it is usually transcribed as [oʊ], even when unstressed. This appears to be quite a contradiction.

No doubt reflecting an earlier perspective, Carrell and Tiffany (1960) state that although the difference between [o] and [oʊ] is easily recognized in American speech, no serious pronunciation problem is likely to arise if the native speaker fails to make this distinction in the use of the sounds. It is satisfactory to follow the convention of using only the symbol [o] in ordinary phonemic transcription.

Edwards (1997) uses the word *boat* as an example of the back mid vowel [o], and then states that the "pure" (nondiphthongized) [o] sound occurs in English mainly in unstressed syllables and in stressed syllables when the following sound is a voiceless consonant, especially a stop. This appears to be somewhat of a contradiction to Small's interpretation because he uses the [oʊ] symbol as in *coke, broke,* and *code* wherein the [o] is followed by a stop consonant. The word *boat* is also transcribed as [bot] by Kenyon and Knott (1953) but as [boʊt] by Ladefoged (1993). Perhaps new insight was gained in those 40 years!

House (1998) describes the [o] as a monophthong and indicates that some speakers pronounce the diphthong [oʊ] depending on the context. She uses only the [o] in the phonetic transcription of [kost], [ot], [stov], [fo], and [fold]. Note that these are all stressed syllables and that the [o] appears in a variety of contexts (stops, fricatives) and in the initial, medial, and final positions in words. This description appears to be considerably different from the others.

MacKay (1987) may be more in agreement with House because he lists such words as *boat, toast,* and *home* as examples of words containing the [o] sound.

Many other variations and interpretations add to this dilemma. The solution may well be provided in the advice of MacKay (1987), who states:

> There are other differences among the systems, but for our purposes it is enough to point out the quality of the long vowels and to be prepared for a possible variety of transcriptions of the same sounds. In all cases it is best to pick one system for one's own use and to stay with it consistently. (p. 75)

The rule that applied to the [e] and [eɪ] sounds also applies throughout this text regarding the [o] and [oʊ] sounds. The [o] symbol is used in the unstressed syllable, and the [oʊ] symbol is used for the stressed syllable, word endings, and one-syllable words.

Different Spellings of the [o] and [oʊ] Sounds

The following may represent dialectic differences. Transcribe the following words. Refer to the Key upon completion of the transcription.

Different Spellings				Key
o	vocation ____ old ____ obey ____			vokeɪʃən, oʊld, obeɪ
	propel ____ Romania ____			proʊpɛl, romeɪnijə
oo	brooch ____			broʊtʃ
oa	coat ____ boat ____			coʊt, boʊt
	gloat ____ coal ____			gloʊt, koʊl
	foam ____ toad ____ coax ____			foʊm, toʊd, koʊks
ow	know ____ snow ____ bow ____			noʊ, snoʊ, boʊ
	slow ____ flown ____			sloʊ, floʊ
oe	toe ____ hoe ____ doe ____ woe ____			toʊ, hoʊ, doʊ, woʊ
eo	yeoman ____			joʊmən
ew	sew ____			soʊ
oh	oh ____			oʊ
eau	beau ____			boʊ
ou	soul ____			soʊl
owe	owe ____			oʊw
ough	though ____ dough ____			ðoʊ, doʊ
os	apropos ____			æprʌpoʊ
au	chauffer ____			ʃoʊfɚ
o-e	rode ____ awoke ____ stove ____			roʊd, əwoʊk, stoʊv
	joke ____ those ____			dʒoʊk, ðoʊz

Different Sounds for the Letters in the [o] and [oʊ] Sounds

Transcribe the following words. Refer to the Key at the right upon completion.

Alphabet Letters	Different Sound	Words		Key
o	[o]	rotate	____	roteɪt
	[oʊ]	obey	____	oʊbe
	[u]	to	____	tu
ough	[oʊ]	though	____	ðoʊ
	[ʌ]	tough	____	tʌf
au	[oʊ]	chauffer	____	ʃoʊfɚ
	[ɑ]	author	____	ɑθɚ/ɔθɚ
os	[oʊ]	apropos	____	æprʌpoʊ
	[ɑ]	lose	____	lɑs
ou	[oʊ]	soul	____	soʊl
	[ɑ]	thought	____	θɑt/θɔt
eau	[oʊ]	beau	____	boʊ
	[i][u]	beauty	____	bijuti
ew	[oʊ]	sew	____	soʊ
	[u]	crew	____	kru

Rules for Spelling and Pronunciation of the [o] Sound

1. In United States English, the [o] becomes diphthongized [oʊ] when the sound occurs in stressed and open syllables, as in *open* [oʊpən] and *note* [noʊt], and at the end of a word, as in *follow* [fɑloʊ].

2. The [o] symbol is used in the unstressed syllable, as in *alone* [ʌlon] and *prohibit* [prohɪbɪt].

3. When o comes before another vowel, as in *float, toe,* and *dough,* the long [o] or [oʊ] is pronounced and the other vowel is silent. The o says its name in this double-vowel context.

Words That Include the Unstressed [o] Sound

Transcribe the following words. Refer to the Key upon completion.

Initial			*Key*
obey _____	obedient _____		obeɪ, obidɪ̈ənt
obituary _____	obese _____		obɪtjuɛri, obis
oasis _____	oblique _____		oaɪəs, oblik
opinion _____			opɪnjən

Medial			*Key*
rotation _____	hallowed _____		roteɪʃən, haʊloəd
vocalic _____	vocation _____		vokælɪk, vokeɪʃən
telephone _____	proclaim _____		tɛlʌfon, prokleɪm
protractor _____	location _____		protrætɚ, lokeɪʃən
automatic _____	biology _____		ɔtomætɪk, baɪɔlodʒi
location _____	donation _____		lokeɪʃən, doneɪʃən

Words That Include the Stressed [oʊ] Sound

Transcribe the following words. Refer to the Key at the right upon completion.

One-Syllable Words			*Key*
own _____	tone _____	grown _____	oʊn, toʊn, groʊn
toast _____	throat _____	goal _____	toʊst, θroʊt, goʊl

Initial			*Key*
open _____	over _____		oʊpən, oʊvɚ
ocean _____	Ohio _____	only _____	oʊʃən, oʊhaɪo, oʊnli

Medial			*Key*
October _____	program _____		oʊktobɚ, proʊgɪæm
Roman _____	moment _____		roʊmən, moʊmɛnt
poem _____	total _____		poʊm, toʊtəl
broken _____	emotion _____		broʊkən, imoʊʃən
chromosome _____	monotone _____		kroʊməsom, mɑnoʊton

Final			*Key*
go _____ no _____ so _____ hello _____			goʊ, noʊ, soʊ, hɛloʊ
ago _____ auto _____ zero _____			əgoʊ, ɔtoʊ, ziroʊ
cargo _____ piano _____			kɑrgoʊ, piænoʊ
potato _____ hero _____ echo _____			pəteɪtoʊ, hiroʊ, ɛkoʊ
volcano _____ below _____ pillow _____			vɔlkeɪnoʊ, biloʊ, pɪloʊ

Auditory Discrimination

Some phoneticians differentiate the use of the [o] and [oʊ] symbols to identify stressed and unstressed sound positions in words. Transcribe the following words using the [oʊ] in the stressed position, single words, and word-ending position. Refer to the Key on the right upon completion.

Contrast Minimal Pairs

[oʊ]	[ɔ]	[oʊ]	[ʌ]	*Key*
low _	law _	home _	hum _	loʊ, lɔ, hoʊm, hʌm
coal _	call _	note _	nut _	koʊl, kɔl, noʊt, nʌt
hole _	hall _	tones _	ton _	hoʊl, hɔl, toʊnz, tʌn
row _	raw _	robe _	rub _	roʊ, rɔ, roʊb, rʌb
know_	gnaw _	bone _	bun _	noʊ, nɔ, boʊn, bʌn
pole _	Paul _	boat _	but _	poʊl, pɔl, boʊt, bʌt
coast _	cost _	stone _	stun _	koʊst, kɔst, stoʊn, stʌn
goes _	gauze_	known _	none _	goʊz, gɔz, noʊn, nʌn

[oʊ]	[ɑ]	[oʊ]	[ʊ]	*Key*
hope _	hop _	stowed _	stood _	hoʊp, hɑp, stoʊd, stʊd
soak _	sock _	pole _	pull _	soʊk, sɔk, poʊl, pʊl
wrote _	rot _	coke _	cook _	roʊt, rɔt, koʊk, cʊk
road _	rod _	broke _	brook _	roʊd, rɑd, broʊk, brʊk
note _	not _	bowl _	bull _	noʊt, nɑt, boʊl, bʊl
known _	non _	code _	could _	noʊn, nɑn, koʊd, kʊd
own _	on _	showed _	should _	oʊn, ɑn, ʃoʊd, ʃʊd

Allophonic and Dialect Variations

When *o, oa-, o-e,* or other spellings associated with [oʊ] occur with [r], as in *far, oar,* and *bore,* the vowel may be spoken or heard as [oʊ], [o], or [ɔ], and dialectically as [ɑ] (Calvert, 1986; Carrell & Tiffany, 1960). Before [r], the [o] is a more lax sound and words like *horse* may be pronounced more like [hɔrs] in most American speech. When the same spelling combinations occur before [l], as in *cold, coal,* and *hole,* either the [oʊ] or [o] may be transcribed according to the listener's judgment.

The pure or monophthong [o] usually occurs in syllables of no more than secondary stress, such as the first syllable in *notation* (Shriberg & Kent, 1995). In syllables with primary stress or when speaking at a slower rate, the diphthong [oʊ] is more likely to occur. The physical contrast between the two sounds distinguishes them from one another. For the [o], the tongue position is slightly lower than for [ʊ] and a distinct rounding of the lips is made.

For the diphthong [oʊ], the tongue makes a raising gesture from [o] and moves toward the [ʊ] position. Phonetic context, stress, and other prosodic variables determine the jaw position that may vary from closed to mid.

Nonnative Speaker Pronunciation

This is a universal sound in languages worldwide and nonnative speakers have no difficulty using the [o] in various contexts in United States English. The [oʊ] presents some problems because of the characteristics of the diphthong with its onset and offset glides and timing.

Speech-Sound Deviations

The [o] and [oʊ] sounds do not present problems to children developing the sounds and they are well established at an early age.

Summary

The [o] is produced with the tongue in the mid, back position. The tongue is tense and the lips rounded. It is classified as a long vowel and has more than 14 different spelling contexts. There is disagreement as to whether the [o] sound exists. To some phoneticians, it appears only as the first sound in the diphthong [oʊ]. Others state it is the sound used in the unstressed position of the [o] context with the [oʊ] diphthong occurring in the stressed and final positions of words. It is a common sound in the languages of the world and nonnative speakers have minimal difficulty with the [o] or [oʊ]. Children also acquire this sound readily, and it seldom appears to be misarticulated.

As a diphthong, the sound proceeds from the vowel nucleus of the [o] mid, back vowel and glides upward to terminate with the high back, lax vowel [ʊ]. The tenseness of the tongue shifts from tense to lax and the lips remain rounded during the movement from one sound to the other.

Competency Quiz

Transcribe the following [oʊ] words. Refer to the Key at the right upon completion.

Set 1

				Key
1. coat	_____	11. dome	_____	koʊt, doʊm
2. foam	_____	12. groan	_____	foʊm, groʊn
3. float	_____	13. home	_____	floʊt, hoʊm
4. remote	_____	14. close	_____	rimoʊt, kloʊs
5. roam	_____	15. molt	_____	roʊm, moʊlt
6. lone	_____	16. toast	_____	loʊn, toʊst
7. quote	_____	17. old	_____	kwoʊt, oʊld
8. holy	_____	18. bolt	_____	hoʊli, boʊlt
9. soap	_____	19. stone	_____	soʊp, stoʊn
10. boast	_____	20. below	_____	boʊst, biloʊ

[oʊ] Transcription Exercises

Remember, the [oʊ] sound is used in stressed syllables, single-syllable words, and word-ending positions.

Set 2

				Key
1. close	_____	11. roam	_____	kloʊz, roʊm
2. wove	_____	12. know	_____	woʊv, noʊ
3. nose	_____	13. gold	_____	noʊz, goʊld
4. boat	_____	14. froze	_____	boʊt, froʊz
5. grow	_____	15. stove	_____	groʊ, stoʊv
6. cold	_____	16. float	_____	koʊld, floʊt
7. drove	_____	17. toe	_____	droʊv, toʊ
8. doze	_____	18. note	_____	doʊz, noʊt
9. lone	_____	19. wrote	_____	loʊn, roʊt
10. coat	_____	20. cloak	_____	koʊt, kloʊk

Set 3

				Key
1. stone	____	11. boast	____	stoʊn, boʊst
2. toad	____	12. own	____	toʊd, oʊn
3. loaf	____	13. coax	____	loʊf, koʊks
4. crow	____	14. row	____	kroʊ, roʊ
5. toes	____	15. folks	____	toʊz, foʊks
6. toast	____	16. hoax	____	toʊst, hoʊks
7. loaves	____	17. croak	____	loʊvz, kroʊk
8. grown	____	18. ghost	____	groʊn, goʊst
9. hose	____	19. most	____	hoʊz, moʊst
10. coal	____	20. phone	____	koʊl, foʊn

Circle the Words with the [oʊ] Sound

Set 4

home	broad	poke
come	loan	gone
love	slow	host
lose	once	goal
soak	sew	whose
glove	sold	most
whole	coach	none

Key: Home, soak, whole, loan, sew, sold, poke, host, goal, most.

Circle the Words with the [oʊ] Sound

Set 5

goat	so	bowl
quote	move	some
sow	blown	cove
scold	one	coast
done	foam	mole
dove	low	drove
globe	smoke	shove

Key: Goat, quote, sow, scold, globe, so, blown, foam, low, smoke, bowl, cove, coast, mole.

This completes the discussion of the long ō [o] and [oʊ] vowel sounds.

PHONETIC SYMBOLS [u] AND [ju]

EXHIBIT 8-5	**Phonetic Symbols [u] and [ju]**	
Phonetic Symbol	[u]	[u] [ju]
Grapheme Symbol	See the section titled "Different Spellings of the [u] Sound," which follows.	
Diacritic Symbol	ōō, ü, ǫǫ	
Phonic Symbol	ū	
Sound Class		
Tongue Position	Position: High-Back Depth: Back Tension: Tense	
Lips	Rounded	
IPA (1999)	[u] #308 Close, Back, Rounded	

A discussion of the long ū [u] sound is now presented.

How the Sound Is Produced

Whenever the [u] is first introduced, some confusion arises regarding its pronunciation and the [ju] sound. Because these two sounds are so closely related, they are presented here in comparison to one another. This approach clarifies the similarities and differences between the two sounds.

How the Sound Is Produced as a Vowel

The airflow from the lungs activates the vibration of the closed (adducted) vocal folds (voiced), and the sound enters the oral cavity because the velopharyngeal port is closed or nearly closed. From its flattened position on the floor of the mouth, the back (back) of the tongue increases in tension (tense) and retracts and rises (high) toward the soft palate (velum). The front of the tongue is in a depressed position, remaining near the floor of the mouth at or below the base of the lower teeth. The lips are protruded and in a "puckered" (rounded) position. During the production of the [u] sound, the tongue usually continues to rise and the lips continue to become more rounded. The [u] is the highest, most tense, and rounded of the back vowels.

How the Sound Is Produced as a Diphthong

The initial sound [j] is produced in one of two tongue postures: (1) the tip of the tongue is positioned behind the lower front teeth and the front-middle of the tongue is raised high toward the palate, or (2) the front of the tongue is raised toward, but not touching, the anterior part of the hard palate.

From either posture, the tongue glides backward and positions itself at points that mark the high back vowel position of [u]. This movement is considered an on-glide because the first sound [j] (vowel-like consonant) of this diphthong is shorter in length than the terminal sound of [u]. This is in contrast to other diphthongs that are considered off-glides because the first sound is more distinct and longer than the terminal or second sound, as in [aʊ] *house* [haʊs].

Commentary

Some phoneticians (Shriberg & Kent, 1995) regard the [ju] combination, as in the words *use* and *you*, to be a diphthong. Frequently, tongue movements from a consonant to [u] are gradual, almost glide-like in character. There is one peculiarity associated with the phoneme [u] and its transcription (Small, 1999). In certain words such as *few*, there are three sounds: [f-j-u]. Without the [j] sound, the word would sound like *foo*. Small (1999) considers the [j] and [u] as two separate monophthongs rather than as a diphthong. One reason to consider [ju] as a diphthong (House, 1998) is because it involves two phonemes, the vowel [u] and the [j], which historically was a version of the [i] sound. House (1998) provides two reasons why it is not a diphthong: (1) it does not involve two vowels; and (2) the nuclei of the diphthong appear at the end, while the shorter-duration phoneme appears at the beginning. The decision on which form is appropriate depends on the formality of the situation and the actual word.

Edwards (1997) elaborates on the processes involved in the production of the [ju]. He indicates that this diphthong is made by gliding from a position just posterior to that for the high front vowels ([i] or [ɪ]) to one that approximates the high back vowels ([u] or [ʊ]), resulting in [ju]. He explains that this is the only distinctive on-glide diphthong in United States English that makes the first sound segment shorter than the second segment.

The first part of a diphthong is usually more prominent than the last, which is often so brief and transitory that it is difficult to determine its exact quality (as in [eɪ] or [ei]) (Ladefoged, 1993). Traditionally, a diphthong does not begin and end with any of the sounds that occur at the end. Ladefoged (1993) states that it is a diphthong because of the way it patterns in English. Historically, the [j] was a vowel, and if it is not a vowel, there is a whole series of consonant clusters in English that can occur before only one vowel. The sounds at the beginning of words like *pew* [pju] and *cue* [kju] occur only before [u]; the [j] is arbitrary. Ladefoged (1993) concludes that, in stating the distributional properties of English sounds, it seems much simpler to recognize [ju] as a diphthong and thus reduce the complexity of the statement one has to make about the English consonant clusters.

According to some phoneticians, there are other words in which the [ju] is not arbitrary. Calvert (1986) offers this comparative analysis between [u] and [ʊ] and the choice of [u] or [ju]. He states that a few words are variable in pronunciation by choice with either [u] or [ʊ], including *roof, hoof,* and *root*, and it is the same with [u] and [ju] as in *new, tune, duke, due,* and *suit*.

There appears to be two prominent trends in the usage of [u] and [ju]. One, they are separate phonemes and thusly transcribed as a consonant + vowel. Example: *new* [n-j-u] CCV = 3 sounds. Second, although unique in its characteristics, the [ju] is a diphthong: *new* /n-ju/ C + Diphthong = 2 sounds. Listeners of United States English speech can understand the semantic meaning of words pronounced differently as *new* [nu] or [nju], and use of [u] and [ju] appears to be a matter of dialect choice in many instances. However, some words require the [j] inclusion, such as *feud* [fjud] to distinguish it from *food* [fud].

Different Spellings of the [u] Sound

Dialect differences may occur with some of the following examples, particularly with the inclusion of the [ju] sound as in *dew* [dju] or [du] and *blue* [blu] and [bəlu]. Transcribe the following words. Refer to the Key at the right upon completion.

Different Spellings				*Key*
u	truly ___ rude ___ presume ___			truli, rud, prizum
ue	true ___ glue ___ rule ___			tru, glu, rul
	blue ___ due ___			blu, du
eu	feud ___			fjud
ui	fruit ___ recruit ___ bruise ___			frut, rikrut, bruz
o	do ___ move ___ tomb ___ lose ___			du, muv, tum, luz
oo	boot ___ hoot ___			but, hut
	school ___ too ___			skul, tu
oe	shoe ___ canoe ___			ʃu, knu
ou	group ___ troupe ___			grup, trup
	soup ___ wound ___			sup, wund
ough	through ___ slough ___			Өru, slu
ous	rendezvous ___			rɑndʌvu
wo	two ___			tu
ew	dew ___ threw ___ crew ___			dju or du, ðru, kru
	grew ___ knew ___			gru, kju or ku
eau	beauty ___			buti or bjutɪ

Different Sounds for the Same Letter(s) for the [u] Sound

The following is representative of the same letters used for different sounds. Dialect variations may be present in individual pronunciation, particularly the [ju] sound as in *dew* [dju] or [du]. Transcribe the following words. Refer to the Key at the right upon completion.

Alphabet Letters	Different Sounds	Words		Key
u	[u]	true	___	tru
	[ʌ]	us	___	ʌs
o	[u]	do	___	du
	[ɑ]	on	___	ɑn
oo	[u]	boot	___	but
	[ʊ]	foot	___	fʊt
ou	[u]	group	___	grup
	[aʊ]	out	___	aʊt
ui	[u]	fruit	___	frut
	[ɪ]	quit	___	kwɪt
oe	[u]	shoe	___	ʃu
	[oʊ]	toe	___	toʊ
ough	[u]	through	___	Өru
	[ɔ] or [ɑ]	thought	___	Өɔt or Өɑt

ous	[u]	rendezvous	___	rɑndʌvu
	[ɪ] or [ə]	nervous	___	n3˞vɪs or n3˞vəs
wo	[u]	two	___	tu
	[ʌ]	won	___	wʌn

Rules for Spelling and Pronunciation of the [u] Sound

1. There are often two vowel letters together when one of them is a long vowel, as in *oe shoe, ue blue, ui fruit, ou group*.
2. There are two options when two *oo*s are adjacent to one another: *oo moon* [mun] (long vowel) or *oo food* [fʊd] (short vowel).
3. When [u] is in a word that ends with an *e*, the *e* is silent.
4. Some dialects include the [j] and [u] combination as in *ew new* [nju].

Transcribe the following words. Refer to the Key at the right upon completion. *Note*: Editors of dictionaries are not in agreement with the preferential pronunciation of words such as *few, view, dew*. Some indicate [fu], [fju], and [vu], [vju] or just the opposite. As mentioned earlier, dialects set the standard for individual differences.

Words That Include the [u] Sound

Initial	*Medial*	*Final*	*Key*
ooze ___	mood ___	who ___	uz, mud, wu
oodles ___	include ___	too ___	udləz, ɪnklud, tu
oozy ___	noodle ___	grew ___	uzi, nudl̩, gru
cruise ___	Sue ___		kruz, su
student ___	do ___		studənt, du
balloon ___	two ___		bəlun, tu

Words That Include the [ju] Sound

Initial	*Medial*	*Final*	*Key*
you ___	beauty ___	few ___	ju, buti, fju or fu
unit ___	humor ___	debut ___	unɪt, humə˞, dɛbu
use ___	review ___	view ___	juz, rivu, vju
usual ___	music ___	value ___	uʒuəl, muzɪk, vælu
unite ___	future ___	due ___	unɪt, futʃə˞, du
union ___	cute ___	drew ___	junjən, kut, dru

Auditory Discrimination

Transcribe the following words. Refer to the Key at the right upon completion.

Contrast Minimal Pairs

[u]		[ʊ]		Key
stewed _____		stood _____		stud, stʊd
pool _____		pull _____		pul, pʊl
fool _____		full _____		ful, fʊl
cooed _____		could _____		kud, kʊd
shoed _____		should _____		ʃud, ʃʊd
wooed _____		would _____		wud, wʊd

Other Pairs

There may be dialect differences with the use of [ju].

[u]		[ju]		Key
fool _____		fuel _____		ful, fjul
booty _____		beauty _____		buti, bjuti
boot _____		butte _____		but, bjut
ooze _____		use _____		uz, juz
moot _____		mute _____		mut, mjut
whose _____		hews _____		wuz, hjuz

[u]		[ʌ]		Key
school _____		skull _____		skul, skʌl
boost _____		bust _____		bust, bʌst
moose _____		muss _____		mus, mʌs
doom _____		dumb _____		dum, dʌm
roost _____		rust _____		rust, rʌst
whom _____		hum _____		ʍum, hʌm

Allophonic and Dialect Variations

Some phoneticians consider the consonant [j] in combination with [ju] as a diphthong in the pronunciation of words such as *use, you,* and *excuse* (Shriberg & Kent, 1995). They indicate that sometimes the tongue movements from a consonant to [u] are gradual, almost glide-like in character. It also has an allophonic variant of a front rounded vowel in words like *commune*.

Different pronunciation using the [u] or [ʊ] occurs in words with the *oo* such as *roof* [ruf] or [rʊf] and *root*

[rut] or [rʊt] (Calvert, 1986). There are dialectic differences in the use of [u] or [ju] as in *new* [nu] or [nju] and *tune* [tun] or [tjun], particularly in Southern and Eastern American speech.

Nonnative Speaker Pronunciation

The voiced affricate [ʤ] may be substituted for the [j] as when *you* [ju] becomes [ʤu] (Edwards, 1997). Generally speaking, nonnative speakers have no significant problems using the [u] and [ju].

Speech-Sound Deviations

None have been noted with the exception of misuse of the [u] and [ju] sounds in certain contexts, as in *few* [fu] for [fju], resulting in diphthong reduction.

Summary

The [u] is a cardinal vowel that indicates the high back apex on the vowel quadrilateral. The position of the tongue is high back, the tongue is tense, and the lips are rounded. The [u] seldom appears in the initial position in words but does occur in the medial and final positions. There are at least 13 different spelling combinations for the [u] sound, and allophonic and dialect variations result from tongue position and sound context. Dialect choices include *roof* [ruf] or [rʊf], and so forth.

The [u] becomes the final sound in the combination of [ju] that is considered by some phoneticians a diphthong. The diphthong [ju] is required in such words as *fuse* [fjuz]; otherwise, the word would be transcribed as [fuz], which is entirely wrong. Other uses of the [ju] are dialectal bound or personal choice, as in *dew* and *do* that are by some speakers differentiated as [dju] and [du].

Nonnative speakers have minimal difficulties with either the [u] or [ju], and neither do these sounds present opportunities for major speech-sound deviations for children and others.

Competency Quiz

Transcribe the following [u] words. Keep in mind any dialect influence in pronunciation throughout these sets of words.

Set I

				Key
1. who	_____	11. whose	_____	hu, whuz
2. broom	_____	12. booze	_____	brum, buz
3. bruise	_____	13. crude	_____	bruz, krud
4. blew	_____	14. roof	_____	blu, ruf
5. spoon	_____	15. fruit	_____	spun, frut
6. Sioux	_____	16. blue	_____	su, blu
7. food	_____	17. troop	_____	fud, trup
8. move	_____	18. Sue	_____	muv, su
9. drew	_____	19. movie	_____	dru, muvi
10. do	_____	20. to	_____	du, tu

[u] Transcription Exercises

Set 2

				Key
1. dune	_____	11. rude	_____	dun, rud
2. blue	_____	12. clue	_____	blu, klu
3. fruit	_____	13. bruise	_____	frut, bruz
4. new	_____	14. crew	_____	nu, kru
5. food	_____	15. bloom	_____	fud, blum
6. flute	_____	16. rule	_____	flut, rul
7. sue	_____	17. glue	_____	su, glu
8. suit	_____	18. cruise	_____	sut, kruz
9. grew	_____	19. drew	_____	gru, dru
10. school	_____	20. cool	_____	skul, kul

Set 3

				Key
1. tube	_____	9. true	_____	tub, tru
2. due	_____	10. screw	_____	du, skwru
3. new	_____	11. roost	_____	nu, rust

				Key
4. few	_____	12. dude	_____	fu, dud
5. moon	_____	13. blew	_____	mun, blu
6. tune	_____	14. hoot	_____	tun, hut
7. moo	_____	15. plume	_____	mu, plum
8. flew	_____	16. grew	_____	flu, gru

This completes the discussion of the long vowels and diphthongs. Chapter 9 provides information regarding the short vowels of United States English.

REFERENCES

Bernthal, J. E., & Bankson, N.W. (1998). *Articulation and phonological disorders*. Englewood Cliffs, NJ: Prentice Hall.

Calvert, D. R. (1986). *Descriptive phonetics*. New York, NY: Thieme Medical Publishers.

Carrell, J., & Tiffany, W. (1960). *Phonetics: Theory and application to speech improvement*. New York, NY: McGraw-Hill.

Edwards, H. T. (1997). *Applied phonetics* (2nd ed.). San Diego, CA: College-Hill Press.

House, L. (1998). *Introductory phonetics and phonology*. Mahwah, NJ: Lawrence Erlbaum.

International Phonetic Association (1999). *Handbook of the International Phonetic Alphabet*. Cambridge: Cambridge University Press.

Kenyon, J. S., & Knott, T. A. (1953). *Pronouncing dictionary of American English*. Springfield, MA: Merriam.

Ladefoged, P. (1993). *A course in phonetics* (3rd ed.). Fort Worth, TX: Harcourt Brace College Publishers.

MacKay, I. R. A. (1987). *Phonetics: The science of speech production*. Boston, MA: Allyn & Bacon.

Shriberg, L., & Kent, R. (1995). *Clinical phonetics* (3rd ed.). Boston, MA: Allyn & Bacon.

Small, L. H. (1999). *Fundamentals of phonetics: A practical guide for students* (3rd ed.). Boston, MA: Allyn & Bacon.

Tiffany, W. R., & Carrell, J. (1977). *Phonetics: Theory and application*. New York, NY: McGraw-Hill.

VanRiper, C. (1979). *An introduction to general American phonetics*. New York, NY: Harper & Row.

Chapter 9

Characteristics of the Short Vowels

PURPOSE

To introduce you to the short vowels and their phonetic symbols.

OBJECTIVES

This chapter will provide you with information regarding:

1. Characteristics of the five short vowels
2. Different spellings for the short vowels
3. Allophonic variations and dialect differences
4. Nonnative speaker pronunciation and speech deviations
5. Transcription exercises

THE SHORT VOWELS

The short vowels are the following:

- ă = [æ] in *ask* [æsk]
- ĕ = [ɛ] in *end* [ɛnd]
- ĭ = [ɪ] in *hid* [hɪd]
- ŏ = [ɑ] in *stop* [stɑp]
- ŭ = [ʌ] (stressed or single syllable) or [ə] (unstressed syllable *above* [əbʌv])

Two generalizations apply to short vowels—but remember that there are always exceptions to the rules: A single vowel that does not conclude a word usually has the short vowel sound as in *ask, at*, and *act*. A single vowel in the medial position usually has the short vowel sound as in *bat, can*, and *fact*.

PHONETIC SYMBOL [æ]

EXHIBIT 9-1	Phonetic Symbol [æ]

		[æ]
Phonetic Symbol	[æ]	
Grapheme Symbol	See the section titled "Different Spellings of the [æ] Sound," which follows.	
Diacritic Symbol	a	
Phonic Symbol	ă	
Sound Class	Short Cardinal Vowel	
Tongue Position	Height: Low-Front Depth: Low-Back Tension: Lax	
Lips	Unrounded	
International Phonetic Alphabet (IPA) (1999)	[æ] #325 Near-Open, Front, Unrounded	

How the Sound Is Produced

The airflow from the lungs activates the vibration of the closed (adducted) vocal folds (voiced), and the sound enters the oral cavity because the velopharyngeal port is closed or nearly closed. The tongue is positioned on the floor of the mouth (low) and with minimal tension (lax). The tip of the tongue is embedded behind the lower front teeth. The remainder of the tongue flexes forward (front) in an upward movement but does not come into contact with the upper molars. The mandible is lowered, and the mouth is opened wider for the [æ] sound than for any of the other front vowels. The lips are in a neutral position (unrounded), and the corners may be slightly retracted. The [æ] sound is positioned below the [ɛ] sound and is the lowest front vowel.

Note: There is some disagreement as to whether [æ] should be considered a tense or lax vowel (Edwards, 1997). Although there is relatively minor muscular tension during its production, it lasts a long time, similar to tense vowels. A simple test is offered by Shriberg and Kent (1995) as a solution: Observe the increased degree of muscular tension felt under the chin during the production of a tense vowel [i] and the [æ] vowel, which appears more lax. In the categories of tense and lax, Singh and Singh (1976) exclude the [æ] and classify it, along with [ʌ] and [ɑ], as "neutral" for the tenseness feature.

Commentary

It is uncertain as to whether or not the [æ] sound is as commonly used today as it was previously when it was considered the standard sound to use in certain words. Over the years, several pronouncing dictionaries have been published with the goal of providing a reference for United States English speech that can serve as a guide to pronunciation. No doubt it was the intention of these lexicographers and phoneticians to provide a standard that reflected the predominant dialect of their period. A pitfall to the establishment of such a narrow perspective is that it does not allow for other dialect differences. Another pitfall is that when something appears in print it is assumed by many to be "frozen" and not subject to change. Such is the case with the [æ] sound. Refer to the sources in **Table 9-1**.

Different Spellings of the [æ] Sound

The following may represent dialectical differences. For example, *prayer* [præjɪr] and [preɪjɪr] and *aunt* [ænt] or [ɑnt]. Transcribe the following words. Refer to the Key at the right upon completion. As you complete the transcription exercises, refer to the key provided in the Sound/Symbol Reference Guide on the inside cover of this book or to your own sound/symbol reference cards.

Different Spellings					*Key*
a	at	_____	have _____	sat _____	æt, hæv, sæt
au	laugh	_____	aunt _____		læf, ænt
	guarantee	_____			gɛrænti
ai	plaid	_____			plæd
i	meringue	_____			məˈæŋ
ei	heir	_____			hær

TABLE 9-1	Early Sources		

Source	Key Words	Pronunciation
Everyman's English (British) Pronouncing Dictionary by Jones, 1917	alphabet algebra	ælfəbɛt ældʒibrə
A Pronouncing Dictionary of American English by Kenyonand Knott, 1944	alphabet algebra	ælfəbɛt ældʒəbrə
Webster's Seventh New Collegiate Dictionary, 1969	alphabet algebra	ælfəbɛt* ældʒəbrə*

*International Phonetic Alphabet (IPA) symbols were used that represent the "key symbols" of the dictionary.

ay   prayer   _____   præɚ

ea   bear   _____   bær

Different Sounds for the Same Letters of the [æ] Sound

The following is a representative sample of the different sound options. Dialect variables may be present. Transcribe the following words. Refer to the Key at the right upon completion.

Alphabet Letters	Different Sounds	Words		Key
a	[æ]	ask	_____	æsk
	[ə]	zebra	_____	zibrə
au	[æ]	aunt	_____	ænt
	[ɔ] or [ɑ]	auto	_____	ɔtoʊ/ɑtoʊ
ai	[æ]	plaid	_____	plæd
	[aɪ]	aisle	_____	aɪl
i	[æ]	meringue	_____	məɚeɪŋ
	[ɪ]	sing	_____	sɪŋ
ea	[æ]	bear	_____	bɛr
	[i]	each	_____	itʃ

Rules for Spelling and Pronunciation of the [æ] Sound

1. Unlike many of the other vowels that have many letters that represent their sound, the [æ] is represented mostly by the *a* letter.

2. The vowel is a short ă [æ] when it is in a closed syllable without the final e as in *sat, cat, man*.

Words That Include the [æ] Sound

The [æ] occurs quite frequently in United States English but not in the final position. Transcribe the following words. Refer to the Key at the right upon completion.

Initial		Medial		Final		Key
axle	_____	grass	_____	baa	_____	æksl̩, græs, bæ
average	_____	factory	_____			ævɝɛdʒ, fæktori
apple	_____	fact	_____			æpl, fækt
atom	_____	contact	_____			ætəm, kɑntækt
action	_____	catch	_____			ækʃən, kætʃ
ant	_____	math	_____			ænt, mæθ
aunt	_____	exact	_____			ænt, ɛgzækt
accident	_____	glad	_____			æksʌdənt, glæd

Auditory Discrimination

Contrast Minimal Pairs

Differences in dialect may occur in the pronunciation of these words. Transcribe the following words. Refer to the Key at the right upon completion.

[æ]		[ɛ]		Key
bad	_____	bed	_____	bæd, bɛd
pat	_____	pet	_____	pæt, pɛt
sat	_____	set	_____	sæt, sɛt
man	_____	men	_____	mæn, mɛn
bag	_____	beg	_____	bæg, bɛg
tan	_____	ten	_____	tæn, tɛn

Other Pairs

[æ]		[ɔ]		Key
cast	_____	cost	_____	kæst, kɔst
at	_____	ought	_____	æt, ɔt
lag	_____	log	_____	læg, lɔg
last	_____	lost	_____	læst, lɔst
sang	_____	song	_____	sæŋ, sɔŋ
rang	_____	wrong	_____	ræŋ, rɔŋ

[æ]		[ɑ]		Key
cap	_____	cop	_____	kæp, kɑp
pad	_____	pod	_____	pæd, pɑd
valley	_____	volley	_____	væli, vɑli
battle	_____	bottle	_____	bætļ, bɑtļ
hat	_____	hot	_____	hæt, hɑt
add	_____	odd	_____	æd, ɑd

Allophonic and Dialect Variations

A wide range of pronunciations is characteristic of the [æ] sound (Tiffany & Carrell, 1977). Allophonic variations occur as a result of tension, height, diphthongization, and nasality. For example, as a nucleus of a syllable or word with nasal consonants [m] and [n], the [æ] projects a nasal quality, as in *tan* [tæn] and *man* [mæn], and a sound closer to the [ɛ] or [e] or [ɪ] may be substituted for the [æ], as in *hang* [hæŋ], [hɛŋ], or [heɪŋ]. A diphthongized [æ] occurs with such words as *cat* [kæt]: [kæɪt] or [kæət] (Shriberg & Kent, 1995).

In New England speech, the [a], a low-front vowel, is a common alternate pronunciation for [æ], as in *bath* [baɵ] for [bæɵ] and *hat* [hat] for [hæt] (Calvert, 1986; Edwards, 1997; House, 1998). The [a] is produced with the jaw more open and with the tongue back somewhat farther than for [æ] (Edwards, 1997). But as VanRiper (1979) observes, the [a] is used selectively by those who speak with a "Harvard accent" as demonstrated by the [a] in *bath* [baɵ]. In addition to the [ɵ] context, this usage occurs frequently before the [f], [s], [n+ another consonant], as in *can't* [kɑnt] or [kant]. Instead of the [ɛr] for *chair* [ʧɛr] and *bear* [bɛr], the [æ] may be used: [ʧær] and [bær]. Another noticeable difference is the appearance of a nasalized [æ] such as in the word *chance*. It may be a result of the nasal [n] that follows the vowel in *chance*. Typically, dialects of the American south-central states have a characteristic pervasive nasality often referred to as a "nasal twang" (MacKay, 1987). The [æ] is highly variable in English and is the only front vowel to be so greatly affected by dialect and phonetic environment (Edwards, 1997).

In the eastern and southern United States, speakers may substitute the [æ] for the [ɛ] sound, such as when *Mary* [mɛrɪ] becomes [mærɪ] (Small, 1999). (Note that the [ɪ] final sound is also consistent with pronunciation in those regions.) VanRiper (1979) has his own solution to the [æ] and [ɛ] usage in this context: "For the word *dare*, some of you may feel that you say [dær] rather than [dɛr] and to be perfectly candid, it is possibly true for you as an individual." (p. 57)

However, because this text deals with general United States phonetics, we will write the word *dare* and all other words that rhyme with it with an [ɛr] ending. Small (1999) cautions against the perception of the [eɪ] substitution for [æ] in such words as *rank* and *bang* and indicates that the [æ] sound is used: [ræŋ] and [bæŋ]. This choice of pronunciation may vary from region to region, and, indeed, an allophone closer to [eɪ] may be spoken in this context. There are enormous dialect variations in the qualities of vowels (MacKay, 1987), and even though the [æ] sound may be used in the word *bang* in some dialects, it may not be used in other dialects.

Nonnative Speaker Pronunciation

The [æ] sound is a problem sound for nonnative speakers of English because of its instability (Edwards, 1997; Tiffany & Carrell, 1977). It is not a common sound in the world's languages and may easily be confused with the low vowels, front or back, or for the central vowels such as [ɐ], a retracted "compromise" vowel between [æ] and [ɑ]; [æ] with a nasalized variant; the higher, more tense [ɛ]-like variant; [æə] or [æjə] variant.

Speech-Sound Deviations

The [æ]sound has been characterized as one of the vowels most frequently incorrect in those with severe phonological disorders (Edwards, 1997). The most frequent substitution is [ɑ] (backing), followed by [a] (low-central). Other deviations include [aɪ] (diphthongization) and [ɛ] (raising). This is consistent with Shriberg and Kent (1995), who indicate that substitutions generally involve a sound near the target sound and on the vowel quadrilateral; the [ɛ] and [a] are in opposite directions but within direct proximity to the [æ] vowel.

Summary

The [æ] is a cardinal vowel that marks the low-front apex of the vowel quadrilateral. It is produced with the tongue in a low-front position. The tongue is lax and the lips are unrounded. It is classified as a short vowel and has more than seven different spelling combinations whose letters also represent other sounds. The [æ] occurs quite frequently but not in the final position of words. There is a wide range of allophonic and dialect variations that are distinct to different regions in the United States. Speech deviations include the substitution of [ɑ] or [ɛ], and it is one of the most frequently incorrect vowels.

Competency Quiz

Transcribe the following [æ] words. Cover the Key at the right side of the page and refer to it upon completion.

Key

1. tax	_____	11. grand	_____	tæks, grænd
2. ask	_____	12. slap	_____	æsk, slæp
3. classic	_____	13. pack	_____	klæsik, pæk
4. pat	_____	14. man	_____	pæt, mæn
5. lad	_____	15. tasks	_____	læd, tæsks
6. land	_____	16. tan	_____	lænd, tæn
7. cat	_____	17. fancy	_____	kæt, fænsi
8. half	_____	18. rack	_____	hæf, ræk
9. hand	_____	19. craft	_____	hænd, kræft
10. add	_____	20. dance	_____	æd, dæns

This completes the discussion of the short vowel ă [æ].

PHONETIC SYMBOL [ɛ]

EXHIBIT 9-2	**Phonetic Symbol [ɛ]**

Phonetic Symbol	[ɛ]	**[ɛ]**
Grapheme Symbol	See the section titled "Different Spellings of the [ɛ] Sound," which follows.	
Diacritic Symbol	e	
Phonic Symbol	ĕ	
Sound Class	Short Vowel	
Tongue Position	Height: Lower Depth: Mid-front Tension: Lax	
Lips	Unrounded	
IPA (1999)	[ɛ] #303 Open-Midfront, Unrounded	

A discussion of the next short vowel ĕ [ɛ] is now presented.

How the Sound Is Produced

The airflow from the lungs activates the vibration of the closed (adducted) vocal folds (voiced), and the sound enters the oral cavity because the velopharyngeal port is closed or nearly closed. The tip of the tongue is centered behind the lower front teeth, and the remaining body of the tongue is shifted forward (front) and elevated (mid) to make contact with the upper molars. The lips are opened to a neutral position (unrounded), and the tongue exhibits minimal tension (lax). The [ɛ] sound is positioned below the [e] and above the [æ] sound.

Different Spellings of the [ɛ] Sound

The following may represent dialectical differences. For example, *egg* [ɛg] or [eɪg] and *men* [mɛn] or [mɪn]. Transcribe the following words. Refer to the Key at the right upon completion.

Different Spellings				Key
e	ebb ___	bed ___	men ___	ɛb, bɛd, mɛn
	egg ___	where ___		ɛg, wɛr or ʍɛr
a	any ___	many ___		ɛni, ɛnɪ, mɛni, mɛnɪ
	bare ___	says ___		bɛr, sɛz
ea	leather ___	head ___		lɛðɚ, hɛd
	bread ___	pear ___		brɛd, pɛr
ai	said ___	again ___	air ___	sɛd, əgɛn, ɛr
ue	guess ___	guest ___		gɛs, gɛst
ie	friend ___			frɛnd
ei	heifer ___	their ___		hɛfɚ, ðɛr
eo	Leonard ___	leopard ___		lɛnɚd, lɛpɚd
ay	says ___			sɛz
u	bury ___			bɛri
ae	aesthetic ___	aerial ___		æsɛtɪk, ɛriəl

Different Sounds for the Same Letters of the [ɛ] Sound

The following is a representative sample of optional sounds for the letters listed. Transcribe the following words. Refer to the Key at the right upon completion.

Alphabet Letters	Different Sounds	Words		Key
ue	[ɛ]	guest ___		gɛst
	[u]	glue ___		glu
ie	[ɛ]	friend ___		frɛnd
	[aɪ]	pie ___		paɪ
eo	[ɛ]	leopard ___		lɛpɚd
	[i]	people ___		pipəl or pipl̩
ay	[ɛ]	says ___		sɛz
	[eɪ]	say ___		seɪ
u	[ɛ]	bury ___		bɛri or bɛrɪ
	[u]	use ___		juz
	[ʌ]	us ___		ʌs

ea	[ɛ]	head ___		hɛd
	[i]	each ___		itʃ
e	[ɛ]	bed ___		bɛd
	Silent	toe ___		toʊ
a	[ɛ]	any ___		ɛni or ɛnɪ
	[æ]	ask ___		æsk

Rules for Spelling and Pronunciation of the [ɛ] Sound

1. In a word or syllable that contains only one vowel, the [ɛ] is usually a short vowel unless it is at the end of a word; the [ɛ] is usually short, as in *ten* [tɛn], *rent* [rɛnt], and so forth, that is between two consonants.

2. In words that begin with the letter *e*, the sound is a short one, as in *egg* [ɛg] and *extra* [ɛkstrə].

3. The [r] and [ɛ] appear in several different vowel combinations, as in "are" in *bare*; "aer" in *aerial*; "ear" in *bear*; "air" in *fair*; "eir" in *their*; "ere" in *where*; and "eir" in *heir*.

4. The [ɛ] cannot appear in stressed open syllables (those without a consonant at the end).

Words That Include the [ɛ] Sound

The [ɛ] is one of the most frequently used sounds, ranking about fourth in United States English. It is classified as an open vowel; therefore, it does not occur in the final position. Transcribe the following words. Refer to the Key at the right upon completion.

Initial		Medial		Final	Key
any	___	general	___	None	ɛni, dʒɛnɚəl
egg	___	head	___		ɛg, hɛd
education	___	mention	___		ɛdʒukeʃən, mɛnʃən
element	___	federal	___		ɛləmɛnt, fɛdɚl
end	___	test	___		ɛnd, tɛst
elegant	___	attention	___		ɛləgʌnt, ətɛnʃən
energy	___	second	___		ɛnɚdʒɪ, sɛkənd
elbow	___	red	___		ɛlboʊ, rɛd

Auditory Discrimination

Contrast Minimal Pairs

Transcribe the following. Refer to the Key at the right upon completion.

[ɛ]		*[eɪ]*		*Key*
debt	_____	date	_____	dɛt, deɪt
best	_____	based	_____	bɛst, beɪst
west	_____	waste	_____	wɛst, weɪst
sell	_____	sale	_____	sɛl, seɪl
wreck	_____	rake	_____	rɛk, reɪk
get	_____	gate	_____	gɛt, geɪt
edge	_____	age	_____	ɛdʒ, eɪdʒ
let	_____	late	_____	lɛt, leɪt

Other Pairs

[ɛ]		*[æ]*		*Key*
net	_____	gnat	_____	nɛt, næt
send	_____	sand	_____	sɛnd, sænd
letter	_____	latter	_____	lɛtɚ, lætɚ (flap)
met	_____	mat	_____	mɛt, mæt
then	_____	than	_____	ðɛn, ðæn
end	_____	and	_____	ɛnd, ænd
led	_____	lad	_____	lɛd, læd
left	_____	laughed	_____	lɛft, læft

[ɛ]		*[ɪ]*		*Key*
bed	_____	bid	_____	bɛd, bɪd
pair	_____	peer	_____	pɛr, pɪr
net	_____	knit	_____	nɛt, nɪt
ten	_____	tin	_____	tɛn, tɪn
set	_____	sit	_____	sɛt, sɪt
head	_____	hid	_____	hɛd, hɪd
well	_____	will	_____	wɛl, wɪl
red	_____	rid	_____	rɛd, rɪd

Allophonic and Dialect Variations

As with other vowels, the precise feature composition of [ɛ] may be considerably altered as a result of the influence of context, rate, stress, and other factors (Carrell & Tiffany, 1960). These factors include the allophonic variations that result from a raised or lowered tongue body or nasalization that still maintains the integrity of the [ɛ] sound but that is not quite as distinct (Shriberg & Kent, 1995).

In some Southern speech, a variant of [ɛ] may be heard that takes the form of a diphthongization transcribed as [ɛə] off-glide, or in some cases, [ɛjə] (Carrell & Tiffany, 1960). The [ɛ] and [ɪ] may be used by Southern and Midland dialects and is found in words such as *pen* [pɛn] or [pɪn], *get* [gɪt] or [gɛt], and *many* [mɛnɪ] or [mɪnɪ]. The word *get* pronounced [gɪt] is also found in informal usage (Edwards, 1997), and because of tensing of the tongue, the [e] may appear in *leg* [leg], *flesh* [fleʃ], and *measure* [meʒɚ]. Both [ɛ] and [æ] are used before *r* as in *chair* [tʃɛr] or [tʃær], *rare* [rɛr] or [rær], but [ɛ] is more common in United States English speech (Shriberg & Kent, 1995). Small (1999) adds that the [ɛr] sequence is also transcribed [ɛɚ] as in *hair* [hɛɚ]. In the northeastern and southeastern United States, the *r*-colored vowel [ɛr] may be pronounced as [er] as in [her], and in the Great Lakes region the [ɛ] sound appears in words such as *pillow* [pɛloʊ] and *milk* [mɛlk].

Nonnative Speaker Pronunciation

Because of the lax, rather indefinite nature of this sound (Carrell & Tiffany, 1960; Edwards, 1997), it is a problem for nonnative speakers of English, who may substitute [e], [æ], [ɑ], or [ʌ].

Speech-Sound Deviations

The most frequent substitution for the [ɛ] is [ɑ] (backed) or a fronted [a] (Edwards, 1997). Several other vowel substitutions, including [æ] (lowering) and [i] (raising), have been observed. Substitutions generally involve an adjacent sound such as the [æ] or [e] (Shriberg & Kent, 1995).

Summary

The [ɛ] is produced with the tongue in a (lower) mid-front position. The tongue is lax and the lips are unrounded. It is classified as a short vowel with more than 11 different spelling combinations. Practically every letter or letter combination that represents the [ɛ] sound can be used to pronounce a different sound. This leads to confusion for both native and nonnative speakers. The [ɛ] is about fourth in frequency of use in United States English. It is an open vowel and does not occur in the final position. It is subject to many dialect variations, and nonnative speakers substitute several different vowels. As might be expected, speech-sound deviations include substitutions of the adjacent vowels and some possible nasality.

Competency Quiz

Transcribe the following [ɛ] words. Refer to the Key at the right upon completion.

Key

1. pet	_____	11. ready _____		pɛt, rɛdi
2. lend	_____	12. any	_____	lɛnd, ɛni
3. dead	_____	13. bell	_____	dɛd, bɛl
4. Thames	_____	14. held	_____	tɛmz, hɛld

5. tent	_____	15. rest	_____	tɛnt, rɛst
6. led	_____	16. many	_____	lɛd, mɛni
7. get	_____	17. ten	_____	gɛt, tɛn
8. men	_____	18. penny	_____	mɛn, pɛni
9. said	_____	19. end	_____	sɛd, ɛnd
10. quest	_____	20. sent	_____	kwɛst, sɛnt

This completes the discussion of the short vowel ĕ [ɛ].

PHONETIC SYMBOL [ɪ]

EXHIBIT 9-3	Phonetic Symbol [ɪ]

Phonetic Symbol	[ɪ]
Grapheme Symbol	See the section titled "Different Spellings of the [ɪ] Sound," which follows.
Diacritic Symbol	ĭ, i
Phonic Symbol	ĭ
Sound Class	Short Vowel
Tongue Position	Position: (Lower) High-Front Lips: Unrounded Tension: Lax
IPA (1999)	[ɪ] #319 Near-Close, Near-Front, Unrounded

[ɪ]

The next short vowel to be discussed is the ĭ [ɪ], as in the word *it* [ɪt].

How the Sound Is Produced

The airflow from the lungs activates the vibration of the closed (adducted) vocal folds (voiced), and the sound enters the oral cavity because the velopharyngeal port is closed or nearly closed. The tip of the tongue is in contact behind the bottom (lower) front teeth. The front portion and body of the tongue decrease in tension (lax) and are elevated and shifted forward (front) and raised (high) toward the hard palate. The sides of the tongue make contact laterally with the molars and sides of the alveolar ridge. The lips are primarily apart and relaxed (lax) and may exhibit slight tension near the corners. The [ɪ] sound is positioned below the [i] sound and above the [ɛ] sound.

Different Spellings of the [ɪ] Sound

The following may represent variations in dialect and usage. For example, *lemon* [lɛmɪn], [lɛmɛn], or [lɛmən]. Transcribe the following. Refer to the Key at the right upon completion.

Different Spellings					*Key*
i in	___	thin	___	it ___	ɪn, Θɪn, ɪt
fish	___	sit	___		fɪʃ, sɪt
o women	___	lemon	___		wɪmɛn, lɛmɪn
e pretty	___				prɪtɪ or prɪti
u busy	___	minute	___		bɪzi, mɪnɪt

ui	build	——	built	——			bɪld, bɪlt
	building	——	guild	——			bɪldɪŋ, gɪld
y	hymn	——	pity	——			hɪm, pɪtɪ or pɪti
	gypsy	——	gypsum	——			ʤɪpsi, ʤɪpsəm
ea	dear	——	hear	——	fear ——		dɪr, hɪr, fɪr
ee	been	——	deer	——	cheer ——		bɪn, dɪr, ʧɪr
ie	pierce	——	sieve	——			pɪrs, sɪv
ei	forfeit	——	weird	——			foʊrfɪt, wɪrd
ia	carriage	——					kɛrɪʤ
ai	fountain	——					faʊntɪn
a	senate	——	surface	——			sɛnɪt, sɝfɪs

Different Sounds for the Same Letters of the [ɪ] Sound

The following is a representative sample of the different sounds and may have different dialect variables. Transcribe the following words. Refer to the Key at the right upon completion.

Alphabet Letters	Different Sounds	Words		Key
i	[ɪ]	bit	——	bɪt
o	[ɪ]	women	——	wɪmɛn
	[oʊ]	so	——	soʊ
e	[ɪ]	pretty	——	prɪti
	[ɛ]	bet	——	bɛt
u	[ɪ]	busy	——	bɪzi
	[ʌ]	us	——	ʌs
y	[ɪ]	gypsy	——	ʤɪpsi
	[j]	yes	——	jɛs
ui	[ɪ]	build	——	bɪld
	[i]	mosquito	——	mɪskito
ea	[ɪ]	fear	——	fɪr
	[i]	each	——	iʧ
ee	[ɪ]	deer	——	dɪr
	[i]	coffee	——	kɔfi or kɑfi
ie	[ɪ]	fierce	——	fɪrs
	[i]	believe	——	biliv

ei	[ɪ]	foreign	——	fɔrɪn
	[i]	receive	——	risiv

Rules for Spelling and Pronunciation of the [ɪ] Sound

There is some doubt about the frequency with which [ɪ] actually ends words in United States English (Edwards, 1997). Such words may end with a sound more closely related to [i]. For example, the word *city* may end with either the [ɪ] or [i] sound, or the final sound may actually be intermediate between the usual [ɪ] or [i] pronunciation. Some authors (Small, 1999; VanRiper, 1979) suggest that in the unaccented endings as in *city* ("even if it sounds like [i] to you" [VanRiper, 1979]), the sound should be transcribed as [ɪ]. The author of this text suggests that the integrity of the transcription can be maintained only when the vowel symbol is used that most resembles the sound that is produced by the speaker.

1. When a single vowel is between two consonants or a syllable, it is usually a short vowel, as in *bit* [bɪt].

2. The letter *y* at the end of a word, such as *city* and *puppy*, in some dialects is the [ɪ] or [i] sound.

Words That Include the [ɪ] Sound

The [ɪ] is one of the most frequently spoken sounds in United States English. Differences in dialect, particularly sound ending, may exist. Transcribe the following words. Refer to the Key at the right upon completion.

Initial		Medial*		Final		Key
instinct	——	children	——	pretty	——	ɪnstɪŋt, ʧɪldrən, prɪti
if	——	history	——	family	——	ɪf, hɪstɔri, fæməli
enjoy	——	thin	——	variety	——	ɪnʤɔɪ, θɪn, vəraɪti
it	——	gypsy	——	nearly	——	ɪt, ʤɪpsi, nɪrli
is	——	cheer	——	lady	——	ɪz, ʧɪr, leɪdɪ
enough	——	forfeit	——	forty	——	ɪnəf, fɔrfɪt, fɔrtɪ
into	——	busy	——	early	——	ɪntu, bɪzi, ɝli
entirely	——	hear	——	sixty	——	ɪntaɪɚli, hɪr, sɪksti

*New England and Southern speech.

Auditory Discrimination

Contrast Minimal Pairs

Transcribe the following words. Refer to the Key at the right upon completion.

[ɪ]	[i]	Key
been _____	bean _____	bɪn, bin
dim _____	deem _____	dɪm, dim
sin _____	seen _____	sɪn, sin
ship _____	sheep _____	ʃɪp, ʃip
live _____	leave _____	lɪv, liv
did _____	deed _____	dɪd, did
rich _____	reach _____	rɪtʃ, ritʃ
bid _____	bead _____	bɪd, bid

Other Pairs

[ɪ]	[i]	Key
pick _____	peak _____	pɪk, pik
bin _____	bean _____	bɪn, bin
dim _____	deem _____	dɪm, dim
ship _____	sheep _____	ʃɪp, ʃip
sin _____	seen _____	sɪn, sin
bit _____	beat _____	bɪt, bit
did _____	deed _____	dɪd, did
ill _____	eel _____	ɪl, il

[ɪ]	[ɛ]	Key
lid _____	led _____	lɪd, lɛd
bid _____	bed _____	bɪd, bɛd
tin _____	ten _____	tɪn, tɛn
bill _____	bell _____	bɪl, bɛl
fear _____	fair _____	fɪr, fɛr
bitter _____	better _____	bɪtɚ, bɛtɚ
knit _____	net _____	nɪt, nɛt
will _____	well _____	wɪl, wɛl

[ɪ]	[æ]	Key
him _____	ham _____	hɪm, hæm
bit _____	bat _____	bɪt, bæt
his _____	has _____	hɪz, hæz

		Key
begin _____	began _____	bigɪn, bigæn
miss _____	mass _____	mɪs, mæs
in _____	an _____	ɪn, æn
sit _____	sat _____	sɪt, sæt
fist _____	fast _____	fɪst, fæst

Allophonic and Dialect Variations

Unstressing of several vowels (Calvert, 1986), especially in New England and Southern speech, results in the use of [ɪ] where another vowel may be used in General American speech; for example, the last unstressed syllable in *Dallas* [əs], which becomes [ɪs], and in *courage* [kɝ-eɪdʒ], which with the long *a* sound or diphthong becomes [kɝ-ɪdʒ]. Also in New England and the Southern speech, the unstressed letter *y*, as in *city* and *army*, is pronounced as an [ɪ], as in [sɪtɪ], whereas the [ɪ] or [i] are used in United States English: [sɪti] or [sɪtɪ]. The use of [ɪ] in unstressed or relatively unstressed syllables may vary in pronunciation to include [ɪ], [i], [ɛ], and [ə], as in *began* [bɪgæn], [bigæn], [bɛgæn], and [bəgæn], and *demand* [dɪmænd], [dimænd], [dɛmænd], and [dəmænd] (Carrell & Tiffany, 1960). Ladefoged (1993) indicates that some dialects use the vowel [ɪ] and other dialects use [i] at the end of *pity, only, taxis*, and nearly everyone pronounces *Texas* as [tɛksəs] instead of [tɛksɪs].

Before [ʃ] in Southern American speech, the [ɛ] may be substituted for the [ɪ] cause of tensing, as in *fish* [fiʃ] for [fɪʃ] (Edwards, 1997). In General American speech, the nasal influence may result in the [ɛ] substitution for the [ɪ], as in *thing* [θɛŋ].

Tiffany and Carrell (1977) make an interesting observation regarding vowel reduction in *-ing* words. The varieties include the tense [iŋ] to lax [ɪŋ], [ɪn] substitution of the [n] for the [ŋ], [ən] substitution in /ɪŋ/, and, finally, deletion of the [ɪ], as when *sitting* [sɪtɪŋ] becomes [sɪtŋ]. Considerable variation in the pronunciation of [ɪ] is a result of contextual influences of stress or tongue height. For example, a stressed word such as *zero* is pronounced either [zɪro] or [ziro]. The tense feature of the [z] may influence the vowel that follows, thereby producing [i] rather than [ɪ].

Nonnative Speaker Pronunciation

For many nonnative speakers, the distinction between [ɪ] and [i] is difficult to make, inasmuch as many languages do not make such a tense/lax distinction (Edwards, 1997; Tiffany & Carrell, 1977).

For example, the speakers of Italian and Spanish dialects of United States English may use a sound that exists somewhere between the [ɪ] and [i], as in *sheep* and *ship*. Nonnative speakers typically substitute the [i] for the [ɪ] in words like *it* [it], *is* [iz], and *hit* [hit]. The vowel is tenser and tends to be longer and more diphthongal than the sound used by native speakers.

Speech-Sound Deviations

Edwards (1997) reports that the [ɪ] sound has been characterized as unstable in those with phonological disorders. The usual substitutions are those sounds that are nearby, the [ɛ], [ɑ], and [i].

Summary

The [ɪ] is a (lower) high front vowel located below the [i] and above the [e]. The tongue is lax and the lips unrounded. It is classified as a short vowel and has at least 13 different spelling combinations whose letters also represent other sounds. The [i] occurs in all positions, initial, medial, and final. There are allophonic variations resulting from context of surrounding sounds, tense, nasality, and so forth and a wide variety of dialect differences. Both native and nonnative speakers may have difficulty in the use of the distinctive [ɪ] sound and may produce a sound that ranges between [ɪ] and [i] in many contexts. Children

acquiring the sound or having difficulty may substitute other surrounding sounds while attempting to establish the appropriate tongue height and tension.

Competency Quiz

Transcribe the following [ɪ] words. Keep in mind that words ending in *y* could be pronounced with either an [i] or [ɪ] vowel sound.

					Key
1. pig	_____	11. busy	_____		pɪg, bɪzi
2. big	_____	12. grit	_____		bɪg, grɛt
3. flit	_____	13. dip	_____		flɪt, dɪp
4. brick	_____	14. cyst	_____		brɪk, sɪst
5. hymn	_____	15. give	_____		hɪm, gɪv
6. bill	_____	16. will	_____		bɪl, wɪl
7. dizzy	_____	17. brisk	_____		dɪzi, brɪsk
8. city	_____	18. built	_____		sɪti, bɪlt
9. dig	_____	19. guilt	_____		dɪg, gɪlt
10. sieve	_____	20. fig	_____		sɪv, fɪg

This completes the discussion of the short vowel ĭ.

PHONETIC SYMBOL [ɑ]

EXHIBIT 9-4	**Phonetic Symbol [ɑ]**
Phonetic Symbol	[ɑ]
Grapheme Symbol	See the section titled "Different Spellings of the [ɑ] Sound," which follows.
Diacritic Symbol	Short ã
Phonic Symbol	ă
Sound Class	Back Vowel
Tongue Position	Position: Low-Back Lips: Unrounded Tension: Lax
IPA (1999)	[ɑ] #305 Open, Back, Unrounded

[ɑ]

The next short vowel to be presented is the ă [ɑ] sound, as in *father*.

How the Sound Is Produced

The airflow from the lungs activates the vibration of the closed (adducted) vocal folds (voiced), and the sound enters the oral cavity because the velopharyngeal port is closed or nearly closed. The tongue rests on the floor of the mouth (low), and the [ɑ] sound travels from the rear portion (back) of the relaxed (lax) tongue and exits through the lips, which are in the unrounded position.

Different Spellings of the [ɑ] Sound

Dialect variations may occur in the pronunciation of these words. Some speakers have a tendency to substitute the [ɔ] such as [ɔn] for *on* [ɑn]. Transcribe the following words. Refer to the Key at the right upon completion.

Different Spellings						Key
a	far	—	part	—	are —	fɑr, pɑrt, ɑr
	barn	—				bɑrn
aa	bazaar	—				bəzɑr
o	on	—	bother	—	rod —	ɑn, bɑðɚ, rɑd
e	sergeant	—				sɑrdʒənt
ua	guard	—				gɑrd
ea	hearth	—	heart	—		hɑrθ, hɑrt
ah	ah	—				ɑ
al	palm	—	calm	—	alms —	pɑlm, kɑlm, ɑlmz
ho	honor	—	honest	—		hɑnɚ, hɑnɛst
ow	knowledge	—				nɑlɛdʒ

Different Sounds for the Same Letters of the [ɑ] Sound

The following is a representative sample and may be influenced by dialect variations. Transcribe the following words. Refer to the Key at the right upon completion.

Alphabet Letters	Different Sounds	Words		Key
a	[ɑ]	part	————	pɑrt
	[æ]	ask	————	æsk
o	[ɑ]	on	————	ɑn or ɔn
	[ʌ]	of	————	ʌv

				Key
e	[ɑ]	sergeant	————	sɑrgənt
	[ɛ]	bet	————	bɛt
ua	[ɑ]	guard	————	gɑrd
	[wei]	quaint	————	kweɪnt
ea	[ɑ]	heart	————	hɑrt
	[i]	each	————	itʃ
al	[ɑ]	palm	————	pɑlm
	[ə]	allow	————	əlaʊ
ow	[ɑ]	knowledge	————	nɑlɛdʒ
	[aʊ]	how	————	haʊ

Rules for Spelling and Pronunciation of the [ɑ] Sound

1. When the letter *a* is followed by the letter *r*, the vowel becomes [ɑ], as in *are, tar, far*.

2. When there is only one vowel in a word, the sound is usually a short [æ] sound.

3. In United States English, the [a] has several different sounds, including the [ɑ] sound.

4. In some dialects, certain words can be pronounced with either the short *a* as in *last* [læst] or the broad *a* as in [lɑst].

5. Words such as *office, water*, and *faucet* are pronounced with a variety of vowels, including [ɑ], [ɔ], or short *o* [ŏ].

6. Words such as *hot, not*, and *got* are often pronounced with the same [ɑ] vowel as in *father* instead of the short ŏ sound.

Words That Include the [ɑ] Sound

Dialect variations may occur for such words as *awful* [ɑfʊl] or [ɔfʊl] and *box* [bɑks] or [bɔks]. Transcribe the following words. Refer to the Key at the right upon completion.

Initial	Medial	Final	Key
honest —	clock —	Utah —	hɑnɛst, klɑk, jutɑ
arm —	calm —	straw —	ɑrm, kɑlm, strɑ
art —	drop —	ah —	ɑrt, drɑp, ɑ
odd —	dollar —	raw —	ɑd, dɑlɚ, rɑ
alms —	mark —	draw —	ɑlms, mɑrk, drɑ
awful —	lot —	hurrah —	ɑfʊl, lɑt, hɝɑ
otter —	box —	Ma —	ɑtɚ, bɑks, mɑ

Auditory Discrimination

Pronunciation may vary. Phoneticians may find it difficult to distinguish or produce the different sounds, particularly the [ɑ] and [ɔ] comparisons.

Contrast Minimal Pairs

Transcribe the following words. Refer to the Key at the right upon completion. *Note:* There may be a difference in the [ɔ] pronunciation. It may sound closer to an [o] sound in some dialects.

[ɑ]		[ɔ]		Key
are	_____	or	_____	ɑr, ɔr
car	_____	core	_____	kɑr, kɔr
star	_____	store	_____	stɑr, stɔr
hock	_____	hawk	_____	hɑk, hɔk
body	_____	bawdy	_____	bɑdi, bɔdi
farm	_____	form	_____	fɑrm, fɔrm

Other Pairs

[ɑ]	[ʌ]	[ɑ]	[æ]	Key
lock __	luck __	rot __	rat __	lɑk, lʌk, rɑt, ræt
shot __	shut __	box __	backs __	ʃɑt, ʃʌt, bɑks, bæks
sock __	suck __	pot __	pat __	sɑk, sʌk, pɑt, pæt
bomb __	bum __	stock __	stack __	bɑm, bʌm, stɑk, stæk
dock __	duck __	cop __	cap __	dɑk, dʌk, kɑp, kæp
calm __	come __	not __	gnat __	kɑlm, kʌm, nɑt, næt

Allophonic and Dialect Variations

The [ɑ] is quite variable in United States English, often interchanged with [ɔ] or [æ] (Calvert, 1986). For example, some Eastern speakers pronounce *aunt* as [ɑnt] rather than [ænt] by using the broad *a* sound. The [ɑ] that is common among New England speakers may be heard in words such as *park* [pɑrk], and instead of [kɑr] for *car*, [kar] is spoken.

Nonnative Speaker Pronunciation

Other than allophonic variations resulting from approximation of tongue position and amount of tension (lax), nonnative speakers can pronounce the [ɑ] sound within acceptable limits. Normal dialect variations using the [æ] may also be present.

Speech-Sound Deviations

The substitution of [æ] may be present, which is the typical pattern for vowel sound deviations. This sound is not usually a problem for children to acquire and is seldom misarticulated.

Summary

The [ɑ] is a cardinal vowel in that it marks the low-back apex of the vowel quadrilateral. It is produced with the tongue in a low-back position. The tongue is lax and the lips are unrounded. It is classified as a short vowel and has more than 10 different spelling combinations whose letters also represent other sounds. The [ɑ] occurs quite frequently in the initial, medial, and final positions in words. There is a wide range of allophonic and dialect variations that are distinct to different regions. For example, [ɔ] or [æ] may be substituted, and Eastern speakers of United States English may use a broad *a* sound for such words as *aunt* [ɑnt] instead of [ænt]. Words such as *hot* [hɑt] become [hɒt], and [ɔ] is substituted, as in *caught* [kɔt] for [kɑt]. Few speech deviations occur and are usually the substitution of [æ] (fronting) or [o] or [ʊ], which maintain the back position similar to [ɑ].

Competency Quiz

Transcribe the following [ɑ] words. Keep in mind that some of these words may also be pronounced with the [ɔ] sound.

				Key
1. guard _____		11. mop _____		gɑrd, mɑp
2. far _____		12. arm _____		fɑr, ɑrm
3. lard _____		13. stop _____		lɑrd, stɑp
4. psalm _____		14. art _____		sɑlm, ɑrt
5. blonde _____		15. from _____		blɑnd, frɑm
6. nod _____		16. calm _____		nɑd, kɑlm
7. heart _____		17. hard _____		hɑrt, hɑrd
8. fox _____		18. tar _____		fɑks, tɑr
9. calm _____		19. market _____		kɑlm, mɑrkɪt
10. flock _____		20. farm _____		flɑk, fɑrm

This completes the discussion of the short vowel ă [ɑ] sound.

PHONETIC SYMBOLS [ʌ] AND[ə]

EXHIBIT 9-5	Phonetic Symbols [ʌ] and [ə]
Phonetic Symbol	[ʌ] [ə]
Grapheme Symbol	See the section titled "Different Spellings and Different Sounds for the Same Letters of the [ʌ] and [ə] Sounds," which follows.
Diacritic Symbol	u, ŭ
Phonic Symbol	ŭ
Sound Class	Central Stressed [ʌ] Central Unstressed [ə]
Tongue Position	Position: Mid-central Depth: Back Tension: Lax Voicing: Plus
Lips	Unrounded
IPA (1999)	Schwa [ə] #322 Midcentral

$$[ʌ] [ə]$$

The next short vowel to be presented is the ŭ [ʌ] sound as in the word *above* [əbʌv] with the [ə] as the unstressed form.

How the Sound Is Produced

The airflow from the lungs passes through the closed vocal folds to create vibration and sound waves (voiced). The velopharyngeal port is closed and the sound waves are directed into the oral cavity. The tongue is somewhat retracted and its sides are closed against the upper molars. The front portion of the tongue is raised toward the palate (midcentral) just behind the alveolar ridge but does not make contact with it.

Commentary on the Schwa [ə] Sound

Julene Fisher, a columnist for the *Salt Lake Tribune*, Salt Lake City, Utah, makes this insightful observation concerning the schwa sound:

Uh, May I Buy a Vowel? No Need to with the Ever-Popular Schwa
Uh. Which vowel sound do English speakers use most? "Uh, . . ." That's right. "Huh?" No, you were right the first time—*uh*. So, how do you spell the *uh*? Give up? It's easy: *a, e, i, o,* or *u.*

Uh is the default vowel sound of our language, the vowel sound in most unstressed English syllables. Listen to the *a* in *attempt,* the *e* in *parent,* the second *i* in *intimate,* the first *o* in *potato,* and the *u* in *until.* Unless you are taking elocution lessons, they all sound like *uh.*

This *uh* sound has a name—*schwa*—and a nifty phonetic symbol [ə]—an upside down *e.* In spite of being ubiquitous, what it does not have is a letter of its own or much pronunciation status. Bill Bryson calls it a "colorless murmur. "

Maybe he does because to utter a schwa you do not have to stretch and tense your lips as you do for the *ee* in a "say *cheese*" smile. You do not circle your lips as for the *o* in *no.* You do not get to look pouty saying *u* as in *true.* You simply relax your lips and everything else connected with your mouth and exhale the lazy sound.

Easy Speaker D.C.F. thinks far too many of us have been relaxing our mouths far too often. The schwa sounds off in places it was never meant to be. How do you say the number 11? Duh! *Eeleven,* of course; so who keeps saying *uhleven* and why?

Eemmediate has become *uhmmediate.* Where will it all end? Will *uh* eventually replace every vowel sound in English, simplifying pronunciation, but further discombobulating spelling?

Adele Smith would like you to take the schwa some of you have been using in *liaison* and stick it in *vinaigrette* where it belongs. Make it *lee-ay-zon*, if you please, and *vin-uh-gret*, NOT *vine-gar-ette*. Easier still, eliminate both from your life and you will not have to worry about pronunciation, scandal or high cholesterol. (Fisher, 1997)

Different Spellings and Different Sounds for the Same Letters of the [ʌ] and [ə] Sounds

Transcribe the following words. Refer to the Key at the end of the transcription.

Different Spellings for the Stressed [ʌ] Sound		Sample of Different Sounds for the Same Letters	
u	cup ____ under ____	[u]	usual ____
ou	rough ____ enough ____	[oʊ]	though ____
o	ton ____ compass ____	[aʊ]	town ____
oe	does ____	[oʊ]	oboe ____
o-e	done ____ come ____	[oʊ]	dome ____
oo	blood ____	[ʊ]	food ____

Key (left to right): kʌp, ʌdɚ, juʒuɔl, rʌf, ənʌf, ðoʊ, tʌn, kʌmpəs, toʊn, dʌz, oʊbo, dʌn, kʌm, doʊm, blʌd, fʊd.

Transcribe the following words. Refer to the Key at the right upon completion.

Different Spellings for the Unstressed [ə] Sound		Sample of Different Sounds for the Same Letters		Key
o lemon	____	[o] oboe	____	lɛmən, oʊbo
oi porpoise	____	[ɔɪ] oil	____	pɔrpəs, oɪl
ou dangerous	____	[oʊ] though	____	deɪnʒɚəs, ðoʊ
a alone	____	[æ] ask	____	əlon, æsk
e moment	____	[eɪ] egg	____	moʊmənt, eɪg
i pencil	____	[ɪ] in	____	pɛnsəl, ɪn
u circus	____	[u] use	____	sɝkəs, juz
ai fountain	____	[aɪ] aisle	____	faʊntən, aɪl
eo pigeon	____	[i] people	____	pɪdʒən, pipəl
ea sergeant	____	[i] each	____	sɑrdʒənt, itʃ
ie conscience	____	[aɪ] pie	____	kɑnʃəns, paɪ
au authority	____	[ɑ] author	____	əθɔrɪti, ɔθɚ

Words That Include the [ʌ] (Stressed) Sound

The [ʌ] does not occur in the final position in words. Transcribe the following words. Refer to the Key at the right upon completion.

				Key
compass	____	hundred	____	kʌmpəs, hʌndrɛd
husband	____	such	____	hʌsbənd, sʌtʃ
come	____	nothing	____	kʌm, nʌθɪŋ
another	____	company	____	ənʌðɚ, kəmpʌni
country	____	once	____	kʌntri, wʌns
something	____	rush	____	sʌmθɪŋ, rʌʃ
fund	____	income	____	fʌnd, ɪnkʌm
suffer	____	trust	____	sʌfɚ, trʌst
front	____	son	____	rʌnt, sʌn
club	____	mother	____	klʌb, mʌðɚ
double	____	production	____	dʌbl̩, prodʌkʃən
judge	____	month	____	dʒʌdʒ, mʌθ
enough	____	sudden	____	inʌf, sʌdn̩
wonderful	____	public	____	wʌndɚfʊl, pʌblɪk
above	____	run	____	əbʌv, rʌn
fun	____	lover	____	fʌn, lʌvɚ

Initial [ʌ]				*Key*
upon	____	usher	____	ʌpɔn, ɔʃɚ
upper	____	ugly	____	ʌpɚ, ʌgli
upward	____	other	____	ʌpwɑrd, ʌðɚ
uncle	____	original	____	ʌŋkl̩, ʌrdʒɪnl̩
observe	____	under	____	ʌbsɚv, ʌndɚ
objection	____	oven	____	ʌbdʒɛkʃən, ʌvən

Medial [ʌ]				*Key*
method	____	money	____	mɛθʌd, mʌni
riot	____	hunt	____	raɪʌt, hʌnt
couple	____	flood	____	kʌpl̩, flʌd
weapon	____	some	____	wɛpʌn, sʌm
blood	____	nothing	____	blʌd, nʌθɪŋ
canyon	____	rough	____	kænjʌn, rʌf

Initial [ə]   *Key*

again _____   əgɛn

away _____   əweɪ

above _____   əbʌv

Medial [ə]   *Key*

table _____   teɪbəl

nation _____   neɪʃən

lemon _____   lɛmən

telephone _____   tɛləfon

Final [ə]   *Key*

banana _____   bənænə

cobra _____   koʊbrə

sofa _____   soʊfə

Auditory Discrimination

Contrast Minimal Pairs

Transcribe the following words. Refer to the Key at the right upon completion.

[ʌ]		[ɑ]		[ʌ]		[ʊ]		Key
putt	___	pot	___	shuck	___	shook	___	pʌt, pɑt, ʃʌk, ʃʊk
come	___	calm	___	tuck	___	took	___	kʌm, kɑm, tʌk, tʊk
sum	___	psalm	___	cud	___	could	___	sʌm, sɑm, kʌd, kʊd
bum	___	bomb	___	huff	___	hoof	___	bʌm, bɑm, hʌf, hʊf
duck	___	dock	___	crux	___	crooks	___	dʌk, dɑk, krʌks, krʊks
cut	___	cot	___	buck	___	book	___	kʌt, kɑt, bʌk, bʊk
nut	___	not	___	lux	___	looks	___	nʌt, nɑt, lʌks, lʊks
gun	___	gone	___	stud	___	stood	___	gʌn, gɑn, stʌd, stʊd

In the following list, the [ɔ] may present some dialect differences. Attempt to pronounce the words with the [ɔ] sound.

[ʌ]		[ɛ]		[ʌ]		[ɔ]		Key
hull	___	hell	___	sung	___	song	___	hʌl, hɛl, sʌŋ, sɔŋ
bun	___	Ben	___	fun	___	fawn	___	bʌn, bɛn, fʌn, fɔn
pun	___	pen	___	cussed	___	cost	___	pʌn, pɛn, kʌst, kɔst
money	___	many	___	ruckus	___	raucous	___	mʌni, mɛni, rʌkəs, rɔkəs

but	___	bet	___	rung	___	wrong	___	bʌt, bɛt, rʌŋ, rɔŋ
mutt	___	met	___	but	___	bought	___	mʌt, mɛt, bʌt, bɔt
nut	___	net	___	done	___	dawn	___	nʌt, nɛt, dʌn, dɔn

Allophonic and Dialect Variations

The [ə] has the shortest duration of any vowel and is the most nearly central in its tongue position (Shriberg & Kent, 1995). In some dialects, particularly Eastern, and some individual usage, the [ə] replaces the final [ɚ], as when *brother* [brʌðɚ] becomes [brʌ<u>ə</u>ə]. In contrast, the [ɚ] may replace the final [ə], as when *Cuba* [kjubə] becomes [kjubɚ]. Calvert (1986) indicates that frequently used, short linking words such as *a* [ei] or [eɪ] are often reduced to [ə] in connected speech and that earlier pronunciations have been replaced, such as *was* [wɑz] becomes [wʌz] and *from* [frɑm] becomes [frʌm]. An [ɑ]-like variation can be heard in certain Eastern and Southern dialects (Tiffany & Carrell, 1977). The unstressed [ə] takes preference over the stressed [ʌ] in conversational speech except for emphasis, such as *government* <u>of</u> [ʌv] *the people*. The [ə] often replaces a more stressed vowel in the last syllable of words such as *lemon* [lɛmən] for [lɛmɛn] and *before* [bifoʊr] for [bəfoʊr]. It appears that in many vowel contexts a vowel can be reduced to the [ə] production. Edwards (1997) notes that the [ə] serves as an allophonic variant of all the nondiphthongized vowels. That may be the reason why it is one of the most frequently occurring sounds in United States English speech.

Tiffany and Carrell (1977) make this timely observation:

> In unstressed syllables there is often such a marked reduction in the duration and energy of the syllable that the vowel tends to lose its characteristic resonance. As a kind of "minimal syllabic" it then retains only that resonance which is allowed by the transition from one consonant to another, which in turn will depend primarily upon the tongue-body position of the adjacent speech sounds. The schwa symbol is, then, a way of indicating that a vowel has been reduced to the status of an indefinite transition. The syllable is still there; the vowel, in its definite contrastive sense, is gone.

The schwa, as this sound is called, has replaced many of the other vowel "slots" in syllables by the process of stress reduction as demonstrated by [ɛ] or [ɪ] in *lemon* [lɛmən]. It is one of the most frequently occurring vowels and may be substituted with the [ɑ], [æ], or as an addition as in vowel insertion in *blue* [bəlu].

Competency Quiz

Remember to allow for dialect differences in the use of the schwa, such as in *reply* [rɪpaɪ] and [rəplaɪ], and that words ending with *y* may have an [ɪ] or [i] sound.

[ʌ]				Key
1. money _____	11. dump _____			mʌni, dʌmp
2. up _____	12. flood _____			ʌp, flʌd
3. result _____	13. rough _____			rəzʌlt, rʌf
4. mutt _____	14. cuff _____			mʌt, kʌf
5. trust _____	15. luck _____			trʌst, lʌk
6. tuft _____	16. tough _____			tʌft, tʌf
7. come _____	17. love _____			kʌm, lʌv
8. does _____	18. hiccough _____			dʌz, hɪkʌp
9. blood _____	19. one (won) _____			blʌd, wʌn
10. cluck _____	20. mumps _____			klʌk, mʌmps

[ə]				Key
1. attempt _____	11. common _____			ətɛmpt, kɑmən
2. enough _____	12. often _____			ənʌf, ɔfən
3. collect _____	13. equal _____			kəlɛkt, ikwəl
4. ability _____	14. accord _____			əbɪlətɪ, əkɔrd
5. system _____	15. upon _____			sɪstəm, əpʌn
6. above _____	16. avoid _____			əbʌv, əvɔɪd
7. ahead _____	17. recent _____			əhɛd, risənt
8. foreign _____	18. medical _____			fɔrən, mɛdəkəl
9. agree _____	19. telephone _____			əgri, tɛləfoʊn
10. sophomore _____	20. lesson _____			sɑfəmɔr, lɛsən

This completes the discussion of the short vowels.

REFERENCES

Calvert, D. R. (1986). *Descriptive phonetics*. New York, NY: Thieme Medical Publishers.

Carrell, J., & Tiffany, W. (1960). *Phonetics: Theory and application to speech improvement*. New York, NY: McGraw-Hill.

Edwards, H. T. (1997). *Applied phonetics* (2nd ed.). San Diego, CA: College-Hill Press.

Fisher, J. E. (1997, September 7). Uh, may I buy a vowel? *Salt Lake Tribune*, p. J8.

House, L. (1998). *Introductory phonetics and phonology*. Mahwah, NJ: Lawrence Erlbaum.

International Phonetic Association. (1999). *Handbook of the International Phonetic Alphabet*. Cambridge: Cambridge University Press.

Jones, D. (1917). *Everyman's english (british) pronouncing dictionary*. 15th ed., ed. by P. Roach/J. Hartman. Cambridge: Cambrige University Press.

Kenyon, J. S. & Knott, T. A. (1944). *A pronouncing dictionary of american english*. Springfield, Mass.: G&C Merriam Company.

Ladefoged, P. (1993). *A course in phonetics* (3rd ed.). Fort Worth, TX: Harcourt Brace College Publishers.

MacKay, I. R. A. (1987). *Phonetics: The science of speech production*. Boston, MA: Allyn & Bacon.

Meriam-Webster (1969). *Webster's seventh new collegiate dictionary*. Springfield, Mass.: Merriam-Webster.

Shriberg, L., & Kent, R. (1995). *Clinical phonetics* (3rd ed.). Boston, MA: Allyn & Bacon.

Singh, S., & Singh, K. (1976). *Phonetics: Principles and practices* (3rd ed.). San Diego, CA: Plural Publishing.

Small, L. H. (1999). *Fundamentals of phonetics: A practical guide for students* (3rd ed.). Boston, MA: Allyn & Bacon.

Tiffany, W. R., & Carrell, J. (1977). *Phonetics: Theory and application*. New York, NY: McGraw-Hill.

VanRiper, C. (1979). *An introduction to general American phonetics*. New York, NY: Harper & Row.

Chapter 10

Other Vowels and Diphthongs

PURPOSE

To introduce you to the remaining vowels and diphthongs used in United States English speech.

OBJECTIVES

This chapter will provide you with information regarding:

1. Characteristics of the remaining vowels and diphthongs
2. Different spellings for each of the vowels and diphthongs
3. Allophonic variations and dialect differences
4. Nonnative speaker pronunciation and speech deviations
5. Transcription exercises

INTRODUCTION

In addition to the five long vowels and five short vowels, there are several other United States English vowels. These vowels and diphthongs are as follows:

- [ʊ] in *book* [bʊk]
- [ɔ] in *caught* [kɔt]
- [ɔɪ] in *oil* [ɔɪl]
- [aʊ] in *how* [haʊ]

These four are discussed in this chapter. The remaining vowel sounds of [ɚ] and [ɝ] that represent the vocalic *r* sound are presented in Chapter 11.

PHONETIC SYMBOL [ʊ]

EXHIBIT 10-1 | Phonetic Symbols [ʊ]

Phonetic Symbol	[ʊ]	**[ʊ]**
Grapheme Symbol	See the section titled "Different Spellings of the [ʊ] Sound," which follows.	
Diacritic Symbol	ŏ, o, ú	
Phonic Symbol	o ŏ	
Sound Class	Short Vowel	
Tongue Position	Height: High Depth: Back Tension: Lax	
Lips	Rounded	
International Phonetic Alphabet (IPA) (1999)	[ʊ] #321 Near Close, Near Back, Rounded	

How the Sound Is Produced

The airflow from the lungs activates the vibration of the closed (adducted) vocal folds (voiced), and the sound waves travel through the pharyngeal cavity. The velopharyngeal port is closed and the sound enters the oral cavity and exits through the mouth. The body of the tongue is shifted back (back) and elevated (high), almost touching the palate, making contact with the upper molars. The tongue exhibits diminished tension (lax) with the tip positioned behind the lower front teeth. The mouth is slightly opened with the lips rounded and somewhat protruded. In the back vowel positions, the [ʊ] is above the /o/ and below the /u/. Its corresponding front vowel is [ɪ].

Different Spellings of the [ʊ] Sound

The following may represent dialectical differences. For example, *stew* [stʊ] or [stu] and *sugar* [ʃugɚ] or [ʃɪgɚ]. Transcribe the following words. Refer to the Key at the right upon completion.

Different Spellings					Key
u	pull ___	put ___	bush ___		pʊl, pʊt, bʊʃ
	sugar ___	bull ___			ʃugɚ or ʃɪgɚ, bʊl
oo	food ___	foot ___	book ___		fʊd, fʊt, bʊk
oul	should ___	would ___	could ___		ʃʊd, wʊd, kʊd
o	woman ___	wolf ___			wʊmən, wʊlf
ew	Lewis ___	stew ___			lʊɪs, stʊ

Different Sounds for the Same Letters of the [ʊ] Sound

Transcribe the following words. Refer to the Key at the right upon completion.

Alphabet Letter(s)	Different Sounds	Words		Key
u	[ʊ]	put	_____	pʊt
	[u]	use	_____	juz
	[ʌ]	us	_____	ʌs
	[ɑ]	pulse	_____	pɑls
o	[ʊ]	wolf	_____	wʊlf
	[ʌ]	of	_____	ʌf
oul	[ʊ]	could	_____	kʊd
	[aʊ]	foul	_____	faʊl
oo	[ʊ]	book	_____	bʊk
	[u]	school	_____	skul
ew	[ʊ]	stew	_____	stʊ
	[u]	ewe	_____	ju

Rules for Spelling and Pronunciation of the [ʊ] Sound

1. In certain contexts, the [ʊ] sound is pronounced for the letter *u*, as in *pull, put,* and *full,* but not in the following words: *but, rug,* or *bust.*

2. The [ʊ] sound is pronounced when two adjacent *oo* letters are present, as in *book, crook, hook,* and *took.*

3. The [ʊ] or [u] sound may be used when the *oo* letters are used, as in *hoof, root*, and *roof*.

4. When the letters *oul* appear in combination, they represent the [ʊ] sound, as in *would, should,* and *could*.

5. The *o* in words such as *woman* and *wolf* may be pronounced with the [ʊ] sound.

6. When the letter *u* appears before the letters *sh*, as in *push, bush,* and *cushion*, the [ʊ] sound is pronounced but not in the words *brush* and *blush*.

7. The [ʊ] sound is pronounced in words that have the *r* letter, as in *cure, detour, mature,* and *poor*.

Words That Include the [ʊ] Sound

Note that the [ʊ] sound does not occur in the initial or final positions in words. Also, the [ʊ] lax vowel can occur only in a closed-syllable context, requiring a consonant at the end (Ladefoged, 1993; Singh & Singh, 1976). However, at the end of words when used in its off-glide form with other sounds, as in the diphthongs [aʊ] and [oʊ], it is pronounced (Edwards, 1997). Transcribe the following words. Refer to the Key at the right upon completion.

Medial			Key
shook _____	wood _____	good _____	ʃʊk, wʊd, gʊd
could _____	push _____	look _____	kʊd, pʊʃ, lʊk
would _____	cook _____	wolf _____	wʊd, kʊk, wʊlf

Auditory Discrimination

Contrast Minimal Pairs

There may be differences in pronunciation because of dialectical variations. Transcribe the following words. Refer to the Key at the right upon completion.

[ʊ]		/u/		Key
hood _____		who'd _____		hʊd, hud
full _____		fool _____		fʊl, ful
look _____		Luke _____		lʊk, luk
could _____		cooed _____		kʊd, kud
should _____		shooed _____		ʃʊd, ʃud

[ʊ]		[ʌ]		Key
puts _____		putts _____		pʊts, pʌts
shook _____		shuck _____		ʃʊk, ʃʌk
took _____		tuck _____		tʊk, tʌk
roof _____		rough _____		rʊf, rʌf
book _____		buck _____		bʊk, bʌk

[ʊ]		[ɝ]		Key
put _____		pert _____		pʊt, pɝt
stood _____		stirred _____		stʊd, stɝd
look _____		lurk _____		lʊk, lɝk
pull _____		pearl _____		pʊl, pɝl
hood _____		heard _____		hʊd, hɝd
shook _____		shirk _____		ʃʊk, ʃɝk

[ʊ]		[oʊ]		Key
brook _____		broke _____		brʊk, broʊk
cook _____		coke _____		kʊk, koʊk
pull _____		pole _____		pʊl, poʊl
should _____		showed _____		ʃʊd, ʃoʊd
bull _____		bowl _____		bʊl, boʊl
could _____		code _____		kʊd, koʊd

Allophonic and Dialect Variations

The [ʊ] vowel seems to present difficulties far out of proportion to its frequency of use, both in speakers attempting to achieve acceptable pronunciation and in phoneticians learning to listen analytically (Tiffany & Carrell, 1977). Many speakers have difficulty distinguishing between the [ʊ] and the [u] sounds even though the [ʊ] appears fewer times than any other stressed vowel in United States English (House, 1998). There are suggestions that this sound could be eliminated without too much damage to the language. Note the contrasts of [u] and [ʊ] in these word pairs: *Luke-look, cooed-could,* and *fool-full*. Shriberg and Kent (1995) indicate that the jaw position usually is closed for the [ʊ] and that lip rounding frequently is not as pronounced as with [u] or may be neglected altogether. These authors also indicate that when English vowels such as the [ʊ] are produced in the context of nasal segments, they are usually nasalized to some degree. The velopharyngeal opening for a preceding nasal segment is maintained during the vowel and is open for a following nasal segment, as in *nook*. So, the nasal context has an allophonic variation on the production of an oral vowel.

The substitution of [u] for [ʊ] may occur in certain regional dialects in the United States, as in the word *push* [puʃ] (Tiffany & Carrell, 1977). The dependence of vowel quality on stress is nowhere more evident than in the pronunciation of the [ʊ] words. Many of these words could be quite acceptably pronounced [ə] where stress is minimal, as it often is in context. Although the speaker may not always be conscious of the following changes when speaking such words as *would* [wʊd]versus [wʌd], *good* [gʊd] versus [gʌd], and *should* [ʃʌd] versus [ʃʊd]. When one listens to a speaker, there is a high probability that the [ʊ] sound is not present. Dialects may also yield differences in such words as *to* and *you*, where the sound used may be [ʊ], [u], or [ʌ] or [ə] in the unstressed position (Shriberg & Kent, 1995). As a comparison, Davenport and Hannahs (1998) indicate that in various areas in England, there is a shift in [ʊ] usage to [u] in words such as *book* and *cook* and that the [ə] is occurring more frequently in the pronunciation of words such as *good, look*, and *could*.

United States English dialect changes use from [ʊ] to [u] when tongue tension is increased, especially before the [ʃ], as when *bush* becomes [buʃ], and in words with *oo*, as in *roof* [rʊf] or [ruf] (Calvert, 1986; Edwards, 1997; House, 1998). Shriberg and Kent (1995) include other words such as *root* and *broom* that may be pronounced with either the [ʊ] or [u] sound. Furthermore, Small (1999) explains that when *oo* is followed by [l], as in *pool* and *tool*, the [u] or [ʊ] may be used depending on the speaker's dialect and especially in the South. He indicates that some eastern speakers may use the [ʊ] in words such as *room* [rʊm] and *broom* [brʊm].

Nonnative Speaker Pronunciation

The [ʊ] sound is generally considered to be a problem sound (Edwards, 1997), but not because it is frequently used in United States English. There are at least six different spelling contexts that contribute to the difficulty nonnative speakers have with this sound. Foreign speakers often have conspicuous difficulty with [ʊ] because in most foreign languages, there is no phonemic distinction between [u] and [ʊ] (Tiffany & Carrell, 1977). Therefore, there is a tendency to substitute [u] for the [ʊ].

Speech-Sound Deviations

The [ʊ] sound is one of the sounds most often used incorrectly in the speech of children with severe phonological disorders (Edwards, 1997). In keeping with the finding that children with speech disorders tend to substitute the back vowels for other back vowels, the most frequent substitution for the [ʊ] sound is [ɔ] (lowering), followed by [u] (simultaneous tensing and raising). Other deviations include [ʌ] and [o].

Summary

The [ʊ] is produced with the tongue in the high back position. The tongue is lax and the lips are rounded. It is classified as a short vowel with more than five different spelling combinations whose letters also represent other sounds. It is unique in that it appears only in the medial position in words and not at the beginning or end. At times, it may be difficult to distinguish [ʊ] from [u], and nasalization influenced by the surrounding sounds may produce allophonic differences. Dialect variations may include the substitution of the [u], [ʌ], or [ə] sound. Those with speech-sound deviations may substitute the [ɔ], [u], or [o] sound. The [ʊ] appears fewer times than other stressed vowels and, when mispronounced, does not interfere with comprehension.

Transcription Exercises

Transcribe the following [ʊ] words. Refer to the Key at the right upon completion.

				Key
1. looked	_____	11. bull	_____	lʊkt, bʊl
2. would	_____	12. cook	_____	wʊd, kʊk
3. crooked	_____	13. put	_____	krʊkɪd, pʊt
4. wolf	_____	14. full	_____	wʊf, fʊl
5. good	_____	15. could	_____	gʊd, kʊd
6. book	_____	16. pulley	_____	bʊk, pʊlɪ
7. bullet	_____	17. stood	_____	bʊlɪt, stʊd
8. brook	_____	18. foot	_____	brʊk, fʊt
9. fulfill	_____	19. rook	_____	fʊlfɪl, rʊk
10. mistook	_____	20. wood	_____	mɪstʊk, wʊd

This completes the discussion of the [ʊ] vowel.

PHONETIC SYMBOL [ɔ]

The [ɔ] as in *caught* [kɔt] is now presented. Keep in mind that the sound of [ɔ] may have great dialectical variances and may be pronounced in a range from a definite [ɔ] sound to that of the [ɑ] sound as in *father*.

EXHIBIT 10-2	Phonetic Symbol [ɔ]
Phonetic Symbol	[ɔ]
Grapheme Symbol	See the section titled "Different Spellings of the [ɔ] Sound," which follows.
Diacritic Symbol	o, ä
Phonic Symbol	ŏ
Sound Class	Back Vowel
Tongue Position	Height: Lower-Mid
	Depth: Back
	Tension: Tense
Lips	Rounded
IPA (1999)	[ɔ] #306
	Open, Midback, Rounded

How the Sound Is Produced

The airflow from the lungs activates the vibration of the closed (adducted) vocal folds (voiced), and the sound waves travel through the pharyngeal cavity. The velopharyngeal port is closed and the sound enters the oral cavity and exits through the mouth. The back and middle sections of the tongue are slightly raised (low-mid) and usually do not make contact with the upper back teeth. The tip of the tongue is positioned behind the lower front teeth and the remainder of the tongue is toward the back (back) of the oral area. Lip and tongue tension (tense) is present with lip rounding (rounded), and the mandible is lowered, resulting in a wide mouth opening. In the back vowel positions, the [ɔ] is below the [o] and above the [ɑ]. Acoustically, the [ɔ] generates a great amount of energy and is one of the longest in duration.

Different Spellings of the [ɔ] Sound

The following may represent dialectical differences such as *ball* [bɔl] or [bɑl] and *caught* [kɔt] or [kɑt]. Transcribe the following words. Refer to the Key at the right upon completion.

Different Spellings							*Key*
a	ball	___	fall	___	tall	___	bɔl, fɔl, tɔl
o	soft	___	cloth	___	off	___	sɔt, klɔθ, ɔf
	strong	___	broad	___			strɔŋ, brɔd
	gone	___	cough	___			gɔn, kɔf
au	fault	___	Paul	___	vault	___	fɔlt, pɔl, vɔlt
	auto		laundry	___			ɔtoʊ, lɔndri
augh	taught	___	caught	___			tɔt, kɔt
aw	law	___	jaw	___	yawn	___	lɔ, dʒɔ, jɔn
	hawk	___	awe	___			hɔk, ɔw
hau	exhaust	___					ɛksɔst
ough	thought	___	ought	___			θɔt, ɔt
	bought	___	cough	___			bɔt, kɔf
ah	Utah	___					jutɔ
oa	broad	___					brɔd
al	talk	___					tɔlk

Different Sounds for the Same Letters of the [ɔ] Sound

There are possible dialect variations in the pronunciation of some of these words. Transcribe the following words. Refer to the Key at the right upon completion.

Different Letters	Different Sounds	Words		Key
a	[ɔ]	ball	_____	bɔl
	[æ]	ask	_____	æsk
o	[ɔ]	off	_____	ɔf
	[ʌ]	of	_____	ʌv
au	[ɔ]	auto	_____	ɔto
	[aʊ]	sauerkraut	_____	saʊɚkraʊt
augh	[ɔ]	caught	_____	kɔt
	[æ]	laugh	_____	læf
ough	[ɔ]	ought	_____	ɔt
	[oʊ]	though	_____	ðoʊ
oa	[ɔ]	broad	_____	brɔd
	[oʊ]	toad	_____	toʊd
al	[ɔ]	talk	_____	tɔk
	[ə]	allow	_____	əlaʊ

Rules for Spelling and Pronunciation of the [ɔ] Sound

To identify the [ɔ] sound verbally and in written form is exceedingly difficult because of variations in pronunciation practices (Carrell & Tiffany, 1960). For example, *cot* [kɑt] and *caught* [kɔt]. Many speakers do not make a distinction between the pronunciation of these two words. According to Edwards (1997), the [ɔ] sound is one of the most interesting United States English sounds. He states that many speakers do not use the [ɔ] sound and that considerable variation has been found among speakers who do use it. This may be because of the fact that individuals have great difficulty in perceiving it as a distinctive sound.

Words That Include the [ɔ] Sound

The [ɑ] sound may be used by those of a different dialect, or an allophonic sound may be spoken that is somewhere between the [ɔ] sound and the [ɑ] sound. Transcribe the following words using the [ɔ] sound. Refer to the Key at the right upon completion.

Initial	Medial	Final	Key
almost ____	cloth ____	jaw ____	ɔlmost, klɔθ, dʒɔ
ought ____	caught ____	claw ____	ɔt, kɔt, klɔ
already ____	walk ____	draw ____	ɔlrɛdi, wɔlk, drɔ
auto ____	dawn ____	gnaw ____	ɔto, dɔn, nɔ
awning ____	thought ____	jaw ____	ɔnɪŋ, θɔt, dʒɔ
autumn ____	hawk ____	straw ____	ɔtəm, hɔk, strɔ
often ____	fault ____	thaw ____	ɔftən, fɔlt, θɔ

Auditory Discrimination

Contrast Minimal Pairs

Because the [ɔ] may be an uncommon sound for some people, particular attention should be given to its acceptable pronunciation.

[ɔ]	[ɑ]	[ɔ]	[oʊ]	Key
auto ___	Otto ___	call ___	coal ___	ɔto, ɑtoʊ, kɔl, koʊl
caller ___	collar ___	taught ___	tote ___	kɔlɚ, kɑlɚ, tɔt, toʊt
taught ___	tot ___	bawl ___	bowl ___	tɔt, tɑt, bɔl, boʊl
core ___	car ___	fawn ___	phone ___	kɔr, kɑr, fɔn, foʊn
wrought ___	rot ___	fall ___	foal ___	rɔt, rɑt, fɔl, foʊl
caught ___	cot ___	bought ___	boat ___	kɔt, kɑt, bɔt, boʊt
naught ___	not ___	paws ___	pose ___	nɔt, nɑt, pɔz, poʊz

[ɔ]	[ʌ]	[ɔ]	[o]	Key
caught ___	cut ___	hauled ___	hold ___	kɔt, kʌt, hɔld, hɑld
pawn ___	pun ___	called ___	cold ___	pɔn, pʌn, kɔld, kɑld
wrought ___	rut ___	clause ___	close ___	rɔt, rʌt, klɔz, klɑz
naught ___	nut ___	naught ___	note ___	nɔt, nʌt, nɔt, nɑt
lost ___	lust ___	gnaws ___	nose ___	lɔst, lʌst, nɔwz, nɑz
bawdy ___	buddy ___	awning ___	owning ___	bɔdi, bʌdi, ɔnɪŋ, ɑnɪŋ
log ___	lug ___	caught ___	coat ___	lɔg, lʌg, kɔt, kɑt

Allophonic and Dialect Variations

Considerable variation has been found among speakers who use the [ɔ] vowel (Edwards, 1997). For example, the [ɔ] is used in *dog* but not in *log* or it is nasalized, as in *ought* [ɔt]. Many speakers do not use the [ɔ] and have great difficulty in perceiving it as a distinctive sound (Edwards, 1997). According to Calvert (1986), the [ɔ] is one of the most inconsistently used vowels in United States English speech. Its acoustic distinctiveness depends on lip rounding and protrusion, which, with some tongue elevation, is its primary difference from [ɑ]. House (1998) agrees that because the [ɔ] requires a distinct lip-rounded posture, the [ɑ] is used as an alternative by some speakers who use little or no lip rounding. Edwards (1997) indicates that speaker variability in the tenseness of lip shaping and dialectic differences in usage lead to a continuum of lip rounding and protrusion ranging from almost total absence of the vowel to universal substitution of [ɑ]. Some United States English speakers substitute the [ɑ] in many of the contexts that used to be reserved for the [ɔ], such as when *law* [lɔ] becomes [lɑ], and *awful* [ɔfəl] becomes [ɑfəl]. The [ɒ] or [ɑ] may be used in United States English speech rather than the [ɔ], as in *caught* [kɔt], [kɒt], or [kɑt], because there is a great deal of dialectal variation regarding the occurrence of [ɔ] (Calvert, 1986; Edwards, 1997). It appears that the dialectical difference is not critical to word meaning.

A word such as *on* is pronounced as [ɔn] in Southern speech, [ɑn] by most United States English speakers, and [an] in New England (Calvert, 1986). Words that contain *-og* exhibit similar variability. In the South, *dog* and *log* have a definite [ɔ] vowel whereas the [ɑ] is generally used elsewhere. Words that include the *o(r)* have very high variability even within a dialect group. For example, for words such as *or, born*, and *origin*, the *or* options are [ɔ], [o], [ou], and [ɑ]. In New England and Southern dialects, *for* may be pronounced as [fɔə] or [fɔr].

Principally in New England, using a slightly rounded [ɔ] or [ɑ] of rather short duration, the [ɒ] may be spoken in such words as *top, not, rock,* and *coffee* (Calvert, 1986). Also, a nasalized [ɔ] sound may occur in such words as *coffee* in a New York City dialect: [kɔfɪ] or [kɔfi] (Edwards, 1997).

Nonnative Speaker Pronunciation

The pronunciation of the vowel that represents the [ɔ] sound varies with the degree of self or formal instruction. Because the [ɔ] is quite regional in usage, those who reside in areas where it is used may acquire the sound. Others may use the [ɑ] sound or an allophone between [ɔ] and [ɑ]. Word meaning is usually not influenced by the choice of the vowel, so lack of the [ɔ] does not present problems.

Speech-Sound Deviations

The [ɔ] has been found to be stable in the speech of children who speak dialects in which it is used (Edwards, 1997). Along with [i] and [u], it is most often correct even in children with phonological disabilities. Some individuals may diphthongize the sound to approximate [aɪ]. If it becomes unrounded, it resembles the [ɑ] sound.

Summary

The [ɔ] is produced with the tongue in a lower-mid back position. The tongue is tense and the lips are rounded. It appears in the initial, medial, and final positions in words. It is not a common sound in United States English, and there are many variations in pronunciation, including [o], [ou], and [ɑ]. Children whose dialect includes the [ɔ] have little difficulty in acquiring it. It may be diphthongized as [aɪ] or become unrounded and substituted with the [ɑ] sound.

Transcription Exercises

Transcribe the following [ɔ] words. Keep in mind that some dialect differences may occur, resulting in more of an [ɑ] sound. Transcribe the words as they are spoken with the [ɔ] sound. Refer to the Key at the right upon completion.

					Key
1. awl	_____	11. sauce	_____		ɔl, sɔs
2. frost	_____	12. fought	_____		frɔst, fɔt
3. wrought	_____	13. walk	_____		rɔt, wɔk
4. squaw	_____	14. soft	_____		skwɔ, sɔft
5. office	_____	15. talk	_____		ɔfɪs, tɔk
6. cough	_____	16. brought	_____		kɔf, brɔt
7. ball	_____	17. gone	_____		bɔl, gɔn
8. caught	_____	18. law	_____		kɔt, lɔ
9. hawk	_____	19. all	_____		hɔk, ɔl
10. fawn	_____	20. brawl	_____		fɔn, brɔl

This completes the discussion of the [ɔ] vowel sound.

PHONETIC SYMBOL [ɔɪ]

EXHIBIT 10-3 | **Phonetic Symbol [ɔɪ]**

Phonetic Symbol	[ɔɪ]	**[ɔɪ]**
Grapheme Symbol	See the section titled "Different Spellings of the [ɔɪ] Sound," which follows.	
Diacritic Symbol	ó, ói	
Phonic Symbol	ô	
Sound Class	Diphthong	
Tongue Position	Height: Lower-Mid to High Depth: Midback to Front Tension: Tense to Lax Voice: Plus Voice	
Lips	Rounded to Unrounded	
IPA (1999)	[ɔ] Open-Mid, Back, Rounded [ɪ] Near Closed, Near Front, Unrounded	

The next sound is the diphthong [ɔɪ], as in *oil* [ɔɪ]. Keep in mind that there may be considerable dialectal variances in the pronunciation of both the [ɔ] and the [ɪ]. The production range might extend from the definite pronunciation of the beginning sound with a glide into the ending sound to an allophonic representation in which the sounds become less distinct but are still recognizable. Also, the beginning sound may be more of an [ɑ] sound and the ending sound closer to the high front [i] sound.

How the Sound Is Produced

The airflow from the lungs activates the vibration of the closed (adducted) vocal folds (voiced), and the sound waves travel through the pharyngeal cavity. The velopharyngeal port is closed and the sound enters the oral cavity and exits through the mouth. The glide that produces the [ɔɪ] diphthong is from a lowback vowel [ɔ] to a highfront off-glide [ɪ] or [i] vowel depending somewhat on how open the mouth is for the pronunciation of the second vowel in the diphthong.

Different Spellings of the [ɔɪ] Sound

The following spellings may represent variations in dialect and usage. Transcribe the following words. Refer to the Key at the right upon completion.

Different Spellings				*Key*
oy boy	__ toy	__ joy __	oyster __	bɔɪ, tɔɪ, ʤɔɪ, ɔɪstɚ
oi oil	__ boil	__ toil __		ɔɪl, bɔɪl, tɔɪl
	coin	__ voice __		kɔɪn, vɔɪs

eu Freud __	frɔɪd
a lawyer __	lɔɪjɚ

Different Sounds for the Same Letters for the [ɔɪ] Sound

The following are just two examples of many possibilities of different sounds. Transcribe the following words. Refer to the Key at the right upon completion.

		Key
eu [ju] feud _____		fjud
a [æ] ask _____		æsk

Rules for Spelling and Pronunciation of the [ɔɪ] Sound

1. When an *i* or *y* follows an *o*, the letter combination is usually pronounced as a diphthong.

2. There is dialect variance of either [ɪ] or [i] as the terminating off-glide vowel.

3. Speakers may tend to insert a [j], as in *jam*, between the two vowels, as in *oil* [ɔjɪl].

Words That Include the [ɔɪ] Sound

Transcribe the following words. Refer to the Key at the right upon completion.

Initial		*Key*
ointment _____ oil _____		ɔɪntmənt, ɔɪl
oiler _____ oyster _____		ɔɪlɚ, ɔɪstɚ

Medial   *Key*

soil ___   foil ___   boycott___   sɔɪl, fɔɪl, bɔɪkɔt

coin ___   royal ___   loin ___   kɔɪn, rɔɪəl, lɔɪn

thyroid ___   Өaɪrɔɪd

mastoid___   join ___   voice ___   mæstɔɪd, dʒɔɪn, vɔɪs

appoint ___   goiter ___   əpɔɪnt, gɔɪtɚ

boil ___	ball ___	bɔɪl, bɔl
noise ___	gnaws ___	nɔɪz, nɔz
soy ___	saw ___	sɔɪ, sɔ
cloy ___	claw ___	klɔɪ, klɔ
loin ___	lawn ___	lɔɪn, lɔn

Final   *Key*

joy ___   poi ___   toy ___   boy ___   dʒɔɪ, pɔɪ, tɔɪ, bɔɪ

soy ___   coy ___   Roy ___   sɔɪ, kɔɪ, rɔɪ

Troy ___   enjoy ___   deploy ___   trɔɪ, ɛndʒɔɪ, diplɔɪ

destroy ___   cloy ___   dɪstrɔɪ, klɔɪ

Auditory Discrimination

Contrast Minimal Pairs

Transcribe the following words. Refer to the Key at the right upon completion.

[ɔɪ]		*[aɪ]*		*Key*
toys	___	ties	___	tɔɪz, taɪz
voice	___	vice	___	vɔɪs, vaɪs
loin	___	line	___	lɔɪn, laɪn
lawyer	___	liar	___	lɔɪjɚ, laɪɚ
oil	___	aisle	___	ɔɪl, aɪl
poise	___	pies	___	pɔɪz, paɪz
boy	___	buy	___	bɔɪ, baɪ
foil	___	file	___	fɔɪl, faɪl
[ɔɪ]		*[ɝ]*		*Key*
boy	___	burr	___	bɔɪ, bɝ
foist	___	first	___	fɔɪst, fɝst
voice	___	verse	___	vɔɪs, vɝs
loin	___	learn	___	lɔɪn, lɝn
oil	___	earl	___	ɔɪl, ɝl
Boyd	___	bird	___	bɔɪd, bɝd
coy	___	cur	___	kɔɪ, kɝ
[ɔɪ]		*[ɔ]*		*Key*
joy	___	jaw	___	dʒɔɪ, dʒɔ
oil	___	awl	___	ɔɪl, ɔl
toil	___	tall	___	tɔɪl, tɔl

Allophonic and Dialect Variations

An [ɔɪ] for [ɝ], as *girl* [gɔɪl], and the opposite substitution of [ɝ] in *oil* [ɝl] for [ɔɪl] occur in some New York City dialects. Pronunciation may vary toward the [oɪ] or [oi], and in some dialects the [aɪ] as in [haɪst] for *hoist* may occur. Speakers who do not distinguish between the words *cot* and *caught* also produce a less distinct [ɔɪ] sound.

Nonnative Speaker Pronunciation

The same variations occur among nonnative speakers regarding the pronunciation of this sound. Dialect variations of a broad range occur, and in many instances the [ɑ], [oi], or [oɪ] substitutes for the [ɔɪ].

Speech-Sound Deviations

Diphthong reduction characterizes the error pattern of children with phonological disorders that involve the vowels (Edwards, 1997). The most frequent error with regard to [ɔɪ] is [o] substitution. Other substitutions include [ɔ] and [ʌ].

Summary

The [ɔɪ] diphthong begins its on-glide near the [ɔ] nucleus depending on dialect and other factors such as context and speaking rate. The off-glide ending can vary, with the [ɪ] or [i] termination depending on the height of the front of the tongue. Only a few different alphabet letters represent this sound, and these letters also represent other sounds. This could be confusing for nonnative speakers who also exhibit variations in pronunciation similar to native speakers. Children may substitute the [o], [ɔ], or [ʌ] as a part of diphthong reduction.

Transcription Exercises

Transcribe the following [ɔɪ] words. Keep in mind that dialect differences may occur and the pronunciation may be more of an [oi] sound. Also, words ending in *y* may have either an [i] or [ɪ] sound depending on dialect.

Key

1. coin	_____	11. Hoyle	_____	kɔɪn, hɔɪl	
2. oily	_____	12. boil	_____	ɔɪli, bɔɪl	
3. employ	_____	13. convoy	_____	ɛmplɔɪ, kɑnvɔɪ	
4. envoy	_____	14. voiced	_____	ɛnvɔɪ, vɔɪst	
5. invoice	_____	15. Roy	_____	ɪnvɔɪs, rɔɪ	

6. poison	_____	16. buoy	_____	pɔɪsɪn, bɔɪ
7. boy	_____	17. voiceless	_____	bɔɪ, vɔɪslɛs
8. toil	_____	18. void	_____	tɔɪl, vɔɪd
9. destroy	_____	19. noise	_____	dɪstrɔɪ, nɔɪz
10. spoil	_____	20. poise	_____	spɔɪl, pɔɪz

This completes the discussion of the diphthong [ɔɪ] sound.

PHONETIC SYMBOL [aʊ]

Next is discussion of the United States English diphthong [aʊ] as in *how* [haʊ].

EXHIBIT 10-4	Phonetic Symbol [aʊ]

Phonetic Symbol	[aʊ]
Grapheme Symbol	See the section titled "Different Spellings of the [aʊ] Sound," which follows.
Diacritic Symbol	ou, aú
Phonic Symbol	ou, ow
Sound Class	Diphthong
Tongue Position	Height: Low to Midhigh Depth: Front to Back Tension: Lax to Lax
Lips	Unrounded to Rounded
IPA (1999)	Diphthongs are not specified by IPA.

How the Sound Is Produced

The airflow from the lungs activates the vibration of the closed vocal folds (voiced), and the sound waves enter the oral cavity because the velopharyngeal port is closed, except in nasal context. The position of the mandible begins in a midopen to open posture for the on-glide and often closes slightly for the off-glide. The middle and back portions of the tongue are raised slightly (on-glide) from a low-back or low-mid back position that is similar to that used for [ɑ] or [ɔ] toward an off-glide midback [o] or high midback position closer to that used for the [ʊ] sound. The tip of the tongue is behind the lower front teeth and may move back slightly as the [ʊ] sound is initiated. Thus, the movement is from an open, front, unrounded, tense vowel to a near-close, back, rounded, lax (off-glide) vowel. The [a] portion is the nucleus of the diphthong and its duration is longer (stressed) than the [ʊ], which is shorter in duration and unstressed.

Different Spellings of the [aʊ] Sound

Transcribe the following words. Refer to the Key at the right upon completion.

Different Spellings				*Key*
ou	ouch	_____	mouse _____	aʊtʃ, maʊs
	found	_____	out _____	faʊnd, aʊt
ow	cow	_____	clown _____	kaʊ, klaʊn
ough	drought	_____		draʊt

au	sauerkraut	_____	saʊɚkraʊt
-h	hour	_____	haʊr
ou-e	house	_____	haʊs

ourselves	_____	outback	_____	aʊrsɛlvz, aʊtbæk
outline	_____	outfit	_____	aʊtlaɪn, aʊtfɪt
output	_____	ours	_____	aʊtpʊt, aʊrz

Different Sounds for the Same Letters of the [aʊ] Sound

The following is a sample of the sound options of the [aʊ] and other sounds. Transcribe the following words. Refer to the Key at the right upon completion.

Alphabet Letter(s)	Different Sounds	Words		Key
ou	[aʊ]	out	_____	aʊt
	[oʊ]	though	_____	ðoʊ
ow	[aʊ]	tower	_____	taʊɚ
	[oʊ]	tow	_____	toʊ
ough	[aʊ]	drought	_____	draʊt
	[u]	through	_____	Өru
au	[aʊ]	sauerkraut	_____	saʊɚkraʊt
	[ɑ] or [ɔ]	autumn	_____	ɔtəm
-h	[aʊ]	hour	_____	haʊr
	+h	house	_____	haʊs

Rules for Spelling and Pronunciation of the [aʊ] Sound

1. The [aʊ] sound is not usually spelled as *ough* or *au*.
2. The [aʊ] sound may occur in the spelling *ou*, as in *sound, doubt, ground*.
3. The [aʊ] sound is often spelled as *ow*, as in *plow, now, towel*.
4. "How now brown cow!"

Words That Have the [aʊ] Sound

Dialect variations may occur in the pronunciation of some of the following words. Transcribe the following words. Refer to the Key at the right upon completion.

Initial				*Key*
output	_____	hour		aʊtpʊt, haʊr
owl	_____	ouch		aʊl, aʊʧ
ounce	_____	outlook		aʊns, aʊtlʊk

Medial				*Key*
towel	_____	count		taʊwəl, kaʊnt
doubt	_____	town		daʊt, taʊn
aloud	_____	found		əlaʊd, faʊnd
scout	_____	amount		skaʊt, əmaʊnt
mountain	_____	council		maʊntən, kaʊnsəl
gown	_____	brown		gaʊn, braʊn

Final				*Key*
thou	_____	vow		ðaʊ, vaʊ
allow	_____	endow		əlaʊ, ɛndaʊ
cow	_____	sow		kaʊ, saʊ
bough	_____	how		baʊ, haʊ
somehow	_____	now		sʌmhaʊ, naʊ
eyebrow	_____	prow		aɪbraʊ, praʊ

Auditory Discrimination
Contrast Minimal Pairs

Dialect variations may occur in the pronunciation of some of these words. Transcribe the following words. Refer to the Key at the right upon completion.

[aʊ]		[ɑ]		[aʊ]		[ɔ]		*Key*
spout	__	spot	__	owl	__	awl	__	spaʊt, spɑt, aʊl, ɔl
scout	__	Scott	__	cloud	__	clawed	__	skaʊt, skɑt, klaʊd, klɔd
doubt	__	dot	__	brown	__	brawn	__	daʊt, dɑt, braʊn, brɔn
shout	__	shot	__	found	__	fawned	__	ʃaʊt, ʃɑt, faʊnd, fɔnd
hour	__	are	__	town	__	tawn	__	aʊr, ɑr, taʊn, tɔn
down	__	don	__	now	__	gnaw	__	daʊn, dɑn, naʊ, nɔ
pound	__	pond	__	howl	__	haul	__	paʊnd, pɑnd, haʊl, hɔl
gout	__	got	__	louse	__	loss	__	gaʊt, gɑt, laʊs, lɔs

[aʊ]		[oʊ]		[aʊ]		[ʌ]		*Key*
noun	__	known	__	pout	__	putt	__	naʊn, noʊn, paʊt, pʌt
ground	__	groaned	__	down	__	done	__	graʊnd, groʊnd, daʊn, dʌn
couch	__	coach	__	noun	__	nun	__	kaʊʧ, koʊʧ, naʊn, nʌn

crowd _ crowed _ town _ ton _ kraʊd, kroʊd, taʊn, tʌn

thou _ though _ gown _ gun _ ðaʊ, ðoʊ, gaʊn, gʌn

now _ know _ cowl _ cull _ naʊ, noʊ, kaʊl, kʌl

town _ tone _ found _ fund _ taʊn, toʊn, faʊnd, fʌnd

[aʊ]		[aɪ]		Key
how	_____	high	_____	haʊ, haɪ
mouse	_____	mice	_____	maʊs, maɪs
down	_____	dine	_____	daʊn, daɪn
spout	_____	spite	_____	spaʊt, spaɪt
noun	_____	nine	_____	naʊn, naɪn
bow	_____	by	_____	baʊ, baɪ
loud	_____	lied	_____	laʊd, laɪd
fowl	_____	file	_____	faʊl, faɪl

Allophonic and Dialect Variations

Probably the most frequent pronunciation is [a], a vowel quality ranging somewhere between the [æ] and [ɑ] (Tiffany & Carrell, 1977). For some speakers, including those from the Midwest, the nucleus may be closer to [ɑ], as in *father* [fɑðɚ] and when *out* [aʊt] becomes [ɑʊt] (Calvert, 1986). Also, the glide may terminate closer to the high back [u] sound. The substitution of the [æʊ] or [ɜʊ] as in *house* [hæʊs] or [hɜʊs] may occur in Eastern and Southern speech (Edwards, 1997). (The [ɜ] sound is used in words such as *bird* [bɜd] when the [r] is not pronounced, as for some British and American speakers.) The pronunciation of the [aʊ] may vary depending on adjacent phonemes and dialect variations such as nasalization in the [m], [n], or [ŋ] context (House, 1998).

In some United States English speech, the second element of this diphthong, [ʊ], may be neglected, and words such as *cloud* [klaʊd] may sound like [klɑd] (Tiffany & Carrell, 1977). Also, because of the weaker nature of the glide, the [ʊ] may become obtrusive and more noticeable than, for example, the ending sound in other diphthongs such as [aɪ] and [ɔɪ]. Some speakers have a complicated movement, making a substitution sequence of sounds beginning with [ɛ] as in *bed* [bɛd], [ʌ] as in *bud* [bʌd], and [u] as in *food* [fud] (Ladefoged, 1993). Ladefoged (1993) offers this exercise: "Say [ɛ-ʌ-u] in quick succession. Now say *how now brown cow* using a diphthong of this type."

Nonnative Speaker Pronunciation

Nonnative speakers have very little difficulty with the pronunciation of this sound (Edwards, 1997).

Speech-Sound Deviations

The substitution of [ɑ] and [æ] is the most frequent error (Edwards, 1997).

Summary

The nucleus of the [aʊ] diphthong is near [a] or [ɑ] and glides back and upward toward the mid to high [ɔ], [ʊ], or [u], depending on dialect. The movement is from an open, front, unrounded, tense vowel to a near-close, back, rounded, lax vowel. There are at least six different letter(s) that represent the [aʊ] sound, and these letters also represent other sounds. It appears in the initial, medial, and final positions in words, and Southern and Eastern United States English are particularly affected with dialect variations. It is not a difficult sound for nonnative speakers to acquire and use, other than for the usual influences of dialect, and children may substitute the [ɑ] or [æ] for the initial sound in the diphthong.

Transcription Exercises

Transcribe the following words with the [aʊ] sound. Refer to the Key at the right upon completion.

				Key
1. house	_____	11. mouse	_____	haʊs, maʊs
2. down	_____	12. sprout	_____	daʊn, spraʊt
3. out	_____	13. outline	_____	aʊt, aʊtlaɪn
4. about	_____	14. pound	_____	əbaʊt, paʊnd
5. sound	_____	15. spout	_____	saʊnd, spaʊt
6. count	_____	16. amount	_____	kaʊnt, əmaʊnt
7. cow	_____	17. power	_____	kaʊ, paʊɚ
8. brown	_____	18. drought	_____	braʊn, draʊt
9. Faust	_____	19. owl	_____	faʊst, aʊl
10. gown	_____	20. hour	_____	gaʊn, haʊɚ

This completes the discussion of the [aʊ] diphthong. Chapter 11 discusses the remaining vocalic *r* sounds that occur in the [ɚ] and [ɜ] central vowel sounds.

REFERENCES

Calvert, D. R. (1986). *Descriptive phonetics*. New York, NY: Thieme Medical Publishers.

Carrell, J., & Tiffany, W. (1960). *Phonetics: Theory and application to speech improvement*. New York, NY: McGraw-Hill.

Davenport, M., & Hannahs, S. J. (1998). *Introducing phonetics and phonology*. Oxford, England: Oxford University Press.

Edwards, H. T. (1997). *Applied phonetics* (2nd ed.). San Diego, CA: College-Hill Press.

House, L. (1998). *Introductory phonetics and phonology*. Mahwah, NJ: Lawrence Erlbaum.

International Phonetic Association. (1999). *Handbook of the International Phonetic Alphabet*. Cambridge: Cambridge University Press.

Ladefoged, P. (1993). *A course in phonetics* (3rd ed.). Fort Worth, TX: Harcourt Brace College Publishers.

Shriberg, L., & Kent, R. (1995). *Clinical phonetics* (3rd ed.). Boston, MA: Allyn & Bacon.

Singh, S., & Singh, K. (1976). *Phonetics: Principles and practices* (3rd ed.). San Diego, CA: Plural Publishing.

Small, L. H. (1999). *Fundamentals of phonetics: A practical guide for students* (3rd ed.). Boston, MA: Allyn & Bacon.

Tiffany, W. R., & Carrell, J. (1977). *Phonetics: Theory and application*. New York, NY: McGraw-Hill.

The Three Rs: Two Vowels and a Consonant

PURPOSE

To introduce you to the consonant [r] and the central vowels [ɝ] and [ɚ].

OBJECTIVES

This chapter will provide you with information regarding:

1. Characteristics of the consonant [r]
2. Characteristics of the two central vowels [ɝ] and [ɚ]
3. Relationship among these three sounds
4. Transcription exercises

THE LETTER *R* AND ITS THREE SOUNDS

Because the orthographic alphabet letter *r* represents three *different* sounds, including the consonant [r] in *radio*, the stressed central vowel [ɝ] in *bird* [bɝd], and the unstressed [ɚ] central vowel in the second syllable of *murder* [mɝdɚ], it makes sense that they should be introduced and discussed together. This approach can help you understand the different contexts in which the alphabet letter *r* and its three different phonetic symbols occur.

But, in reality, there are *four r* symbols to consider! Before 1996, the International Phonetic Association used the [r] symbol for the consonant *r* in such words as *car, radio*, and *right*. In 1996, the association revised the International Phonetic Alphabet (IPA) and changed from using the [r] symbol to using the [ɹ] symbol, referred to as the "turned R," to represent the voiced, dental, or alveolar approximant consonant (#151; IPA, 1999). The turned R symbol has yet to be used much in printed text. Indeed, most phoneticians resist its use. Most of the publications previously printed contain the original [r] symbol, and it seems practical to maintain that symbol. As you read the literature, keep in mind that the [r] and [ɹ] may be used interchangeably in works published after 1996. It takes some time for revisions to occur, particularly in assessment instruments and books. This text uses the original [r] symbol throughout. Note that the [r] as it is currently used represents a "trilled *r*" sound, not the traditional consonant [r] of the past.

All three symbols [r], [ɝ], and [ɚ] contain the "r" sound. For example, the consonant [r] in *ran* [ren], and the two other "r" sounds in the stressed and unstressed syllables such as *murder* [mɝdɚ].

The two different central vowels, the stressed [ɝ] and the unstressed [ɚ], are discussed first, and then the consonant [r] is discussed.

PHONETIC SYMBOLS [ɝ] AND [ɚ]

EXHIBIT 11-1	Phonetic Symbols [ɝ] and [ɚ]	
Phonetic Symbols	[ɝ][ɚ]	[ɝ] [ɚ]
Grapheme Symbols	ir, er, ear, or, urr, ur, yr	
Diacritic Symbols	ǝr, ǝ, ûr, îr	
Phonic Symbol	r	
Sound Class	Central Stressed [ɝ] and Unstressed [ɚ] Vowels	
Tongue Position	Depth: Mid-central Tension: Tense	
Lips	Unrounded	
IPA (1999)	[ɝ] #326 Open, Midcentral, Unrounded [ɚ] #327 R-colored, Midcentral	

How the Sounds Are Produced

The airflow from the lungs activates the vibration of the closed vocal folds (voiced), and the sound enters the oral cavity because the velopharyngeal port is closed. The tip and front of the tongue are raised toward the palate (midcentral) and are positioned behind the alveolar ridge without contact. The sides of the (tense) tongue press against the upper molars or sides of the rear portion of the alveolar ridge in a retracted posture.

For the [ɚ] sound, the tongue is more relaxed and the energy of the sound both in loudness and duration is less than for the [ɝ] sound. The lips are basically unrounded, but there is a degree of lip rounding (**Figure 11-1**).

Commentary

Ladefoged (1993) indicates that [ɝ] cannot be described simply in terms of the features high–low, front–back, and so forth, although it appears to be a midcentral vowel such as [ɜ]. It involves an additional feature called *rhotacization*, which describes the auditory property, the *r*-coloring, of the vowel. In other words, how the vowel sounds. Ladefoged (1993) and Tiffany and Carrell (1977) state that rhotacized vowels are often called *retroflex vowels*, but there are at least two distinct ways in which a rhotacized quality can be produced. A very similar auditory effect occurs even though speakers may use different gestures to produce the sound. For example, some speakers have the tip of the tongue raised, as in a retroflex consonant.

Other speakers keep the tip down and produce a high bunched tongue position. The fact is there is wide variation in tongue posture used in the production of the [ɝ] and [ɚ] sounds.

House (1998) offers some interesting insight, stating that the vowel plus [r] combinations such as [ɪr], [ɛr], [ɑr], [ɔr], [jur], [aɪr], and [aʊr] are often referred to as *centering diphthongs*. She notes that the [jur] as in *pure* [pjur] in formal speech may be pronounced as [pɝ] in everyday conversation and that speaker choice occurs with such words as *fire* as a monosyllabic [faɪr] or bisyllabic [faɪjɚ]. The [ɝ] differs from the consonant [r] in the following ways: (1) the [ɝ] has greater duration, (2) it is a vowel, and (3) it is never voiceless (Calvert, 1986). The lightly stressed or unstressed counterpart of [ɝ] is [ɚ]. In contrast to the [ɝ], during the production of the [ɚ], the tongue is more relaxed and duration is noticeably shorter.

The purpose of this text is to offer an introduction to the study of phonetics. In-depth discussion of the use of the [ɝ] and [ɚ] and all of the extensions, exceptions, and varieties, including the diphthongization of these sounds, is readily available for advance study from other sources.

Different Spellings of the Stressed [ɝ] Sound

Transcribe the following words. Refer to the Key at the right upon completion.

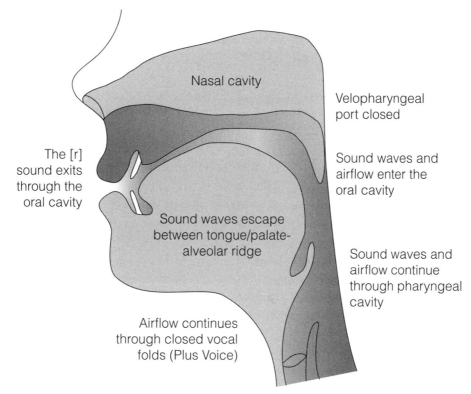

Figure 11-1 [r] production.

Different Spellings							Key
ir	bird	__	girl	__	first	__	bɝd, gɝl, fɝst
	shirk	__	circus	__	sir	__	ʃɝk, sɝkəs, sɝ
ur	burn	__	fur	__	murmur	__	bɝn, fɝ, mɝmɚ
	curb	__	hurry	__			kɝb, hɝi/hɝɪ
er	her	__	fern	__	herd	__	hɝ, fɝn, hɝd
	were	__	camera	__			wɝ, kæmɝə
ear	earth	__	learn	__	earn	__	ɝθ, lɝn, ɝn
or	word	__	worth	__			wɝd, wɝθ
	world	__	work	__			wɝld, wɝk ·
urr	burr	__	purr	__			bɝ, pɝ
our	journey	__	courage	__			dʒɝni, kɝɪdʒ
aur	restaurant	__					rɛstɝɑnt
yr	myrtle	__					mɝtl̩
olo	colonel	__					kɝnəl

Different Spellings of the Unstressed [ɚ] Sound

Transcribe the following words. Refer to the Key at the right upon completion.

Different Spellings				Key
ar	dollar	__	sugar __	dɑlɚ, ʃʊgɚ
ir	confirmation	__		kɑnfɚmeʃən
er	teenager	__		tineɪdʒɚ
ur	murmur	__	surprise __	mɝmɚ, sɚpraɪz
or	opportunity	__	liquor __	ɑpɚtunɪti, lɪkɚ
	information	__		ɪnfɚmeʃən

Different Sounds for the Same Letters of the [ɝ] Sound

Transcribe the following words. Refer to the Key at the right upon completion.

Alphabet Letters	Different Sounds	Words		Key
ir	[ɝ]	first	___	fɝst
	[ɚ]	desire	___	dizaɪɚ
	[aɪ]	iron	___	aɪɝn
ur	[ɝ]	fur	___	fɝ
	[ɚ]	surprise	___	sʌpraɪz
	[u]	uranium	___	jurenijəm
er	[ɝ]	her	___	hɝ
	[ɚ]	suffer	___	sʌfɚ
	[ir]	erase	___	ireɪs
ear	[ɝ]	earn	___	ɝn
	[ɛɪ]	year	___	jɛɪr
or	[ɝ]	word	___	wɝd
	[ɚ]	doctor	___	dɑktɚ
	[oʊr]	order	___	ordɚ
our	[ɝ]	journey	___	dʒɝni
	[aʊ]	hour	___	aʊr/aʊɚ
aur	[ɝ]	restaurant	___	rɛstɝrənt
	[ə]	aurora	___	ərɔrə
ar	[ɚ]	grammar	___	græmɚ
	[ɑr]	art	___	ɑrt

Medial				Key
worm ___		dirt ___		wɝm, dɝt
learn ___		turn ___		lɝn, tɝn
hurt ___		bird ___		hɝt, bɝd
work ___		girl ___		wɝk, gɝl
curl ___		turf ___		kɝl, tɝf
first ___		heard ___		fɝst, hɝd

Final				Key
fur ___		purr ___		fɝ, pɝ
sir ___		her ___		sɝ, hɝ
spur ___		fir ___		spɝ, fɝ
cur ___		blur ___		kɝ, blɝ
recur ___		infer ___		rikɝ, ɪnfɝ
stir ___		burr ___		stɝ, bɝ

Words That Include the Stressed [ɝ] Sound

Transcribe the following words. Refer to the Key at the right upon completion.

Initial				Key
urge ___		early ___		ɝdʒ, ɝli
irk ___		herb ___		ɝk, ɝb
urn ___		earn ___		ɝn, ɝn
Ernest ___		ermine ___		ɝnɛst, ɝmən
erstwhile ___		earth ___		ɝstʍaɪl, ɝθ
urban ___		earnest ___		ɝbən, ɝnɛst

Words That Include the Unstressed [ɚ] Sound

Transcribe the following words. Refer to the Key at the right upon completion.

				Key
answer ___		opportunity ___		ænsɚ, ɑpɚtunɪti
gather ___		brother ___		gæðɚ, brʌðɚ
daughter ___		lower ___		dɑtɚ, lowɚ
labor ___		later ___		leɪbɚ, leɪtɚ
mister ___		teacher ___		mɪstɚ, titʃɚ
liquor ___		neighbors ___		lɪkɚ, neɪbɚz
river ___		energy ___		rɪvɚ, ɛnɚdʒi
summer ___		information ___		sʌmɚ, ɪnfɚmeɪʃən
modern ___		older ___		mɑdɚn, oʊldɚ
remember ___		understand ___		rimɛmbɚ, ʌndɚstænd
junior ___		either ___		dʒunjɚ, iðɚ
sugar ___		November ___		ʃɪgɚ, novɛmbɚ
government ___		soldier ___		gʌvɚnmənt, soldʒɚ
character ___		dinner ___		kɛrɪktɚ, dɪnɚ

Auditory Discrimination

Contrast Minimal Pairs

Pronunciation may differ because of dialect variations. Transcribe the following words.

Refer to the Key at the right upon completion.

[ɝ]	[ʊ]	[ɝ]	[ʌ]	Key
gird ___	good ___	burn ___	bun ___	gɝd, gʊd, bɝn, bʌn
stirred ___	stood ___	hurt ___	hut ___	stɝd, stʊd, hɝt, hʌt
curd ___	could ___	stern ___	stun ___	kɝd, kʊd, stɝn, stʌn
Turk ___	took ___	burrs ___	buzz ___	tɝk, tʊk, bɝz, bʌz
furl ___	full ___	shirk ___	shuck ___	fɝl, fʊl, ʃɝk, ʃʌk
word ___	wood ___	circle ___	suckle ___	wɝd, wʊd, sɝkļ, sʌkļ
shirk ___	shook ___	third ___	thud ___	ʃɝk, ʃʊk, Ɵɝd, Ɵʌd
lurk ___	look ___	girl ___	gull ___	lɝk, lʊk, gɝl, gʌl

[ɝ]	[ɔɪ]	Key
verse ___	voice ___	vɝs, vɔɪs
early ___	oily ___	ɝli, ɔɪli
learn ___	loin ___	lɝn, lɔɪn/loin
sir ___	soy ___	sɝ, sɔɪ/soɪ
verge ___	voyage ___	vɝʤ, vɔɪʤ
curl ___	coil ___	kɝl, kɔɪl/koiļ
hurt ___	Hoyt ___	hɝt, hɔɪt/hoit
burrs ___	boys ___	bɝz, bɔɪz/boiz

[ɝ]	[r]	Key
curried ___	creed ___	kɝid, krid
terrain ___	train ___	tɝeɪn, treɪn
corrode ___	crowed ___	kɝod, kroʊd
beret ___	bray ___	bɝeɪ, breɪ
duress ___	dress ___	dɝɛs, drɛs
thorough ___	throw ___	Ɵɝoʊ, Ɵroʊ
caressed ___	crest ___	kɝɛst, krɛst

Allophonic and Dialect Variations

For the most part, it is not difficult to differentiate the [ɝ] and [r] in United States English (Tiffany & Carrell, 1977).

For example, the glide [r] either initiates or terminates a syllable, as in *rivet* [rɪvɛt] and *before* [bifoʊr]. Notice that it does not produce major resonance or the nucleus of the syllable. The [ɝ] sound obviously functions as the nucleus, as in *early* [ɝli] and *farmer* [fɑrmɚ].

Tiffany and Carrell (1977) indicate that the way the various *r*-colored vowels are used accounts for one of the most distinctive differences among dialects. In general, speakers of Eastern and Southern speech drop their *r*s and replace them with the [3] or schwa sound, as when *murmur* [mɝmɚ] becomes [mɝmə] and *refer* [rɪfɝ] becomes [rɪf3]. Speakers of United States English who do not use the [ɝ] substitute a [3] or a diphthongized [3ɪ] for [ɝ], especially in the Deep South and in areas of New York City, such when *heard* becomes [hoɪd] in a Brooklyn accent (Edwards, 1997). The vowel plus *r* combinations [ɪr], [ɛr], [ær], [ɑr], [ɔr], and [ʊr] are substituted with the [ɝ] as when *far* [fɑr] becomes [fɝ] and *here* [hɪr] becomes [hɝ]. Also, the opposite may occur, as in *learn* [lɑrn] for [lɝn] and *heard* [hɪrd] for [hɝd]. Other examples include the use of [ʌ] in *hurry* [hʌri] and *worry* [wʌri], and *syrup* may be either [sɪrəp] or [sɝəp] (Edwards, 1997; Tiffany & Carrell, 1977).

Nonnative Speaker Pronunciation

The [ɝ] appears to be one of the most easily recognized vowels in the United States English sound system (Tiffany & Carrell, 1977).

Speech-Sound Deviations

The [ɝ] is typically the last sound children learn (Tiffany & Carrell, 1977), and it often gives them great difficulty. For the consonant [r], a [w] substitution is frequent. For the [ɝ] and [ɚ], either [3] or [ə] is substituted. Children may also substitute a labialized or lip-rounded sound such as [u], [ʊ], or [ʌ]. Another type of *r* distortion may occur in children and adults when the [ɝ] takes on an [i] quality and the [r] sounds like a [j].

Summary

The stressed [ɝ] and unstressed [ɚ] are two of the four central vowels. The other two are the stressed [ʌ] as in *up* and unstressed [ə] as in *above* [əbʌv]. The [ɝ] and [ɚ] *r*-like vowels are distinguished from the consonant [r] by their auditory property called rhotacization that makes the sound of the [r] different from the consonant [r] as in (vowel *r*) *bird* [bɝd] and (consonant

r) *repeat* [ripit]. The stressed [ɝ] is used in stressed syllables and in single words. The [ɚ] symbol is used in lesser stressed syllables such as *computer* [kɑmputɚ] and *confirmation* [kɑmfɚmeɪʃən] and in unstressed syllables, as in *verbal* [vɚbɑl]. There are numerous allophonic and dialect variations including substitutions of other vowels. Children develop this sound later and have difficulty with it.

PHONETIC SYMBOLS [r] AND [ɹ]

EXHIBIT 11-2   **Phonetic Symbols [r] and [ɹ]**

$$[r]\ [ɹ]$$

Phonetic Symbols	[r] and [ɹ]
Grapheme Symbol	r
Diacritic Symbol	r
Phonic Symbol	r Cognate: None
Homorganic	Lingua-Palatal [ʃ], [ʒ], [j], [h]
Sound Class	Consonant
Tongue Position	Height: Mid Depth: Central Tension: Plus
IPA (1999)	[ɹ] #151 Voiced Dental or Alveolar Approximant

How the Sound Is Produced

The [r] can be produced in two ways. The more common method involves raising of the tip of the tongue (lingua) and curling it back in a retroflexed position toward the anterior portion of the palate (palatal). The sides of the tongue may touch the upper molars and the alveolar ridge but generally do not contact the palate. The second method produces the [r] with the sides of the tongue against the upper molars, the front of the tongue raised toward the palate with the tip neutral or in a downward position, and the blade of the tongue (lingua) closely approximating the hard palate (palatal). In both methods, the velopharyngeal port is closed and the voiced (voicing) air stream escapes between the tongue and the palate–alveolar ridge and exits through the oral cavity.

Different Spellings of the [r] Sound

Transcribe the following words. Refer to the Key at the right upon completion.

Different Spellings			Key
r	rose ___ troupe ___ through ___		roʊz, trup, θru
	oar ___ surprise ___		ɔr, sɝpraɪz
rr	borrow ___		bɑroʊ
rh	rhyme ___ rhythm ___		raɪm, rɪðəm/rɪðm
wr	wrote ___ write ___ wroth ___		roʊt, raɪt, rɔθ
rrh	catarrh ___		kətɑr
rt	mortgage ___ sort ___ part ___		morgɪdʒ, sort, pɑrt
rps	corps ___		kər

Different Sounds for the *r* Letter

The alphabet letter *r* represents both the consonant [r] sound and the *r* that functions as a vowel. The *r* letter that functions as a vowel appears as two different symbols depending on whether it appears in the stressed or unstressed position in the word:

■ [r] Consonant *free* [fri], *ride* [raɪd], *hair* [hɛr], *tear* [tɪr]

■ [ɝ] Vowel *fur* [fɝ] and *earnest* [ɝnɛst] (stressed position)

■ [ɚ] Vowel *mother* [mʌðɚ] and *labor* [leɪbɚ] (unstressed position)

Rules for Spelling and Pronunciation of the [r] Sound

I. The *r* in the consonant context is pronounced [r] as in *red*.

2. The *h* in *rhythm* and the *w* in *write* are both silent.

3. The *r* is usually pronounced [r] when it is in the initial position of a word: *ripe*. In the medial position, as in *corn*, and in the final position in words such as *car, for, chair*, the *r* is pronounced mainly because the vowel has already been designated.

4. The consonant [r] is used in blend combinations as in *train, broke*.

There are two vowels with [r] qualities. The accented [ɝ], as in *fur* and *bird*, and the unaccented [ɚ], as in *mother*. Spelling combinations for the vowel [ɝ] quality in the accented position include *ur: turn; ir: bird; or: word; ear: heard; er: herd;* and *yr: Myrtle*. The *ir: elixir; our: glamour; re: centre; ure: pleasure;* and *yr: martyr* combinations occur in the unaccented position.

Words That Include the [r] or [ɹ] Sound

The [r] sound occurs in all three positions, initial, medial, and final. Transcribe the following words. Refer to the Key at the right upon completion.

Initial		Medial		Final ·		Key
reap	—	very	—	or	—	rip, vɛri, ɔr/or
rose	—	borrow	—	are	—	roʊz, bɑroʊ, ɑr
read	—	around	—	chair	—	rid, əraʊnd, tʃɛr
rate	—	orange	—	more	—	raɪt, ɔrɛnʒ, moʊr
rabbit	—	arrive	—	your	—	ræbɪt, əraɪv, jɔr/jɑr
reed	—	wearing	—	near	—	rid, wɛrɪŋ, nɛr
rock	—	terrible	—	bar	—	rɑk, tɛrɪbl̩, bɑr
rhythm	—	story	—	fore	—	rɪðm, stori, foʊr
robe	—	arouse	—	dear	—	roʊb, əraʊz, dɛr

Initial Blend		Final Blend		Key
crack	—	fears	—	kræk, fɛrz
brow	—	carts	—	braʊ, kɑrts
grow	—	parts	—	groʊ, pɑrts
drive	—	horn	—	draɪv, hɔrn
press	—	bark	—	prɛs, bɑrk
friend	—	marks	—	frɛnd, mɑrks
strain	—			straɪn
scream	—			skrim
thrust	—			θrʌst

Auditory Discrimination

Contrast Minimal Pairs

Transcribe the following words. Refer to the Key at the right upon completion.

[r]		[w]		[r]		[l]		Key
rail	—	wail	—	grow	—	glow	—	reɪl, weɪl, groʊ, gloʊ
red	—	wed	—	rain	—	lain	—	rɛd, wɛd, reɪn, leɪn
train	—	twain	—	ram	—	lamb	—	treɪn, tweɪn, ræm, læm
run	—	won	—	rare	—	lair	—	rʌn, wʌn, rɛr, lær
rest	—	west	—	crowd	—	cloud	—	rɛst, wɛst, kraʊd, klaʊd
rate	—	wait	—	pray	—	play	—	reɪt, weɪt, preɪ, pleɪ
array	—	away	—	brew	—	blew	—	əreɪ, əweɪ, bru, blu
wreak	—	week	—	correct	—	collect	—	wrik, wik, kərɛkt, kəlɛkt

[r]		[ɝ]		Key
dress	—	duress	—	drɛs, dɝɛs
creed	—	curried	—	krid, kɝid
throw	—	thorough	—	θroʊ, θɝoʊ
crowed	—	corrode	—	kroʊd, kɝoʊd
crest	—	caressed	—	krɛst, kɝɛst
bray	—	beret	—	breɪ, bɝeɪ

[r]		[j]		Key
crew	—	cue	—	kru, kju
rung	—	young	—	rʌŋ, jʌŋ
roar	—	yore	—	rɔr, jɔr

ram _____	yam _____	ræm, jæm
Ruth _____	youth _____	ruθ, juθ
rear _____	year _____	rɛr, jɛr
rue _____	you _____	ru, ju
raw _____	yaw _____	rɑ, jɑ

Allophonic and Dialect Variations

The [r] sound may be devoiced and become a fricative [r] in a voiceless blend as when *train* [traɪn] becomes [ʧraɪn] (Edwards, 1997). It also becomes a fricative following the [d] sound, as in *drop, dry*. The [t] and [d] are lingua-alveolar **cognates**. The [r] is voiced when it initiates a syllable and when it is preceded by a voiced consonant as in *bread, grin*, and *dream* in the same syllable (Calvert, 1986). It is given partially without voice, especially near the point of juncture, when it is preceded by a voiceless consonant in the same syllable, as in *prince, tree, cream*, and *free*, except in clusters, as in *scratch, sprint, strong* where the stop is unreleased.

In Eastern and Southern American English, when the [s] sound is in the postvocalic position or is followed by [a] or [ɑ], the final [r] is substituted, as when *floor* [flour] becomes [floʊə], or is omitted, as when *car* [kɑr] becomes [kɑ] (Edwards, 1997; Small, 1999). It is also omitted in African American speech, as when *berry* [bɛri] becomes [bɛɪ] and *door* [doʊr] becomes [doʊ]. In blends, as when *professor* [proʊfɛsɚ] becomes [pɚfɛsə], the intrusive [r] appears in Eastern American English. Edwards (1997) gives the example of *idea of it* [aɪ'dirʌv ɪt]. In New England and Southern speech, the General American preconsonantal [r] as in *park* or *first* and the final [r] as in *bar* or *more* are either omitted or replaced by a vowel (Calvert, 1986) .

Carrell and Tiffany (1960) indicate that the reason for the complexity of the United States English [r] and [ɝ] sounds is that they represent an evolutionary weakening of a strong trilled sound believed to be the forerunner of the present glide. The historically older sound, still standard in many languages and dialects, has weakened to a single tap in certain British dialects and to no obstruction at all in most American dialects.

Speech-Sound Deviations

Children normally acquire the [r] sound between the ages of 3 and 6 years (Sander, 1972). The most common problem with the [r] sound involves labialization (Calvert, 1986; Edwards, 1997). This results in the substitution of the [w] glide or, occasionally, the [d] sound. For reasons not entirely clear, the [r] sound and the *r*-colored vowels [ɝ] and [ɚ] appear to be among the most difficult sounds for children to learn, and children may make such errors as when *Peter Rabbit* [pitɚ ræbɪt] becomes [pitə wæbət] (Carrell & Tiffany, 1960).

Nonnative Speaker Pronunciation

The United States English [r] poses genuine difficulties for nonnative speakers, almost without exception (Edwards, 1997). Substitution of the flap *r* or trilled *r* occurs when the lips are not slightly rounded but rather spread in an unrounded posture. Some foreign speakers may use a one-tap trill of the British intervocalic [r], which may make *very* [vɛrɪ] or [vɛri] sound like [vɛdɪ]. Asians may produce an [r] sound with the tongue point touching behind the alveolar ridge, giving the impression of an [l] substitution. This is because the [r] is like a glide as well as the [l] sound. Nonnative speakers have a multitude of problems with the [r] sounds (Carrell & Tiffany, 1960). The main reason is that many modern languages have *r*s that differ conspicuously from the United States English [r] sound, which should be pronounced as a glide rather than as a fricative, tap, or trill, which characteristically are represented by the letter *r* in other languages.

The following seven languages spoken prominently in the United States do not have the [r] sound or its allophonic variation (devoicing, etc.) but include the trill *r*: Arabic, tap-flap *r*; Hindi, alveolar or retroflex; Japanese, flap-postalveolar; German, French, uvular, fricative *r*; Portuguese, tap *r*, alveolar; Korean and many other Asian sound systems do not include the [r] sound.

Summary

The [r] is one of the four oral-resonant sounds. The others are [l], [j], and [w]. It does not have a cognate and is **homorganic** (lingua-palatal) with [ʃ], [ʒ], [h], and [j]. It is consistent in its spelling; however, the *r* letter also represents the *r*-sounding vowels [ɝ] (stressed) and [ɚ] (unstressed). In certain contexts, the [r] sound becomes devoiced, particularly in blends such as *br-, gr-*, and so forth. There are considerable dialect differences and nonnative speaker difficulties. The [r] is almost unique to United States English in comparison to other sound systems of world languages, although variations in the form of a trill or flap *r* occur in many of these other sound systems. Speech defects in children include substitutions of other vowels and consonants and/or deletion of the sound. It is one of the more difficult sounds to remediate.

The contemporary phonetic symbol [ɹ] has replaced the traditional [r] symbol, according to the International

Phonetic Association. During the transition period, either symbol may appear.

Transcription Exercises

Transcribe the following words. Refer to the Key at the right upon completion.

[r]

				Key
1. rake	_____	6. resist	_____	reɪk, rɪsɪst
2. star	_____	7. repeat	_____	stɑr, ripit
3. rough	_____	8. fear	_____	rʌf, fɪr
4. hair	_____	9. wreck	_____	hɛr, rɛk
5. raft	_____	10. run	_____	ræft, rʌn

[ɝ]

				Key
1. curve	_____	11. burst	_____	kɝv, bɝst
2. heard	_____	12. were	_____	hɝd, wɝ
3. term	_____	13. irk	_____	tɝm, ɝk
4. colonel	_____	14. bird	_____	kɝnəl, bɝd
5. person	_____	15. early	_____	pɝsən, ɝlI
6. hurt	_____	16. word	_____	hɝt, wɝd
7. purr	_____	17. pearl	_____	pɝ, pɝl
8. work	_____	18. cur	_____	wɝk, kɝ
9. sir	_____	19. insert	_____	sɝ, ɪnsɝt
10. her	_____	20. worse	_____	hɝ, wɝs

[ɚ]

				Key
1. speaker	_____	11. worker	_____	spikɚ, wɝkɚ
2. sister	_____	12. opportunity	_____	sɪstɚ, ɑpɚtunətɪ
3. upper	_____	13. murder	_____	ʌpɚ, mɝdɚ
4. rector	_____	14. disorder	_____	rɛktɚ, dɪsɔrdɚ
5. suffered	_____	15. winter	_____	sʌfɚd, wɪntɚ
6. dipper	_____	16. rubber	_____	dɪpɚ, rʌbɚ
7. river	_____	17. under	_____	rɪvɚ, ʌndɚ
8. proper	_____	18. number	_____	prɑpɚ, nʌmbɚ
9. perturb	_____	19. sleeper	_____	pɚtɝb, slipɚ
10. farmer	_____	20. order	_____	fɑrmɚ, ɔrdɚ

NOW FOR THE *REAL* CHALLENGE: THE *R* POTPOURRI!

The following words include one of the *r* sounds discussed in this chapter. Transcribe the following words. Refer to the Key at the right upon completion.

Key

1. urge ____ 2. doctor ____ 3. parents ____ ɝdʒ, dɑktɚ, pɛrənts

4. teacher ____ 5. curb ____ 6. steer ____ titʃɚ, kɝb, stɛr

7. art ____ 8. urn ____ 9. upper ____ ɑrt, ɝn, ʌpɚ

10. foreign ____ 11. summer ____ 12. sir ____ fɔrɪn, sʌmɚ, sɝ

13. lower ____ 14. fear ____ 15. work ____ loʊɚ, fɛr, wɝk

16. sugar ____ 17. berry ____ 18. circus ____ ʃɪgɚ, bɛri, sɝkəs

19. gather ____ 20. Gary ____ 21. dipper ____ gæðɚ, gɛri, dɪpɚ

22. burn ____ 23. tourist ____ 24. junior ____ bɝn, toʊrəst, dʒunjɚ

25. earth ____ 26. fir ____ 27. star ____ ɝθ, fɝ, stɑr

28. her ____ 29. answer ____ 30. arrow ____ hɝ, ænsɚ, ɛroʊ

31. hurry ____ 32. modern ____ 33. forest ____ hɝɪ, mɑdɚn, fɔrəst

34. winter ____ 35. herald ____ 36. bird ____ wɪntɚ, hɛrold, bɝd

37. forum ____ 38. infer ____ 39. world ____ fɔrəm, ɪnfɚ, wɝld

SUMMARY

The United States English vowels and diphthongs discussed in this text are as follows:

Long Vowels

1. [e] and [eɪ] long ā as in *rotate* [roʊtet] and *rotation* [roteɪʃən]
2. [i] long vowel ē as in *beet* [bit]
3. [aɪ] long vowel ī as in *ice* [aɪs]
4. [o] and [oʊ] long ō as in *rotation* [roteɪʃən] and *ocean* [oʊʃən]
5. [u] and [ju] long ū as in *do* [du] and *you* [ju]

Short Vowels

1. [æ] short vowel ă as in *ask* [æsk]
2. [ɛ] short vowel ĕ as in *bed* [bɛd]
3. [ɪ] short vowel ĭ as in *it* [ɪt]
4. [ɑ] short vowel ŏ as in *stop* [stɑp]
5. [ʌ] and [ə] short vowel ŭ as in *above* [əbʌv]

Other Vowels and Diphthongs

1. [ʊ] as in *book* [bʊk]
2. [ɔ] as in *caught* [kɔt]
3. [ɔɪ] as in *boil* [bɔɪl]
4. [aʊ] as in *out* [aʊt]
5. [ɝ] and [ɚ] as in *murder* [mɝdɚ]

There is a total of 14 vowels and 4 diphthongs. In the vowel quadrilateral matrix, there are five front vowels: [i], [ɪ], [e], [ɛ], and [æ]; four central vowels: [ʌ], [ə], [ɝ], and [ɚ]; and five back vowels: [u], [ʊ], [o], [ɔ], and [ɑ].

One function of vowels and diphthongs is to serve as the nucleus of a syllable. In most contexts, they are abutted by consonants such as the series of consonant-vowel-consonant (CVC) in the word *pet*.

REFERENCES

Calvert, D. R. (1986). *Descriptive phonetics*. New York, NY: Thieme Medical Publishers.

Carrell, J., & Tiffany, W. (1960). *Phonetics: Theory and application to speech improvement*. New York, NY: McGraw-Hill.

Edwards, H. T. (1997). *Applied phonetics* (2nd ed.). San Diego, CA: College-Hill Press.

House, L. (1998). *Introductory phonetics and phonology*. Mahwah, NJ: Lawrence Erlbaum.

International Phonetic Association. (1999). *Handbook of the International Phonetic Association*. Cambridge, England: Cambridge University Press.

Ladefoged, P. (1993). *A course in phonetics* (3rd ed.). Fort Worth, TX: Harcourt Brace College Publishers.

Sander, E. (1972). When are speech sounds learned? *Journal of Speech and Hearing Disorders, 37*, 55–63.

Small, L. H. (1999). *Fundamentals of phonetics: A practical guide for students* (3rd ed.). Boston, MA: Allyn & Bacon.

Tiffany, W. R., & Carrell, J. (1977). *Phonetics: Theory and application*. New York, NY: McGraw-Hill.

United States English Consonants

PURPOSE

To introduce you to the United States English consonants.

OBJECTIVES

This chapter will provide you with information regarding:

1. The identification of the stop consonants
2. The identification of the fricative consonants
3. The identification of the affricate consonants
4. A summary chart of the characteristics of the United States English consonants according to the phonetic description and the International Phonetic Alphabet description
5. General allophonic variations of consonants

BASIC CHARACTERISTICS: POINT OF REFERENCE

Just as vowels have features that distinguish one from another, so do consonants. Unlike vowels that are identified by their high to low, front to back orientation, lip rounding, and tongue tension, the 25 consonants are referenced by several other methods. Two of these methods are (1) the basic traditional descriptors of (a) manner in which the airflow is modified; (b) placement

of the articulators; and (c) voicing (plus or minus) (Stockwell & Minkova, 2001); and (2) the descriptors developed by the International Phonetic Association. These two methods are described in this chapter.

BASIC PHONETIC METHOD

Each phoneme (sound) is distinguished from all others by a bundle of physiologically and acoustically determined features that make it distinctive (Faircloth & Faircloth, 1973). The basic phonetic features of a phoneme result from the specific articulatory adjustments that modify the breath stream to produce an acoustic result identifiable as a particular speech sound. These primary or basic phonetic features include (1) placement of the articulators; (2) manner in which the airflow is modified; and (3) voicing, plus or minus voice.

Manner of Airflow Modification

For the production of the consonants, the airflow from the lungs is modified in five different ways:

1. *Stop and then release of airflow.* This occurs with the six *stop consonants* [p], [b], [t], [d], [k], and [g]. Notice that as these sounds are produced, there is a blockage of the airflow and a buildup of air pressure to one degree or another, and then a release of that air pressure.

2. *Constriction of airflow.* This occurs with the 10 *fricative consonants* [s], [z], [f], [v], [h], [ʍ] or [hw] as in *when* [ʍɛn], the voiced *th* [ð] as in *the* [ðʌ], and the unvoiced *th* [Θ] as in *three* [Θri], the *sh* [ʃ] as in *shy* [ʃaɪ], and the [ʒ] as in *azure* [æʒjɚ]. Notice that when these sounds are produced there is a "continuance" of the airflow, but it is constricted in one manner or another, as in the production of the [f] and *sh* [ʃ].

3. *Stop followed by a constriction of airflow.* This occurs with the two *affricate consonants* so named because the airflow progresses from a sudden stop to a release, and the remaining airflow to complete the sequence is constricted by the different articulators. The affricates are the combination of [t] and [ʃ] that results in the sound *ch* [ʧ] as in *church*, and the combination of [d] and [ʒ], also considered one sound, as the initial sound in *jam* [ʤæm].

4. *Oral cavity resonation.* The airflow and sound waves are modified by the surfaces of the oral cavity with minimal interference by the articulators. The four *oral resonant consonants* are [l], [r], [w], and [j] as in *yell* [jɛl].

5. *Nasal cavity resonation.* The airflow and sound waves are modified mainly by the surfaces of the nasal cavity. The three *nasal resonant consonants* are [n], [m], and *ng* [ŋ] as in *sing* [sɪŋ].

Table 12-1 lists the consonants and the different ways the airflow is modified to produce the individual sounds.

Placement of the Articulators

Placement of the various articulators distinguishes several consonants from one another. Some consonants have the *same* placement but different features

of manner of airflow modification or voicing. When the placement is the same, the word *homorganic* is used to describe this common feature. The following placement of the articulators is used for the consonants:

1. *Lingua-alveolar (tongue and upper gum ridge).* The eight sounds for which contact is made between the tongue and upper gum ridge are [t], [d], [s], [z], [ʧ], [ʤ], [l], and [n]. Note that the [t], [d], [l], and [n] use approximately the same placement of the tongue on the upper gum ridge. This is an example of the homorganic feature of the same placement of the articulators.

2. *Linguadental (tongue and teeth).* The two sounds for which contact is made between the tongue and *upper* front teeth are the voiceless *th* [Θ] in *thin* [Θɪn] and the voiced *th* [ð] in *the* [ðʌ]. Many speakers also produce the [s] and [z] as linguadentals with the tip of the tongue embedded behind the *lower* front teeth.

3. *Linguapalatal (tongue and palate).* The five sounds for which contact is made between the tongue and different areas of the palate are the *sh* [ʃ] in *shy* [ʃaɪ], [ʒ] as in *azure* [æʒjɚ], [r], [j] in *yell* [jɛl], and [h]. The placement of the articulators for [h] is actually linguapalatal, lingua-velar and should be considered as such.

4. *Lingua-velar (tongue and velum).* In addition to the [h], four other sounds are considered lingua-velar: [k], [g], [ŋ], and [sɪŋ]. Two sounds, the [w] and *wh* [ʍ] in *white* [ʍaɪt], have dual placement of the articulators in the lingua-velar and bilabial (two lips) positions.

5. *Bilabials (two lips).* The three sounds for which contact is made between the two lips are the [p],

TABLE 12-1	Categorical Summary According to Manner of Airflow Modification
Manner of Modification of Airflow	**Consonants**
6 Stops	[p], [b], [t], [d], [k], [g]
10 Fricatives	[f], [v], [s], [z], [Θ], [ð], [h], [ʍ], [ʃ], [ʒ]
2 Affricates	[ʧ], [ʤ]
4 Oral Resonants	[l], [r], [j], [w]
3 Nasal Resonants	[m], [n], [ŋ]

TABLE 12-2	Placement of the Articulators (Homorganic)

Placement of Articulators	Consonants
3 Bilabial	[b], [p], [m]
8 Lingua-alveolar	[t], [d], [l], [n], [s], [z], [dʒ], [tʃ]
6 Lingua-velar	[k], [g], [ŋ], [h], [w], [ʍ]
4 Labiodental	[f], [v], and linguapalatal [tʃ], [dʒ]
5 Linguapalatal	[ʃ], [h], [ʒ], [r], [j] bilabial
4 Linguadental	[θ], [ð], [s], [z]

Note: Alternative placement for [s] and [z] is indicated as lingua-alveolar or linguadental. In the linguadental position, the tongue tip is lowered behind the bottom front teeth instead of elevated and making contact with the alveolar ridge.

[b], and [m]. As mentioned earlier, the [w] and [ʍ] also involve the two lips.

6. *Labiodental (lower lip and upper teeth).* The two labiodental sounds are [f] and [v] for which contact is made between the lower lip and upper front teeth. The [s] and [z], as noted previously, are also produced as labiodentals by speakers who lower the tip of the tongue (labio) behind the inside bottom of the lower teeth (dental).

Table 12-2 groups the consonants according to placement of the articulators.

Voicing

When the vocal folds are closed together (abducted), voicing is produced and the sound waves continue to be acted on by the articulators. When the vocal folds are opened (adducted), no sound waves are produced and the airflow moves unobstructed through the glottis (open space) of the larynx. When a pair of sounds such as [t] and [d] share the common features of placement of the articulators (linguadental) and manner of airflow modification (stops) but *differ* in voicing, they are called a **cognate pair**. The following sets of sounds each share the same placement and manner but differ in voicing. To assist you in understanding this concept, begin by producing the [v] sound and then "cut off" the voice and you will automatically move into the [f] sound: *vvvvvvvvvvffffffff.* Same placement and manner, different voicing feature. **Table 12-3** shows how the consonants are categorized as voiced or voiceless.

TABLE 12-3	Voicing Characteristics of Consonants

Cognate Pairs		*Noncognate Sounds*	
Voice (+)	Voice (−)	Voice (+)	Voice (−)
[b]	[p]	[m]	[ʍ]
[d]	[t]	[n]	[h]
[g]	[k]	[ŋ]	
[z]	[s]	[l]	
[ð] the	[θ] thin	[r]	
[v]	[f]	[j] *yell*	[jɛl]
[dʒ] jam	[tʃ] chin	[w]	
[ʒ] azure		[ʃ] ship	

Table 12-4 lists the three basic features of United States English consonants grouped according to (1) placement of articulators, (2) manner of modification of airflow, and (3) voicing.

TABLE 12-4	Summary of the Basic Phonetic Features of Consonants

Consonant	Placement of Articulators	Manner of Modification of Airflow	Voicing
1. [p]	Bilabial	Stop	Minus
2. [b]	Bilabial	Stop	Plus
3. [t]	Lingua-alveolar	Stop	Minus
4. [d]	Lingua-alveolar	Stop	Plus
5. [k]	Lingua-velar	Stop	Minus
6. [g]	Lingua-velar	Stop	Plus
7. [f]	Labiodental	Fricative	Minus
8. [v]	Labiodental	Fricative	Plus
9. [s]	Lingua-alveolar or linguadental	Fricative	Minus
10. [z]	Lingua-alveolar or linguadental	Fricative	Plus
11. [ʃ]	Linguapalatal	Fricative	Minus
12. [ʒ]	Linguapalatal	Fricative	Plus
13. [Θ]	Linguadental	Fricative	Minus
14. [ð]	Linguadental	Fricative	Plus
15. [h]	Linguapalatal *and* lingua-velar	Fricative	Minus
16. [ʍ]	Lingua-velar *and* bilabial	Fricative	Minus
17. [ʧ]	Lingua-alveolar *to* linguapalatal	Affricative	Minus
18. [ʤ]	Lingua-alveolar *to* linguapalatal	Affricative	Plus
19. [l]	Lingua-alveolar	Oral resonant	Plus
20. [r]	Linguapalatal	Oral resonant	Plus
21. [j]	Linguapalatal	Oral resonant	Plus
22. [w]	Lingua-velar *and* bilabial	Oral resonant	Plus
23. [m]	Bilabial	Nasal resonant	Plus
24. [n]	Lingua-alveolar	Nasal resonant	Plus
25. [ŋ]	Lingua-velar	Nasal resonant	Plus

INTERNATIONAL PHONETIC ASSOCIATION

The International Phonetic Association uses similar descriptors for United States English consonant sounds, the International Phonetic Alphabet (IPA). The latest revision (updated 1996) of the symbols and descriptors is shown in **Table 12-5**, where the consonants are listed in numerical order with their coordinate identification number, symbol name, and description.

Although widely used and generally accepted, the IPA has not always found favor among scholarly phoneticians. For example, Steton (1951) states:

> In spite of its provisions and the fact that it is the basis of phonics, the International Phonetic Alphabet (IPA) is an unsatisfactory collection of symbols. It was thrown together when the problem of phonetics was believed to be the determination of a fixed position for each sound and speech was thought of as a series of such sounds.

Steton indicates that the fundamental differentiation of vowel and consonant is not recognized and that there is no distinction between compound consonants with a single syllable function and abutting consonants that function in two different syllables.

A sample comparison in **Table 12-6** gives (1) basic traditional method (a) manner in which the airflow is modified, (b) placement of the articulators, and (c) voicing; and (2) International Phonetic Alphabet.

You should become aware of the different descriptions of United States English consonants and the settings in which they are used.

GENERAL ARTICULATION VARIATIONS

In discussion of the consonants in the following chapters, description of allophonic and dialect variations is useful for each specific sound and its variations in the production. In addition, some general placement variations occur as a result of the point of articulation, which might affect a "cluster" of consonants in the same manner. The bilabials [p] and [b] and the nasal [m] make contact with the lower lip as the articulator and the upper lip as the point of articulation. The placement may actually become labiodental when it comes before [f] or [v]. For example, produce the [p] in *cupful* and *rupture*, the [m] in *comfort* and *compass, symphony* and

sympathy, and the [b] in *obvious* and *obnoxious*. Bilabial consonants tend to become labiodental when they are followed immediately by a labiodental consonant. Another alternate change may occur with the addition of a sound such as the addition of [p] in com*p*fort and sym*p*hony.

Notice the slight or obvious difference in the placement of the tip of the tongue in the sound context of the italicized sounds: *bid* and *width, at bat* and *at that, esteem* and *esthetic, ten* and *tenth, is it* and *is that*. Some of these sounds may occur at a more postalveolar position of a word. Also compare the placement of the [n] when it precedes the [tʃ] and [dʒ] sounds, as in *branch* and *lunge* to *tent* and *lend*.

The lateral consonant [l] has two different placements. The "light" [l] is produced with the front of the tongue high in the mouth and the back of the tongue low. A "dark" [l] is made with the back of the tongue raised; the center is low and the front of the tongue may be raised. The variation depends mostly on the position of the [l] in a syllable and only partly on what kind of phoneme follows. Notice the slight difference in the placement of the [l] in such words as *leaf, feel, feeling, simple, clean*, and *milk*.

The [k], [g], and [ŋ] vary in articulation from a more frontal placement (palatal or prevelar) to a more back (velar) position depending on the influence of the placement of the preceding vowel. For example, alternate a front and back vowel context and notice the difference in the effect they have on the degree of velarization of the [k], [g], and [ŋ] in *lick:look, cool:kill, dig:dog, geese:goose, sing:song*.

The [r] may take on a "friction-like" characteristic in such consonant clusters as *drain, train, strain*. The [t] and [d] are assimilated to [r] by moving backward along the horizontal axis of the oral chamber, and thus the change from a frictionless to a fricative-like [r] sound is produced. It is interesting to note the variation that occurs in lip shape of a consonant as the following vowel influences roundness of the lips. Notice the "roundness" or "unroundness" of the lips for the [n] sound in the following vowel context: *noose:neice, too:tea, goose:geese, doom:deem*. Such lip roundness also occurs with [w] as in *twin:tin*.

In most contexts, the [l], [r], and [w] are considered *voiced* consonants. However, notice what happens to the voicing feature in the following contexts: the [l] in *blade* and *glass* has more voicing to it than in *play, class*, and *slow* as a result of the voiceless feature of the preceding sounds [b] and [g]. Likewise, the [r] in *crazy*

TABLE 12-5 **International Phonetic Association Depiction of United States English Consonants**

IPA Number	Symbol	Symbol Name	Phonetic Description
101	[p]	Lowercase P	Voiceless, bilabial plosive
102	[b]	Lowercase B	Voiced, bilabial plosive
103	[t]	Lowercase T	Voiceless dental or alveolar plosive
104	[d]	Lowercase D	Voiced dental or alveolar plosive
109	[k]	Lowercase K	Voiceless velar plosive
110	[g]	Open-tail G	Voiced velar plosive
114	[m]	Lowercase M	Voiced bilabial nasal
116	[n]	Lowercase N	Voiced dental or alveolar nasal
119	[ŋ]	Eng	Voiced velar nasal
128	[f]	Lowercase F	Voiceless labiodental fricative
129	[v]	Lowercase V	Voiced labiodental fricative
130	[θ]	Theta	Voiceless dental fricative
131	[ð]	Eth	Voiced dental fricative
132	[s]	Lowercase S	Voiceless alveolar fricative
133	[z]	Lowercase Z	Voiced alveolar fricative
134	[ʃ]	Esh	Voiceless postalveolar fricative
135	[ʒ]	Ezh; Tailed Z	Voiced postalveolar fricative
146	[h]	Lowercase H	Voiceless glottal fricative
151	[ɹ]	Turned R	Voiced dental or alveolar approximant (*Note*: the [ɹ] symbol has replaced the [r] symbol and to adhere strictly to the IPA, the [ɹ] should be used.)
153	[j]	Lowercase J	Voiced palatal approximant
155	[l]	Lowercase L	Voiced dental or alveolar lateral approximant
169	[ʍ]	Turned W	Voiceless labial-velar fricative
170	[w]	Lowercase W	Voiced labial-velar approximant
213	[tʃ]	T-esh ligature	Voiceless postalveolar affricate
214	[dʒ]	D-esh ligature	Voiced postalveolar affricate

TABLE 12-6	Sample of Two Different Methods to Describe the United States English Consonants	

Consonant	Basic Description (Traditional)	IPA
[ʃ]	Voiceless Linguapalatal Fricative	Voiceless Postalveolar Fricative
[n]	Lingua-alveolar Nasal resonant alveolar Voiced	Dental orvoiced nasal
[h]	Lingua-velar Voiceless	Glottal Voiceless

and *try* has less voicing than the [r] in *gravy* and *dry*. Which of the following words have a more voiceless [w] sound: *Gwen, dwindle, queen, swell,* or *twin*?

Stop consonants are noted for three phases, onset, hold, and release of the airflow. Produce the following stops and note these phases: [p], [b], [t], [d], [k], and [g]. Now produce these sounds in the following contexts and notice how vague these phases may become: *caption, uptown, rubdown, nightgown, meatball,* and *actor.* There is only one onset and release in "combined consonants" such as *ten nights, bad day, unknown,* and *ripe peach.* Contrast this hold phase with the separate holds in compound words such as *bookcase* and *homemade* and cognate pairs (same placement and airflow modification, different voicing): *round tire, soup bowl, five fingers.*

You should note that variations in the production of consonants can occur in placement of the articulators, liprounding, onset and release, and duration. Such variations do not change the recognition of the sound by a listener, but there is some allophonic difference in the overall production as a result of these variations.

SUMMARY

You need to understand at least two basic principles. One, not all phoneticians use the same descriptors or method to identify the United States English consonants. Second, you need to have a working knowledge and understanding of the terminology used by different phoneticians to see the relationship of the various terms and the possible settings for their use. Such differences of terminology exist both in printed research materials and in the clinical application of phonetics.

Ideally, everyone would use the same descriptors, but unfortunately not everyone comes from the same orientation. Lengthy debates among professional phoneticians occur over the terms used to describe a sound. In many instances, a majority of scholars, rather than a consensus of the whole group of these phonetic scholars, determine the end results.

Skill-Building Activity

Fill in the blanks for the 25 consonant sounds in the matrix. Place a + or – mark next to the phonetic symbol to indicate plus or minus voicing.

Symbol	Placement	Manner	Voicing
[b]			
[d]			
[f]			
[g]			
[h]			
[j]			
[k]			
[l]			
[m]			
[n]			
[p]			
[r]			
[s]			
[t]			
[v]			
[w]			
[z]			

[θ]	_____	_____	_____
[ð]	_____	_____	_____
[ʃ]	_____	_____	_____
[ʒ]	_____	_____	_____
[tʃ]	_____	_____	_____
[dʒ]	_____	_____	_____
[ʍ]	_____	_____	_____
[ŋ]	_____	_____	_____

Note: Alternative placement for [s] and [z] is indicated as lingua-alveolar or linguadental. In the linguadental position, the tongue tip is lowered behind the bottom front teeth instead of elevated and making contact with the alveolar ridge.

REFERENCES

Faircloth, S. R. & Faircloth, M. A. (1973). *Phonetic science, a program of instruction.* Englewood Cliff, NJ: Prentice Hall.

International Phonetic Association. (1999). *Handbook of the International Phonetic Association.* Cambridge, England: Cambridge: University Press.

Steton, R. H. (1951). *Motor phonetics.* Amsterdam: North-Holland Publishing Company.

Stockwell, R., & Minkova, D. (2001). *English words: History and structure.* Cambridge, England: Cambridge University Press.

Familiar Phonetic Symbols: Stop Consonants Analysis and Transcription

PURPOSE

To provide an introduction to the six stop consonants that use the same symbols as the alphabet letters and to transcribe these phonetic symbols.

OBJECTIVES

This chapter will provide you with information regarding:

1. The identification of and description of how the United States English stop consonants are produced

2. Different spellings for each stop sound and different sounds for each of the corresponding orthographic letters

3. Rules for spelling and pronunciation of each sound

4. Various contexts in which each sound occurs

5. Examples of cognates and other minimal pairs for auditory discrimination

6. Examples of allophonic variations, dialect differences, and nonnative speaker difficulties

7. Normal development and disordered production of each sound

8. Phonetic transcription exercises throughout the chapter and self-quiz

IDENTIFICATION OF STOP CONSONANTS

The stop consonant phonemes of United States English speech are the following cognate pairs:

Voiceless	Voiced	Placement
[p]	[b]	Bilabial
[t]	[d]	Lingua-alveolar
[k]	[g]	Lingua-velar

In addition to being called *stops*, the term *plosives* or *aspirates* are also associated with these sounds. Some phoneticians include the affricate cognate pair of [ʧ] as in *chin* [ʧɪn] and [ʤ] as in *jam* [ʤæm] as stops because the initial sounds are the stop cognates [t] and [d]. These two affricate sounds are discussed in a later chapter.

GENERAL PRODUCTION OF THE STOP CONSONANTS

For stop consonants, the airflow travels from the lungs through the pharyngeal area where the velopharyngeal port is closed so that the airflow proceeds to the oral cavity. The essential action of stop consonant production is an interruption of the air stream, whether voiced or voiceless, by a closure within the oral cavity (Calvert, 1986; Small, 1999). The closing and opening movements for stops tend to be quite fast, usually the fastest movements in speech (Shriberg & Kent, 1995). This interruption action consists of three phases (Ball, 1993).

First, in the shutting phase, the articulators briefly form a complete obstruction of the outgoing air stream. Second, in the closure phase, the articulators form the necessary stop with its rapid closure that causes the implosion (intraoral air pressure) of air to remain in the oral cavity. The length of closure time is approximately 50–60 milliseconds, during which the articulators are kept closed. This closure phase is a period of silence for voiceless stops and a vocal fold "buzz" for fully voiced stops.

The third, release phase is a variable aspiration plosive phase when the impounded air is loosed and a burst of noise is released as the air pressure equalizes as a result of its release. There are two possible sources of this noise: turbulence at the glottis that produces an *h*-like sound, and turbulence generated as the breath rushes through the aperture (opening) created by release of the articulatory constriction (Tiffany & Carrell, 1977).

ALLOPHONIC VARIATIONS

Some allophones of these stops are made without aspiration or are made with varying degrees of diminished aspiration (House, 1998). The superscript ^{h} is used in narrow transcription to denote aspiration, as in *pep*: [p^{h}ɛp]. A given segment or phoneme cannot be pronounced in an unchanging way because of its environment (MacKay, 1987). Individual speech sounds are thus pronounced differently depending on the neighboring sounds. For example, the [p] in the initial position in the word *pen* is released with more aspiration and explosion than the [p] in the medial position in *open*. Place a thin sheet of paper in front of your mouth and say these two words in a natural manner: *pen, open*. Notice the displacement of the paper for the initial [p] in *pen* and the diminished or total lack of movement of the paper when you speak the word *open*. You can also notice a difference between the amount of aspiration of air when the [p] sound is at the final position of a word as in *pop, pup, peep*, and *pep*. The characteristics of the surrounding sounds play major roles in determining which features of the target sound prevail. Usually, stop consonant sounds—or any other sounds—are not produced in isolation (Davenport & Hannahs, 1998). When oral stops are produced in ordinary connected speech, the closing stage and/or the release stage may be missing as a result of the influence of neighboring sounds. Only the closure stage is necessary for all stops in all positions. If there is no period of closure, a stop sound is not produced. Notice that the voiceless stops [p], [t], and [k] can be said with only aspiration and do not incorporate a following vowel sound. However, the voiced stops [b], [d], and [g] always have the [ə] schwa sound at the end: [bʌ], [dʌ], and [gʌ]. These allophonic variations are discussed for each of the stop consonants presented in this chapter.

INTEGRITY OF THE SPEECH MECHANISM

Production of the stop consonants depends very much on the integrity of the speech mechanism (Zemlin, 1998). Zemlin explains that the articulators, including the lips, tongue, and velum, must be brought into full contact, firmly, to resist the air pressure being generated. It is also essential that there is adequate velopharyngeal seal to prevent the air from escaping into the nasal cavity. It has been generally noted that the air pressures for the voiceless consonants can be significantly greater than for the voiced consonants, at least at the beginning of a stressed syllable (MacKay, 1987). Plosives that have higher intraoral pressure are often called *fortis*, and those with lower pressure are *lenis*, from the Latin words for strong and weak. This plosive burst, which is not present in unreleased, laterally released, and nasal released stops, is relatively short for unaspirated plosives and longer for aspirated plosives (Ball, 1993). Ball (1993) reports that for bilabial [p], [b] plosives the noise is generally distributed through frequencies of approximately 600–800 Hertz (Hz); for velars [k], [g], 1800–2000 Hz; and for alveolars [t], [d], approximately 4000 Hz.

In terms of time, the lenis plosives are generally shorter in duration than the fortis in both the silent phase and the noise burst (Ball, 1993). The silent segment of the plosive can last between 70 and 140 milliseconds, with lenis being at the shorter end of this range and fortis at the longer end. The noise burst is quite short in the lenis stops, approximately 10 to 15 milliseconds, whereas with aspirated stops it can stretch 50 milliseconds, although the precise length is somewhat determined by placement of the articulators and the surrounding sounds.

In Spanish and French, both the voiced and voiceless plosives are lenis and unaspirated, which makes it difficult for English-speaking people to distinguish [p] from [b] and [t] from [d]. Voiceless plosives are lenis when they occur in the medial or final positions in a word.

Ladefoged (1993), MacKay (1987), and Carrell and Tiffany (1960) provide very thorough and detailed accounts of the stop and its functions. These authors include discussion of two other phenomena related to the elements of stop and plosive: the glottal stop and the flap, also known as the "tap" and the "one-tap trill."

THE GLOTTAL STOP

Ladefoged (1993) offers some helpful suggestions regarding understanding the glottal stop. These suggestions are summarized here:

1. Make small coughing noises to get the sensation of the vocal cords being pressed together.

2. Take a deep breath. With the mouth open, let the breath go and listen to the small plosive (cough) sounds that occur.

3. While exhaling the air through the opened mouth, abruptly interrupt and release the airflow, producing short glottal stops.

4. Do step 3 and add the "ahhh" continuous sound with the abrupt interruptions and releases. Produce the glottal stop with the prolongation of other vowel sounds to become acquainted with the production and sound of a glottal stop.

The inclusion in the phonetic alphabet of the glottal stop, transcribed as [ʔ], although not a contrasting phoneme, seems justified by the frequency of its occurrence in English, particularly in certain dialects (Carrell & Tiffany, 1960). For example, the glottal stop regularly replaces [t] in words such as *little, bottle*, and *dental* and in the utterance for "No!" *uh-uh* [ʌʔʌʔ]. The glottal stop has the major features of a stop but is produced by a closure of the glottis rather than by the articulators in the oral cavity.

The glottal stop has three uses in English: (1) as an allophonic realization of [t] and other voiceless stops in certain varieties, as in *mitten* [mɪʔn̩]; (2) it occurs in emphatic pronunciation of vowel-initial words, for example, *I want an apple* [ʔæpl̩] *not a pear*; and (3) as an intrusive element between two vowels when the second vowel is stressed, as in *myopic* [maɪʔpɪk]. The [h] is considered another glottal sound and is discussed in the fricative sound category in this text.

THE FLAP

Ladefoged (1993) reports that most Americans, irrespective of whether they have a lateral plosion or not, do not have a voiceless [t] stop in *little* [lɪtl̩]. Many Americans do not distinguish between pairs of words such as *latter, ladder*. There is a general rule in United States English that whenever [t]

occurs after a stressed vowel and before an unstressed syllable other than [n], it is changed into a voiced sound. For those Americans who have lateral plosion, this is the stop [d]. For those who do not, and for nearly all Americans in words such as *city, better, writer*, the articulation is not really a stop but a quick flap or tap in which the tongue tip is thrown against the alveolar ridge. This sound is represented by the symbol [ɾ] so that *city* can be transcribed as [sɪɾi]. Notice that the [ɾ] replaces the [t] or [d] sound.

Carrell and Tiffany (1960) agree that this stop form known as the flap is common in American speech and is often the medial sound in words such as *water* and *butter*. In words of this type, the flap consists of a single tap or bounce at the point of articulation, rather than a hold; breath flow is interrupted but not occluded to the point where pressure rises high enough for an audible aspirate release.

The flap is an allophone of the [t] and [d] phonemes. Shriberg and Kent (1995) indicate that speakers of English usually produce words such as *patty* [pæɾɪ], *rider* [raɪɾɚ], and *writer* [raɪɾɚ] with the allophonic lingua-alveolar flap [ɾ] in the intervocalic position. The flap is a modified stop sound, in which a rapid stroking or flapping motion of the tongue tip contacts the alveolar ridge very briefly. Shriberg and Kent (1995) regard the flap as a reduced version of [t] and [d] because it can replace both of these phonemes in pairs such as *latter-ladder* [læɾɚ] and *knotting-nodding* [nɔɾɪŋ] or [nɑɾɪŋ]. Although some phoneticians give the flap full phonemic status as a manner of production, Shriberg and Kent (1995) prefer to view it as a variant or modification of the more general stop category.

The ballistic movement that creates the flap (MacKay, 1987) can result in either a rhotic or nonrhotic flap, meaning those that have an *r*-like quality and those that do not. North American English has a nonrhotic flap that occurs as a variety of [t] and [d] when intervocalic and posttonic (between vowels and following the stressed syllable) as in *matter* [mæɾɚ] and *betting* [bɛɾɪŋ]. A rhotic flap is heard in many dialects of British English and, to the American English listener, the word *very* sounds like *veddy*. The rhotic flap is also present in Spanish where there is one orthographic *r*. MacKay (1987) postulates that the articulatory difference between the rhotic and nonrhotic flap probably lies in the tongue root position because the *r*-like quality is very likely associated with some degree of tongue root retraction (narrowing of the pharynx).

The six stop consonants are discussed in sequence of cognate pairs: [p] and [b], [t] and [d], and [k] and [g]. A comprehensive description of each sound and its features is presented followed by a summary and transcription exercises.

PHONETIC SYMBOL [p]

EXHIBIT 13-1 | **Phonetic Symbol [p]**

		[p]
Phonetic Symbol	[p]	
Grapheme Symbols	p, pp, gh, ph	
Diacritic Symbol	p	
Phonic Symbol	p	
Cognate	[b]	
Homorganic	Bilabial [b] [w] [m] [ʍ]	
Sound Class	Consonant	
Basic Phonetic Features	Placement: Bilabial Manner: Stop/Plosive Voicing: Minus Voice	
IPA (1999)	[p] #101 Voiceless, Bilabial, Plosive	

How the Sound Is Produced

The [p] sound is made by impounding the airflow from the lungs by closing the lips (bilabial) firmly together and forcing air into the oral cavity. Pressure is built up during this short period of closure and velopharyngeal closure is complete, or nearly so. Then, the air pressure is released by separating the lips in an explosive (stop/plosive) manner and the [p] sound is heard (voiceless) as a result of the noise created as the released breath stream passes through the lips. The [p] sound is minus voice because the vocal folds are in an open position. The voiced cognate is the [b] sound and it is produced with less aspiration (Shriberg & Kent, 1995) than the [p] sound because the amount of intraoral pressure is greater for voiceless phonemes (Small, 1999). See **Figure 13-1**.

Different Spellings for the [p] Sound

Transcribe the following. Cover the Key at the right until you complete the transcription, and then check your answers.

Different Spellings				Key
p	plan ___	help ___	peanuts ___	plæn, hɛlp, pinəts
	swept ___	splash ___	spring ___	swɛpt, splæʃ, sprɪŋ
pp	mapping ___	apple ___	stepping ___	mæpɪŋ, æpl̩, stɛpɪŋ
gh	hiccough (or hiccup) ___			hɪkəp
ph	shepherd ___			ʃɛphɚd

Different Sounds for the Letter *p*

Transcribe the following words. Refer to the Key at the right upon completion.

				Key
ph = [f]	phonetics ___	photograph ___		fonɛnɪks, fotoʊgræf
	physics ___			fɪzɪks
p = (Silent)	psalm ___	psychology ___		ʤ, sɑm, aɪdɑloʤi
	receipt ___			risit

Rules for Spelling and Pronunciation of the [p] Sound

1. The *p* in most spelling contexts is pronounced [p].

2. Two adjacent *p* letters (*pp*) may be pronounced as a single [p], as in *puppet* (pupp-et) and *pepper* (pepp-er). In some instances, the second *p* may be observed to one degree or another as the initial sound in the second syllable (pep-per).

3. The *p* is silent in *psalms* (salms) and in words of Greek origin such as *psychic* (sychic), *pneumonic* (neumonic), and *psoriasis* (soriasis).

4. The letters *gh* are produced as a [p] sound, as in *hiccough* (hiccoup).

5. The letters *ph* are produced as an [f] sound, as in *telephone* (telephone) and *pheasant* (feasant).

6. The *p* is pronounced in the *ph* context, as in *shepherd*.

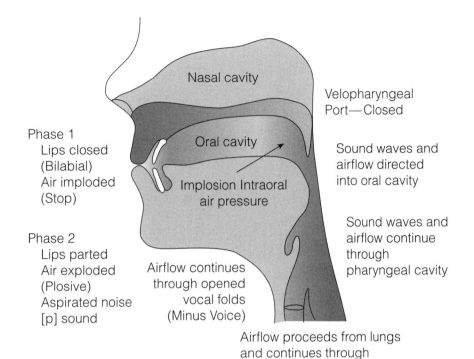

Figure 13-1 [p] pronunciation.

7. In compound words, when the *p* occurs at the end of the first syllable, it may be ignored, such as in the pronunciation of *cupboard* (cuboard). The voiced [b] cognate of [p] may take preference. However, in a word such as *cupcake*, where the [p] sound is followed by a voiceless [k] sound, the integrity of the [p] remains.

8. The *p* is silent, as in *receipt* and *glimpse* (in some dialects).

Words That Include the [p] Sound

The [p] sound occurs in the prevocalic, intervocalic, and postvocalic positions and in the initial, medial, and final positions. Transcribe the following words in which the [p] occurs in different positions within the words. Refer to the Key at the right upon completion of the transcription.

Initial Consonant   *Key*

pea ____ patch ____ perfect ____   pi, pæʧ, pɝfɛkt

post ____ power ____ proper ____   poʊst, paʊwɚ, prɑpɚ

Unstressed Syllable

Medial Consonant

teepee ____ coupon ____ rapid ____   tipi, kupɑn, ræpɪd

oppose ____ staple ____ copy ____   əpoʊz, steɪpl̩, kɔpi

Stressed Syllable

Medial Consonant

napkin ____ apply ____ epic ____   næpkɪn, aplaɪ, ɛpɪk

trapeze ____ happy ____ puppy ____   træpiz, hæpi, pʌpi

Final Consonant

camp ____ stop ____ group ____   kæmp, stɑp, grup

ship ____ deep ____ tape ____   ʃɪp, dip, teɪp

Initial and Final Consonants

peep ____ pop ____ pipe ____   pip, pɑp, paɪp

polyp ____ pomp ____ pup ____   pɔləp, pɔmp, pʌp

Pope ____ pump ____   poʊp, pʌmp

Initial Blends

sp speech ____   pr prey ____   spiʧ, preɪ

pl play ____   spr sprinkle ____   pleɪ, sprɪnkl̩

spl spleen ____   splin

Medial Blends

[None]

Final Blends

ps tips ____   pt crept ____   tɪps, krɛpt

pped tripped ____   mp stamp ____   trɪpt, stæmp

pse relapse _____   _mps_ mumps _____   rilæps, mʌmps

mpt prompt _____   prɑmpt

Auditory Discrimination

Transcribe the following words and listen to the minimal differences in pronunciation. Refer to the Key at the bottom upon completion of the transcription.

Cognates			_Other Minimal Pairs_		
[p] (– Voice)	[b] (+Voice)	[p]	[t]	[p]	[k]
pill _____	bill _____	pin _____	tin _____	lip _____	lick _____
pet _____	bet _____	pop _____	top _____	lap _____	lack _____
pay _____	bay _____	hip _____	hit _____	P	key _____
patch _____	batch _____	pan _____	tan _____	pear _____	care _____
rip _____	rib _____	lip _____	lit _____	pain _____	cane _____
staple _____	stable _____	pen _____	ten _____	part _____	cart _____

Key (left to right): pɪl, bɪl, pɪn, tɪn, lɪp, lɪk, pɛt, bɛt, pɑp, tɑp, læp, læk, peɪ, beɪ, hɪp, hɪt, pi, ki, pætʃ, bætʃ, pæn, tæn, pɛir, kɛir, rɪp, rɪb, lɪp, lɪt, peɪn, keɪn, steɪpl̩, steibl̩, pɛn, tɛn, pɑrt, kɑrt

Allophonic and Dialect Variations

In connected speech, the [p] sound may or may not be released with aspiration (Ball & Rahilly, 1999; Calvert, 1986; Davenport & Hannahs, 1998). The following list describes the influence of aspiration and other factors that bring about the allophonic differences.

The [p] sound is usually released with audible aspiration [pʰ] in the following contexts:

1. Initial consonant in a stressed syllable as in _pupil, power, portion_

2. Final consonant following the homorganic (same place of articulation) [m] as in _stamp, lump, amp_

3. Final consonant following [s] as in _crisp, clasp, grasp_

4. Medial position with less aspiration as in _express, April, interpret_

The [p] sound is usually released without audible aspiration [p] in the following contexts:

1. Final consonant preceded by a vowel as in _drip, crop, clap_

2. In an _sp_ blend in the same syllable as in _sparkle, spell, inspect, prosper_

3. Initial consonant in an unstressed syllable as in _pacific, pajamas, perfection_

Additional conditions also result in allophonic features that influence the production of the [p] sound. For example, the [p] is released into the position of the voiceless consonant as in _crept, lips_, and when followed by a word beginning with a voiceless consonant as in _soda pop can_ and _sportsmanship team_. A nasal release [p] occurs when the [p] sound is followed by a syllabic nasal, as in "Stop now!" and "Shop more." The lips remain closed and the air pressure and sound are released through the nasal cavity. A lengthening of the [p] sound [p:] occurs when it's in the final position, then the [p] is followed by a releasing [p], as in "The antelope play" and "lamp post."

An intrusive [p] may occur when the lips open from the [m] position to the following unvoiced sound, as when _something_ [sʌmɵən] becomes [sʌmpɵɪn] and _comfort_ [kʌmfɚt] becomes [kʌmpfɚt] (Carrell & Tiffany, 1960; House, 1998).

Black American speech sometimes omits the final consonant clusters, as when _grasp_ [græsp] becomes [græ]. When speakers substitute a _p_-like sound for the [b] sound, it becomes difficult for the listener to determine whether the speaker said _bored_ or _poured_. This difficulty is a result of reduced voicing resonance of the [b] sound. Varying degrees of the pressure release of the sound is equated with dialectic differences from a soft release to a very powerful release.

Normal and Deviant Development of the [p] Sound

The [p] sound is usually acquired by age 3 years and is seldom misarticulated (Calvert, 1986; Sander, 1972). It is a relatively easy sound to learn, and in speakers with normal lips and palates it is relatively easily corrected if problems do occur (Tiffany & Carrell, 1977).

Speakers with velopharyngeal closure incompetence, including cleft palate, may experience inability to close off the nasal passageway, and air may escape into the nasal cavity preventing the oral pressure to build to a level for the production of an adequate [p] sound. Quite often these individuals substitute a glottal stop for the [p] sound. Deaf speakers may have articulatory difficulty with the [p] sound because of insufficient pressure for audible plosive feature (MacKay, 1987). They may also have a tendency to voice all of the plosive sounds. In some speech disorders, particularly those associated with disease of or injury to the central nervous system, speakers may have weak labial musculature or difficulty controlling it such as in cerebral palsy, traumatic head injury, stroke, and Parkinson's disease (Carrell & Tiffany, 1960). Certain extreme dental malocclusions that involve abnormal relationships between the upper and lower teeth may present a condition where it is difficult for the speaker to bring the lips together and the placement of the articulators may be more of a labiodental closure for the [p] sound (upper lip and lower teeth or lower lip and upper teeth).

Nonnative Speaker Pronunciation

The allophonic [p] sound occurs in many sound systems worldwide. The [p] sound may be underpronounced because it requires a relatively precise and firm articulatory adjustment (Carrell & Tiffany, 1960) and often a distinct plosive release. Nonnative speakers may tend to weaken the [p] sound, especially in the initial position (Edwards, 1997). This results in the production of a voiceless bilabial fricative or a voiceless labiodental fricative [f]. Meaning may also be changed by degree of aspiration, as in Korean (IPA, 1999), [p] in *pal* means "sucking" and [pʰ] means "arm." Because such distinctive aspiration marks do not appear in United States English, the [p] sound may present some confusion to both speaker and listener when the speaker attempts to adapt such marks to United States English pronunciation. The [p] sound, with some allophonic variations, is present in the 15 other sound systems of languages predominantly spoken in the United States. For example, Ball and Rahilly (1999) describe the Vietnamese *p* as a postnasal oral stop influenced by the [m] sound. It is considered as postnasal because the oral stop might have a brief nasal portion at the end of the closure stage, just before the release. The other sound systems are Spanish, French, German, Italian, Chinese, Tagalog, Polish, Korean, Portuguese, Japanese, Greek, Arabic, Hindi (Urdu), and Russian.

Summary

The [p] sound is one of the three voiceless stop consonants ([t], [p], [k]) and its voiced cognate is the [b] sound. In addition to the [b], it is homorganic (bilabial) with the [w], [ʍ], and [m] sounds. The *p* represents the [p] sound in most contexts except when it is silent, as in *receipt*, or functions as an [f] sound, as in *phonetics*. The [p] sound is one of the first sounds to be acquired because it is easily observed

and appears in many other foreign sound systems. Varying degrees of pressure release occur to create minor dialect or allophonic differences. A degree of voicing may occur making it difficult for a listener to discriminate between the [b] and [p] sounds. Nonnative speakers may weaken the [p] sound, or the placement may result in a voiceless bilabial or labiodental fricative [f] sound. Speakers with impaired velopharyngeal closure or weakened labial strength may have difficulty in accomplishing the pressure buildup and release to adequately produce the [p] sound.

[p] +

Write the orthographic and phonetic spellings of the following words. Refer to the Key at the bottom upon completion.

	Orthographic	Phonetic
1. [p] + 2 sounds: opposite of rich	_____	[_oʊ_]
2. [p] + 3 sounds: something we win	_____	[_ _ aɪ _]
3. [p] + 2 sounds: a man's name	_____	[_i_]
4. [p] + 3 sounds: when wages are received	_____	[_ eɪ _ eɪ]
5. [p] + 1 sound: Winnie the Pooh	_____	[_u]
6. [p] + 7 sounds: Rose Parade and Bowl	_____	[_ æ _ ə _ ɛ _ ə]
7. [p] + 9 sounds: foot doctor	_____	[_ ə _ aɪə _ _ ɪ _ _]
8. [p] + 7 sounds: a fuel	_____	[_ ə _ _ oʊ _ ɛə _]
9. [p] + 8 sounds: hospital ward for babies	_____	[_ i _ iæ _ _ ɪ _]
10. [p] + 9 sounds: to get involved	_____	[_ ɑ _ _ ɪ _ ə _ e _]
11. [p] + 6 sounds: a wooden puppet	_____	[_ ə _ oʊ _ io]

Key: 1. poor [poʊr]; 2. prize [praɪz]; 3. Pete [pit]; 4. payday [peɪdeɪ]; 5. Pooh [pu]; 6. Pasadena [pæsədɛnə]; 7. podiatrist [pədaɪətrɪst]; 8. petroleum [pətroʊlɛəm]; 9. pediatric [pidiætrɪk]; 10. participate [pɑrtɪsəpet]; 11. Pinocchio [pənokio]

PHONETIC SYMBOL [b]

EXHIBIT 13-2	Phonetic Symbol [b]

Phonetic Symbol	[b]	**[b]**
Grapheme Symbols	b, bb	
Diacritic Symbol	b	
Phonic Symbol	b	
Cognate	[p]	
Homorganic	Bilabial [p] [w] [m] [ʍ]	
Sound Class	Consonant	
Basic Phonetic Features	Placement: Bilabial Manner: Stop/Plosive Voicing: Plus Voice	
IPA (1999)	[b] #102 Voiced, Bilabial, Plosive	

How the Sound Is Produced

The [b] sound is produced by impounding the airflow from the lungs by closing the lips (bilabial) firmly together and forcing air into the oral cavity. Pressure is built up during this short period of closure, and velopharyngeal closure is complete, or nearly so. The air pressure is released by separating the lips in an explosive (stop/plosive) manner, and the vocal folds are activated simultaneously to add voicing (voicing) as the released breath stream passes through the lips. The [p] cognate to [b] is produced in the same manner and placement with minus voice and more aspiration than the [b] sound (MacKay, 1987). See **Figure 13-2**.

Different Spellings for the [b] Sound

Transcribe the following words. Refer to the Key at the right upon completion.

Different Spellings			*Key*
b best ___	boast ___	baby ___	bɛst, boʊst, beɪbi
Bob ___	scrub ___		bɑb, skrʌb
bb robber ___	Bobby ___		rɑbɚ, bɑbi
rubber ___	bubble ___		rʌbɚ, bʌbl̩

Different Sounds for the Letter b

			Key
b [b] big ___	b (silent) lamb ___		bɪg, læm

Rules for Spelling and Pronunciation of the [b] Sound

1. The written *b* is pronounced [b].
2. Two adjacent *b* letters (*bb*) may be pronounced as a single [b], and traditionally the [b] sound is assigned to the first syllable (*bubb-le*).
3. The *b* is silent in *lamb, comb, subtle, doubt, debt*.
4. In the context *pb*, as in *cupboard*, the [p] is silent.
5. The consonant blend combinations of *br, bl* occur in the initial, medial, and final positions: br *brown, abroad*; bl *blow, establish, able*; rb *carbon, harbor, curb, adverb*.
6. When the [b] is produced in isolation, it is followed by the schwa [bʌ].

Words That Include the [b] Sound

The [b] sound occurs in all three positions: initial, medial, and final. Transcribe the following. Refer to the Key at the right upon completion.

Initial Consonant			*Key*
bee ___	big ___	beg ___ bag ___	bi, bɪg, bɛg, bæg
bird ___	bud ___	bar ___	bɝd, bʌd, bɑr
boar ___	boot ___	book ___	bɔr, bʊt, bʊk

Unstressed Syllable

Medial Consonant		
habit ___	stubborn ___	hæbət, stʌbɚn
orbit ___	label ___	ɔrbət, leɪbl̩

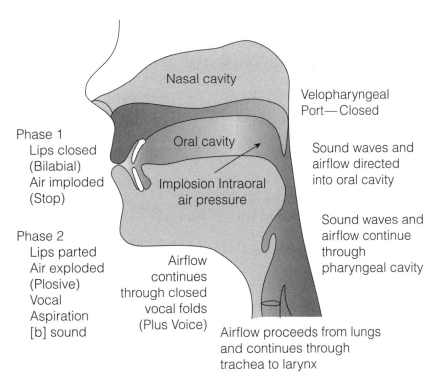

Figure 13-2 [b] pronunciation.

Stressed Syllable

Medial Consonant

above _____ abide _____ əbʌv, əbaɪd

imbibe _____ rebuild _____ ɪmbaɪb, ribɪld

Final Consonant

throb __ rib __ herb __ globe __ ɵrɑb, rɪb, hɝb, gloʊb

Initial and Final Consonants

Bob _____ bib _____ babe _____ bɑb, bɪb, beɪb

Initial Blends

bl blue _____ blown _____ blu, bloʊn

br broke _____ brother _____ broʊk, brʌðɚ

Medial Blends

bs absorbed _____ rb arbor _____ əbsɔrbəd, arbɚ

mb number _____ thimble _____ nʌmbɚ, ɵɪmbl̩

bl obligation _____ ɑbləgeɪʃən

br cobra _____ fabric _____ koʊbrə, fæbrɪk

Final Blends

rb curb _____ bd stabbed _____ kɝb, stæbəd

bl double _____ noble _____ dʌbl̩, noʊbl̩

Auditory Discrimination

Transcribe the following. Listen to the slight difference in pronunciation. Refer to the Key at the bottom of this section upon completion.

Cognates		*Other Minimal Pairs*			
[b] (+)	*[p] (–)*	*[b]*	*[v]*	*[b]*	*[d]*
bee ___	pea ___	cabs ___	calves ___	bet ___	debt ___
big ___	pig ___	best ___	vest ___	bill ___	dill ___
beg ___	peg ___	boat ___	vote ___	ball ___	doll ___
bat ___	pat ___	berry ___	very ___	B ___	D ___
bar ___	par ___	Serb ___	serve ___	lab ___	lad ___
bore ___	pore ___	beg ___	vague ___	rib ___	rid ___

Key (left to right): bi, pi, kæbz, kævz, bɛt, dɛt, bɪg, pɪg, bɛst, vɛst, bɪl, dɪl, bɛg, pɛg, boʊt, voʊt, bɔl, dɔl, bæt, pæt, bɛri, vɛri, bi, di, bɑr, pɑr, sɝb, sɝv, læb, læd, bɔr, pɔr, beɪg, veɪg, rɪb, rɪd

Allophonic and Dialect Variations

The bilabial [b] shows no significant assimilation, typically remaining bilabial irrespective of context (Davenport & Hannahs, 1998). Calvert (1986) notes the following:

1. Voicing begins with the lips closed and the [b] is released into the following voiced sound when it

is the initial sound of an utterance, as in *boy*, or immediately following a voiced consonant, as in *these boys*.

2. Between two voiced sounds, as in *about*, the [b] is a brief closure and release with continued voicing.

3. Immediately before a voiceless consonant, as in *lab coat*, the [b] is closed but not released with voicing.

4. As the final sound, as in *lab*, the [b] is either held without release or is released lightly, as in [læb].

It is interesting to note that the voiced cognate [b] takes preference over the voiceless [p] such as in the word baptize. Have some of your friends repeat the word "baptize" and see how many of them substituted the [b] for the [p] sound. Much of the discussion concerning the allophonic variations of the [p] sound applies to the [b] sound (Tiffany & Carrell, 1977), but certain other variations apply as well:

1. Because [b] is a voiced sound, there is ordinarily no aspiration [b] on the plosive phase of the production of the [b] sound, as in *but* [bʌt].

2. The characteristic weakening of the force of aspiration of [p] to that of the [b] sound may result in the substitution of the [b] for the [p], as in *paper/baber*.

3. A nasal plosion of [b] may be heard when the sound is followed by [m], as in *rob 'em*. The [b] sound acquires a nasal resonance because the soft palate begins to lower while the lips remain closed in preparation for the [m] sound.

4. The lateral plosion is heard when the [b] sound is followed by [l] because of the same principle, that is, the movement of the articulators anticipate the next sound, [l], as the [b] sound is in its completion phase.

Edwards (1997) reports that a lengthening allophonic variation [b:] occurs when the arresting [b] is followed by a releasing [b] sound, as in *rob Bob* [rɑb:ab].

Native English speakers may have many of the same difficulties with [b] that they do with the [p] sound (Tiffany & Carrell, 1977). The tendency to weaken the voicing results in the sound being underpronounced in conversational speech. This does not often occur in the initial position but more often in the medial and final positions, as in *hamburger* and *lobe*, where incomplete voicing or lax lip closure reduces the intelligibility of the [b] sound. In minimal pairs such as *rip/rib, cap/cab* speakers may not make the necessary distinction between the sounds to be clearly understood, particularly out of context. Generally speaking, the vowel before [p] is usually slightly shorter than that before

[b], and this is sometimes the determining cue in the discrimination between the two sounds.

In Black American speech, the [b] is generally affected in the final positions of single-syllable words, usually a consonant-vowel-consonant (CVC) combination. The [b] is substituted with the [p] sound and the vowel is usually lengthened. For example, *cab* becomes *cap*.

Normal and Deviant Development of the [b] Sound

The [b] sound is mastered early, by age 3 years (Sander, 1972) and is seldom misarticulated (Calvert, 1986). It is acquired later than its voiceless cognate, [p]. Deviations for [b] in the initial position are extremely rare (Edwards, 1997), but in the final position the [b] may lack sufficient voicing or be devoiced, thus approximating the [p] sound, or the sound in this final position may be omitted. Shriberg and Kent (1995) report that among the six stops, the [p] and [b] are most stable regarding developmental substitutions.

Nonnative Speaker Pronunciation

The allophonic [b] sound occurs in many sound systems, including Spanish, Korean, Tagalog (Philippines), and Hmong (Vietnam). Spanish speakers may not make the [b] sound with firm closure and may substitute a bilabial fricative sound that to United States English listeners may sound like a [v] sound (Calvert, 1986). This is heard most prominently when [b] occurs in the medial position, as in *cabin* and *labial*. Also, with Spanish speakers, the [b] sound may be substituted for the [v] sound, as in *base* for *vase,* and the final [b] sound may become devoiced which results in a [p] sound as in *tap* for *tab* (Kayser, 1993). German and Russian speakers may pronounce the final [b] as a [p] sound due to the reduced voicing feature as in *about* [əbaʊt] sounds more like *apout* [əpaʊt]. Since there are no labiodentals in Korean (Cheng, 1993), the [b] may be substituted for the [v] sound so that *have* becomes *habe*. This is also a common pronunciation in Tagalog. The other sound systems of languages predominantly spoken in the United States include French, Italian, Chinese, Polish, Portuguese, Japanese, Greek, Arabic, and Hindi (Urdu), all of which contain an allophonic representation of the [b] sound.

Summary

The [b] is one of the three voiced stop consonants ([b], [d], [g]), and its voiceless cognate is the [p] sound. In addition to the [p], it is homorganic (bilabial) with the [w], [m], and [ʍ]. Unlike many of the other orthographic letters that may represent a variety of different sounds, the [b] and [bb] remain constant and no other alphabet letters represent the [b] sound. Although its cognate [p] may be mastered by age 3, the [b] may not be mastered until age 4. Dialect differences are a result of decreased voicing, and reduced intelligibility occurs when such words as *cap* and *cab* are spoken with minimal contextual cues.

The [b] sound and its allophonic variations are present in many of the sound systems worldwide. Nonnative speakers may substitute a bilabial fricative *v*-like sound, and reduced voicing produces an allophone that may sound more like a [p] sound. The [b] and [p] sounds have few developmental errors. For speakers with disordered speech, the feature of voicing may be a problem. Lack of sufficient velopharyngeal closure and labial muscle strength, endurance, and precision may result in a weakened or nasal resonant distorted [b] sound.

[b] +

Write out the words using both the orthographic spelling and phonetic symbols. Refer to the Key at the bottom upon completion.

	Orthographic	Phonetic
1. [b] + 2 sounds: a two-wheeler	_____	[_ aɪ _]
2. [b] + 2 sounds: small red vegetable	_____	[_ i _]
3. [b] + 2 sounds: put on a fishing hook	_____	[_ eɪ _]
4. [b] + 2 sounds: it sails	_____	[_ oʊ _]
5. [b] + 2 sounds: a color in U.S. flag	_____	[_ _ u]
6. [b] + 6 sounds: to watch young children	_____	[_ eɪ _ i _ ɪ _]
7. [b] + 6 sounds: second-story porch	_____	[_ aʊ _ _ ə _ i]
8. [b] + 5 sounds: a fruit	_____	[_ ə _ æ _ ə]
9. [b] + 6 sounds: a barrier	_____	[_ ɛ _ ɪ _ e _]
10. [b] + 6 sounds: arched legs	_____	[_ oʊ _ ɛ _ ɪ _]

Key: 1. bike [baɪk]; 2. beet [bit]; 3. bait [beɪt]; 4. boat [boʊt]; 5. blue [blu]; 6. babysit [beɪbisɪt]; 7. balcony [baʊlkəni]; 8. banana [bənænə]; 9. barricade [bɛrɪked]; 10. bowlegged [boʊlɛgɪd]

PHONETIC SYMBOL [t]

EXHIBIT 13-3 | **Phonetic Symbol [t]**

Phonetic Symbol	[t]	**[t]**
Grapheme Symbols	t, tt, ed, th, z	
Diacritic Symbol	t	
Phonic Symbol	t	
Cognate	[d]	
Homorganic	Lingua-Alveolar [s], [z], [d], [l], [n] Initial Sound in [tʃ] and [dʒ]	
Sound Class	Consonant	
Basic Phonetic Features	Placement: Lingua-Alveolar Manner: Stop/Plosive Voicing: Minus Voice	
IPA (1999)	[t] #103 Dental or Alveolar, Plosive, Voiceless	

How the Sound Is Produced

The airflow from the lungs is directed into the oral cavity because the velopharyngeal port is closed. The [t] sound is made by placing the tongue (lingua) against the upper gum (alveolar) ridge. These two articulators form a seal, and air pressure builds up (stop/implosion) in the oral cavity between the surface of the tongue and the roof of the mouth. When the air is expelled (plosive) by the release of the tongue, an audible aspirated noise is produced that results in the [t] sound. The [t] sound is voiceless (minus voice) because the vocal folds are in an open position. The voiced cognate is the [d] sound, and it is produced with less aspiration than the [t] sound. See **Figure 13-3**.

Different Spellings for the [t] Sound

Transcribe the following. Refer to the Key at the right upon completion.

Different Spellings					*Key*
t	top __	stone __			tɑp, stoʊn
	tilt __	tasty __	two __		tɪlt, teisti, tu
tt	mitten __	bitter __	butter __		mɪtŋ, bitɚ, bʌtɚ
bt	debt __	doubt __			dɛt, daʊt
ed	picked __	fenced __	fished __		fɪkt, fɛnst, fɪʃt
pt	ptomaine __				toʊmen

				Key
pteropod __	receipt __			tə-roʊpɑd, risit
phth	phthisic __ (but not phthisis)			tɪsɪk
th	thyme __	Thomas __		taɪm, tɑməs
	Thames __			teɪmz
ght	bought __	thought __	fought __	bɔt, ðɔt, fɔt
cht	yacht __			jɑt
ct	indict __	precinct __		Indaɪt, prisɪnk
z	pizza __			pitsə

Different Sounds for the Letter t

Transcribe the following words. Refer to the Key at the right upon completion.

						Key
th [ð] (Voiced)	the __	them __				ðʌ, ðɛm
	that __	there __	these __			ðæt, ðɛr, ðiz
	mother __	bathe __				mʌðɚ, beɪð
th [Θ] (Voiceless)	thin __	thirty __				Θɪn, Θɝti
	thorn __	health __				Θɔrn, hɛlΘ
	month __	ninth __				mʌnΘ, nəɪnΘ
(Silent)	listen __	castle __				lɪstən, kæsļ
	whistle __	often __				ʍɪsļ, ɔfən

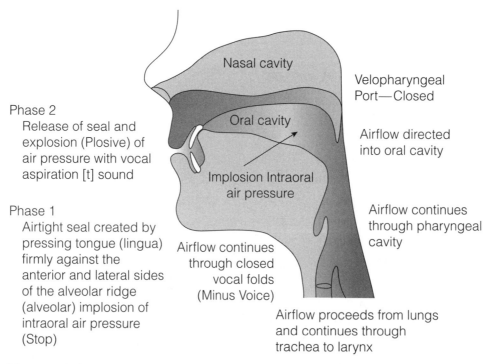

Phase 2
Release of seal and explosion (Plosive) of air pressure with vocal aspiration [t] sound

Phase 1
Airtight seal created by pressing tongue (lingua) firmly against the anterior and lateral sides of the alveolar ridge (alveolar) implosion of intraoral air pressure (Stop)

Nasal cavity

Velopharyngeal Port—Closed

Oral cavity

Airflow directed into oral cavity

Implosion Intraoral air pressure

Airflow continues through pharyngeal cavity

Airflow continues through closed vocal folds (Minus Voice)

Airflow proceeds from lungs and continues through trachea to larynx

Figure 13-3 [t] pronunciation.

Rules for Spelling and Pronunciation of the [t] Sound

1. The *t* in most spelling contexts is written *t*: *time, recital, coat*.

2. Two adjacent *t*s in the final position, as in *mutt*, are pronounced as a [t] sound. When the *tt* occurs in the medial position, as in *butter, stutter*, a sound is produced that is considered neither a [t] nor a [d] sound but an allophone of the [t] caused by a brief, voiced flap of the tongue that sounds somewhat like "bud-er" and "stud-er."

3. In words such as *dou**bt*** and *de**bt***, the *b* is silent. The final sound is [t].

4. For verbs that end in a voiceless consonant, as in *pop, lau**gh*** (f), or *pic**k***, the letters *ed* are added to indicate past tense: *popped, laughed*, or *picked*; the *d* becomes a [t] sound.

5. The *p* is silent and the *t* becomes the initial sound in such unusual scientific words such as *pteropod, pteridology*, and *ptomaine*.

6. The initial sound in the word *phthisic* is [t] but is the voiced *th* [ð] sound in *phthisis*.

7. The *th* is the [t] Greek sound as in *thyme* and *Thomas* but not in such wordsas *that* and *thin*.

8. In the *ght* context, the *gh* is silent and only the [t] sound is pronounced, as in *thought, bought, caught*.

9. In the *ct* context, the *c* is silent and the [t] sound is pronounced, as in *indict*.

10. One of the most unusual pronunciations occurs with the [t] sound in the *zz* context in the word *pizza*. In other contexts, such as *drizzle*, the [z] sound is pronounced.

Words That Include the [t] Sound

The [t] sound appears in all three positions, initial, medial, and final. Transcribe the following. Note the position in which the [t] sound occurs. Refer to the Key at the right upon completion.

Initial Consonant

				Key
tick ____	tub ____	table ____		tɪk, tʌb, teɪbḷ
tea ____	tube ____	Texas ____		ti, tub, tɛksəs
turkey ____	Thomas ____	tax ____		tɝki, tɔməs, tæks

Unstressed Syllable (Less Aspiration)

Medial Consonant

freighter ____			freɪtɚ
guitar ____	duty ____	eaten ____	kʌtɑr, duti, itən

Stressed Syllable (More Aspiration)

Medial Consonant

until ____	utensil ____		ʌntɪl, utɛnsəl
return ____	football ____	determine ____	ritən, fʊtbɔl, ditɝmən
protect ____	notation ____	potato ____	protɛt, noteɪʃən, pəteɪto

Final Consonant

belt ____	thrust ____	scent ____	bɛlt, ɵrʌst, sɛnt
meat ____	detect ____	comet ____	mit, ditɛt, kɔmət
dent ____	last ____	picked ____	dɛnt, læst, pɪkt

Initial and Final Consonant (More/Less Aspiration)

tight ____				taɪt
tipped ____	taught ____	tot ____	tent ____	tɪpt, tɔt, tɔt, tɛnt

Initial Blends

<u>tw</u> twin ____	twelve ____		twɪn, twɛlv
twilight ____	twig ____	twister ____	twaɪlaɪt, twɪg, twɪstɚ
<u>tr</u> trade ____	trip ____	troupe ____	treid, trɪp, trup
<u>st</u> stay ____	stop ____	store ____	steɪ, stɑp, stɔr

Medial Blends

<u>ft</u> rafter ____	thrifty ____	fifty ____	ræftɚ, ɵrɪfti, fɪfti
leftovers ____	<u>kt</u> active ____	practice ____	lɛftovɚz, æktɪv, prætəs
necktie ____	<u>tl</u> atlas ____	outlaw ____	nɛktaɪ, ætləs, aʊtlɔ
settler ____	outline ____	<u>lt</u> alter ____	sɛtlɚ, aʊtlaɪn, ɔltɚ
delta ____	filter ____	multiply ____	dɛltə, fɪltɚ, mɔltɪplaɪ
<u>nt</u> painting ____	rental ____	ninety ____	peɪntɪŋ, rɛntəl, naɪnti
county ____	printer ____		kaʊnti, prɪntɚ
<u>ts</u> Betsy ____	pizza ____	<u>st</u> coastal ____	bɛtsi, pitsə, koʊstəl
instant ____	abstain ____	distance ____	ɪnstənt, æbsteɪn, dɪstəns
<u>tr</u> introduce ____	actress ____		ɪntroʊdus, æktrəs
introduction ____			ɪntrodʌkʃən
<u>rt</u> departed ____	courtesy ____		dipɑrtəd, kɝtɪsi
comfortable ____			kəmfɝtəbḷ

Final Blends

<u>rt</u> airport	___	insert	___	yogurt	___	ɛrpɔrt, Insɝt, joʊgɚt
<u>st</u> therapist	___	soloist	___			Ɵɛrʌpɪst, soʊloɪst
nest	___	frost	___			nɛst, frɔst
<u>ts</u> rates	___	carrots	___	oats	___	reɪst, kɛrəts, oʊts
debts	___	putts	___	<u>nt</u> want	___	dɛts, pʌts, wɑnt
event	___	vibrant	___			ivɛnt, vaɪbrənt
<u>lt</u> belt	___	fault	___	adult	___	bɛlt, fɔlt, ədʌlt
<u>tl</u> parental	___	rattle	___	title	___	pɛrɛntəl, rætl̩, taɪtl̩
hotel	___	<u>ct</u> strict	___	conduct	___	hoʊtɛl, strɪkt, cəndʌkt
reflect	___	<u>ft</u> soft	___	thrift	___	riflɛkt, sɔft, Ɵrɪft
laughed	___	swift	___			læfət, swɪft
<u>pt</u> stepped	___	kept	___	shopped	___	stɛpt, kɛpt, ʃɑpt
<u>sht</u> pushed	___	rushed	___	crashed	___	pʊʃt, rʌʃt, kræʃt

Clusters

<u>str</u> strong	___	straight	___	stray	___	strɔŋ, streɪt, streɪ
<u>rcht</u> marched	___	searched	___			mɑrtʃət, sɝtʃɪd,
starched	___					stɑrtʃɪd
<u>rkt</u> parked	___	sparked	___	worked	___	pɑrkt, spɑrkt, wɝkt
<u>lts</u> malts	___	belts	___	melts	___	mɔlts, bɛlts, mɛlts
<u>rst</u> forced	___	first	___	endorsed	___	fɔrst, fɝst, ɛndɔrsɪd
<u>rts</u> parts	___	exports	___			pɑrts, ɛkspɔrts
quarts	___					kwɑrts
<u>sts</u> beasts	___	roasts	___	vests	___	bists, roʊsts, vɛsts
<u>mpt</u> lumped	___	stamped	___	dumped	___	lt, stæmpt, dʌmpt
<u>nts</u> fenced	___	tents	___	prints	___	fɛnts, tɛnts, prɪnts
[ŋkt] spanked	___	thanked	___			speɪŋkt, Ɵeɪŋkt,
ranked	___					reɪnkt

Auditory Discrimination

Transcribe the following words and note the slight difference in pronunciation of each set. Refer to the Key at the bottom upon completion.

Cognates				*Other Minimal Pairs*					
[t] (–)		*[d] (+)*		*[t]*		*[k]*		*[t]*		*[Ɵ]*

[t] (–)	*[d] (+)*	*[t]*	*[k]*	*[t]*	*[Ɵ]*
tick ___	Dick ___	late ___	lake ___	tie ___	thigh ___
to ___	do ___	lot ___	lock ___	tree ___	three ___
cart ___	card ___	tall ___	call ___	team ___	theme ___
ten ___	den ___	tame ___	came ___	tick ___	thick ___

touch	___	Dutch	___	mate	___	make	___	pat	___	path	___	
ate	___	aid	___	tea	___	key	___	boat	___	both	___	

Key (left to right): tɪk, dɪk, leɪt, leɪk, taɪ, Ɵaɪ, tu, du, lɑt, lɑk, tri, Ɵri, kɑrt, kɑrd, tɔl, kɔl, tim, Ɵim, tɛn, dɛn, taɪm, kaɪm, tɪk, Ɵɪk, tʌtʃ, dʌtʃ, meɪt, meɪk, pæt, pæƟ, eɪt, eɪd, ti, ki, boʊt, boʊƟ

Allophonic and Dialect Variations

The allophones within the [t] sound vary considerably (Carrell & Tiffany, 1960). They may be classified as follows: (1) variants in place of articulation resulting from assimilation, elision, consonant clustering, and dialect; (2) variants in articulatory tension or force that result from differences in stress, rhythm, and juncture; (3) variants in release mechanisms, related to stress and context; and (4) variants of articulatory type, largely related to stress and rhythm. Many of the allophonic variations of the [t] sound are similar to its cognate, the [d] sound (Davenport & Hannahs, 1998). The [t] sounds somewhat different depending on the position in which it occurs and the surrounding sounds (Edwards, 1997). The four positions are initial: *time*; medial: *total* and *brittle*; final: *caught, tight*; and cluster: *steeple, stream*. When the [t] sound occurs in connected speech, the feature of aspiration is particularly varied (Calvert, 1986). The following is a summary of the allophonic variations:

1. The flapped, intervocalic [ɾ]. One of the most unusual and yet logical variations occurs with what is termed the flap sound [ɾ] that replaces the more distinct [t] sound in words where the letters *tt* occur in the medial position, as in *butter* and *bitter*. This phenomenon of "flapping" found in many North American accents neutralizes the distinctiveness of the [t] sound because of the influence of the vowel (voiced) sounds on both sides of the [t] (voiceless) sound.

   Most American speakers, irrespective of whether they have lateral plosion or not, do not have a voiceless stop in *little* and do not distinguish between words such as *latter* and *ladder* (Ladefoged, 1993). Whenever [t] occurs after a stressed vowel and before an unstressed syllable other than [ŋ], it is changed into a voiced sound. For most Americans who have lateral plosion, in words such as *city, better, writer*, the articulation is not really a stop but a quick flap or tap in which the tongue tip is thrown against the alveolar ridge, thus *city* [sɪti] becomes [sɪɾi].

Phoneticians refer to the sound that is produced as a flap and transcribe it as *butter*: [bʌɾɚ]. Because of this allophonic definition, such a pronunciation is not to be considered as a [d] substitution for a [t] sound, although, acoustically, it may sound like the [d] sound. The pronunciation is somewhere between the two (Small, 1999), and the term *tap* is used interchangeably with *flap*. Tap articulation involves a very rapid movement of the tongue tip against the alveolar ridge creating a very brief stop consonant. The motion associated with a tapped stop consonant is more rapid than the traditional stop articulation of [t] or [d]. It generally occurs in words with an intervocalic *t* or *d* digraph in which the first syllable is stressed, as in *bitter, battle*, and *stutter*, and when the intervocalic [t] is at the end of a stressed syllable, as in *static, photos*, and *vital*.

It is interesting to note that most published articulation tests used by speech pathologists do not address the flap. Neither do they include the *tt* in the medial position or the flap [t] in the stimuli items. They usually consider the flap in *pity* [pidy] as a [d] substitution of the [t] sound. In teaching phonics, Hull and Fox (1998) indicate in their discussion of the [t] sound that only one *t* is sounded in such words as *letter*. Perhaps this is the case in the most precise pronunciation of the word *letter*, but it is doubtful that when reading aloud such precision is maintained.

2. Audible aspiration [tʰ]. (a) The initial consonant in a stressed syllable, as in *tie, retire, until, attest*; (b) the final consonant following consonants that are homorganic, having the same or nearly the same place of articulation, as in *want, cart, salt*; (c) following voiceless consonants in the final position, as in *kept, act, finished, watched*, or a medial consonant, as in *after, luster, sitting*; (d) the [t] is released into the position of the following voiceless consonant, as in *pats, that sign, that part*, and *that ship*.

3. Without audible aspiration [t]. (a) The final consonant followed by a vowel, as in *at, bit, hot, let*; (b) after [s] in the same syllable, as in *stop* (compare aspirated *top* with *stop*), *steam, restore*. However, the [t] is released with aspiration when it initiates a syllable. Compare *the store* with *this tore*.

4. Unreleased. Weakening of the final stop in certain clusters may result in its complete omission. Such as when *act* [ækt] becomes [æk] and *ghosts* [goʊsts] becomes [gos].

5. Dentalized. The [t] is made as a linguadental sound with the tongue tip in contact with the teeth rather than with the alveolar ridge. Examples include *eighth* [eɪtθ] and phrases such as *at them* [æt θəm].

6. Nasal release. A nasal after the [t] may lead to a nasal release, as in *button* [bʌtn̩].

7. Glottal stop [ʔ]. Before a syllabic [n̩] or [l̩], as in *bottle* [bɔʔl̩].

8. Intrusive. The addition of [t], as in *dance* [dænts]. Notice that there is no difference in the pronunciation of *tense/tents* [tɛns], but because of the proximity of the *n-t-s*, a [t] may be slightly pronounced.

9. Lengthening. When an arresting [t] is followed by a releasing [t], as in *not time* [nɑt:aɪm].

Some languages have a plosive produced by placing the tip or apex of the tongue against the forward part of the palatal region (MacKay, 1987). The term **retroflex** is used to describe the place of articulation because the tongue is bent (or flexed) back on itself. MacKay indicates that in some dialects of English, when a [t] occurs at the beginning of a word before an *r* sound, both the plosive and the *r* may be retroflex, as in the word *train*.

Words with the *tr* blend may produce an affrication of the [t], and such words as *train* would be pronounced as [tʃreɪn] and *trap* [tʃræp]. Omission may occur within consonant clusters that are somewhat difficult to pronounce, as in *fists* [fɪs:]. Black American speakers may omit the final consonant blend, as in *guest* [gʌɛ:], and in consonant clusters *str*, the velar [k] (backing) may occur as in *strong* [skrɑŋ]. Also, the [d] may be substituted for the [t], as in *they* [deɪ]. The voiceless *th* [θ] becomes [t] initially as in *thumb* [tʌm] and after a lingua-alveolar [n], as in *month* [mʌnt]. Typical of some New York City speakers is the use of the glottal stop before [l̩], as in *battle* [bæʔl̩] and *bottle* [bɑʔl̩], and dentalization of the [t] as in *total* [toʊtl̩].

Normal and Deviant Development of the [t] Sound

The [t] sound is the last of the stop consonants to be acquired (Sander, 1972). It is mastered by age 6, two years after the other stops, and is one of the most frequently occurring consonants in United States English speech (Calvert, 1986). During the developmental period of acquisition, the [t] may be omitted or have a different sound substitution such as –at for *cat* or *dat*.

Nonnative Speaker Pronunciation

Test for strength of production, especially in initial position, so that [t] is produced with aspiration (Edwards, 1997). A dentalized [t] may have little aspiration and may be heard by a listener as a [d] sound (Tiffany & Carrell, 1977). A number of Asian languages, as well as French and Italian, exhibit a more "fronted" dental [t] sound. On the other hand, excessive aspiration of [t] may occur in the speech of persons with a foreign dialect. In some Eastern dialects and in British English, the [t] has a more strident release and words such as *butter* and *bitter* are pronounced with much more [t] precision. The allophones are very important for this sound, especially the voiced intervocalic [t]. It is not a problem otherwise. Europeans may make the [t] with insufficient aspiration in the initial and final positions, and they may make closure with the tip of the tongue on the inside surface of the upper front teeth rather than on the alveolar ridge (Calvert, 1986).

The [t] sound, with some allophonic variations, is present in the 15 other sound systems of languages predominantly spoken in the United States. These sound systems are Spanish, French, German, Italian, Chinese, Tagalog, Polish, Korean, Portuguese, Japanese, Greek, Vietnamese, Arabic, Hindi (Urdu), and Russian.

Summary

The [t] sound is one of the three voiceless stop consonants ([t], [p], [k]), and its voiced cognate is the [d] sound. In addition to [d], it is homorganic (lingua-alveolar) with the [s], [z], [l], [m], and with the first sounds in the affricatives [ʧ] and [ʤ]. There are at least 10 different orthographic letters or set of letters of a wide variety that represent the [t] sound, including *ct, pt, ed, z*, and at least three entirely different functions of the *t* wherein the [t] sound is not present. For example, the letters *th* represent the voiced *th* [ð] in *the* and the voiceless *th* [Ө] in *thin* and *t* is silent as in *castle* and *listen*. The [t] sound, acquired by age 6, is the last of the stops to be mastered, taking up to 2 years after the others have been established. The flapped [ɾ] intervocalic symbol is used to

indicate the sound that is produced in words such as *butter* [bʌɾɚ] and *pity* [pɪɾi], and it is difficult for a listener to distinguish between such words as *latter* and *ladder*. Dialect differences may occur with the affrication of the [t] sound, resulting in [tʃreɪn] for *train*. Consonant clusters such as *sts* as in *infests* may be difficult to pronounce, resulting in the deletion of the [t] sound. Some New York City speakers substitute the glottal stop. Nonnative and foreign speakers may either under- or overaspirate the [t] sound and have a tendency to dentalize it.

Individuals with impaired velopharyngeal closure may experience difficulty in the production and maintenance of the stop phase of the [t] sound, and a portion of the aspiration may escape through the nasal passageway.

[t] +

Write out the words using both orthographic spelling and phonetic symbols. Refer to the Key at the bottom upon completion of the transcription.

	Orthographic	Phonetic
1. [t] + 2 sounds: opposite of give	_____	[_eɪ_]
2. [t] + 3 sounds: one of our senses	_____	[_eɪ__]
3. [t] + 2 sounds: a large East Indian tree	_____	[_i_]
4. [t] + 3 sounds: crisp slice of bread	_____	[_oʊ__]
5. [t] + 1 sound: one plus one	_____	[_u]
6. [t] + 2 sounds: comes in at night at the beach	_____	[_aɪ_]
7. [t] + 6 sounds: a wild wind	_____	[_ɔ__eɪ_o]
8. [t] + 5 sounds: a fruit	_____	[_ə_eɪ_o]
9. [t] + 7 sounds: a car for hire	_____	[_æ__ɪ_æ_]
10. [t] + 6 sounds: famous sunken ship	_____	[_aɪ_æ_ɪ_]

Key: 1. take [teɪk]; 2. taste [teɪst]; 3. teak [tik]; 4. toast [toʊst]; 5. two [tu]; 6. tide [taɪd]; 7. tornado [tɔrneɪdo]; 8. tomato [təmeɪto]; 9. taxicab [tæksikæb]; 10. *Titanic* [taɪtænɪk]

PHONETIC SYMBOL [d]

EXHIBIT 13-4 **Phonetic Symbol [d]**

Phonetic Symbol	[d]	**[d]**
Grapheme Symbols	d, dd, ed, ld	
Diacritic Symbol	d	
Phonic Symbol	D	
Cognate	[t]	
Homorganic	Lingua-Alveolar [s], [z], [t], [l], [n] Initial Sound in [tʃ] and [dʒ]	
Sound Class	Consonant	
Basic Phonetic Features	Placement: Lingua-Alveolar Manner: Stop/Plosive Voicing: Plus Voice	
IPA (1999)	[d] #104 Dental or Alveolar, Plosive, Voiceless	

How the Sound Is Produced

The [d] sound is made by placing the tongue (lingua) against the upper gum (alveolar) ridge. These two articulators form a seal, and air pressure builds up (implosion-stop) in the oral cavity between the surface of the tongue and the roof of the mouth. When the air is expelled (explosion-plosive) by the release of the tongue, an audible aspirated voiced (plus voice) [d] sound is produced by the activation of the adducted (closed) vocal folds by the air stream from the lungs. The voiceless cognate [t] is produced with more aspiration than the [d]. See **Figure 13-4**.

Different Spellings for the [d] Sound

Transcribe the following. Refer to the Key at the right upon completion.

Different Spellings			*Key*
d deed ___ bold ___			dɪd, boʊld
dictionary___ rider ___			dɪkʃənɛri, raɪdɚ
dd fiddle ___ meddle ___	ladder ___		fɪdl̩, mɛdl̩, lædɚ
wedding ___ pudding ___			wɛdɪŋ, pʊdɪŋ
ed shaved ___ plowed ___	played ___		ʃeɪvd, plowd, pleɪd
rubbed ___ tried ___			rʌbd, traɪd
ld could ___ would ___	should ___		kʊd, wʊd, ʃʊd

Different Sounds for the Letter *d*

Transcribe the following words. Refer to the Key at the right upon completion.

		Key
di [j] soldier ___		soʊldʒɚ
ed [t] jumped ___ waited ___ picked ___		dʒʌmpt, weɪtɪd, pɪkt
dg [dʒ] edge ___ ridge ___		ɛdʒ, rɪdʒ

Rules for Spelling and Pronunciation of the [d] Sound

1. The written *d* is pronounced as [d] in most contexts.

2. Two adjacent *d* letters (*dd*) may be pronounced as a single [d], and traditionally the [d] sound is assigned to the first syllable (*todd-ler*).

3. The [d] sound maintains its integrity when used in word endings (suffixes) when it occurs after a *voiced* consonant such as the [g] in *tugged* and *returned*. However, its voiceless cognate [t] is substituted when the *ed* suffix occurs after a *voiceless* consonant, as in *mixed, picked*.

4. In words such as *judge* and *ridge*, the [dʒ] such as the first sound in the word *jam* [dʒæm] is spoken rather than the [d] sound.

5. In the *ld* context, the *l* is silent as in *could, would* but not in *mold* and *cold*.

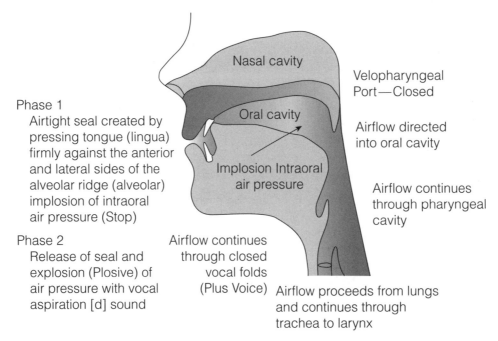

Phase 1
Airtight seal created by pressing tongue (lingua) firmly against the anterior and lateral sides of the alveolar ridge (alveolar) implosion of intraoral air pressure (Stop)

Phase 2
Release of seal and explosion (Plosive) of air pressure with vocal aspiration [d] sound

Nasal cavity

Velopharyngeal Port—Closed

Oral cavity

Airflow directed into oral cavity

Implosion Intraoral air pressure

Airflow continues through pharyngeal cavity

Airflow continues through closed vocal folds (Plus Voice)

Airflow proceeds from lungs and continues through trachea to larynx

Figure 13-4 [d] pronunciation.

6. The first sound in the word *yellow* [jɛlo] has the distinction of the peculiar pronunciation of *soldier* [soʊljɚ].

Words That Include the [d] Sound

The [d] sound occurs in all three positions, initial, medial, and final. Transcribe the following words and note the position of the [d] sound. Refer to the Key at the right upon completion.

Initial Consonant   *Key*

deed _____ dig _____ dead _____   did, dɪg, dɛd

dagger _____ dirty _____ dug _____   dægɚ, dɝɾɪ, dʌg

dart _____ door _____   dɑrt, dɔr

Unstressed Syllable

Medial Consonant

indicate _____ sturdy _____   ɪndɪket, stɝdi

modern _____ fading _____ lady _____   mɔdɚn, feɪdɪŋ, leɪdi

Stressed Syllable

Medial Consonant

produce _____ today _____   proʊdus, tudeɪ

reduction _____   ridʌkʃən

Final Consonant

cloud _____ need _____ loved _____ klaʊd, nid, lʌvd

odd _____ add _____   ɔd, æd

Initial and Final Consonants

did __ dead __ deed __ dad __   dɪd, dɛd, did, dæd

Initial Blend

drop __ drew __ drum __ dread __   drɔp, dru, drʌm, drɛd

Final Blends

<u>nd</u> round _____   <u>ld</u> told _____   raʊnd, toʊld

<u>rd</u> card _____   <u>md</u> tamed _____   kɑrd, teɪmd

<u>gd</u> rigged _____   <u>zd</u> sneezed _____   rɪgd, snizd

<u>bd</u> robbed _____   <u>vd</u> shaved _____   rɑbd, ʃeɪvd

<u>gd</u> judged _____   banged _____   dʒʌdʒd, beɪŋd

<u>rds</u> curds _____   <u>thd</u> soothed _____   kɝdz, suðd

Auditory Discrimination

Transcribe the following. Note the slight difference in the pronunciation of the pairs of words. Refer to the Key at the end upon completion.

Cognates		*Other Minimal Pairs*			
[d] (+)	*[t] (–)*	*[d]*	*[b]*	*[d]*	*[n]*
Dee __	tea __	Dan __	ban __	D __	knee __
door __	tore __	did __	bid __	dot __	not __
do __	to __	deed __	bead __	main __	made __
doe __	toe __	dead __	bed __	dear __	near __
bad __	bat __	darn __	barn __	mad __	man __
had __	hat __	cad __	cab __	done __	none __

Key (left to right): di, ti, dæn, bæn, di, ni, dɔr, tɔr, dɪd, bɪd, dɑt, nɑt, du, tu, did, bid, meɪn, meɪd, doʊ, toʊ, dɛd, bɛd, dɛr, nɛr, bæd, bæt, dɑrn, bɑrn, mæd, mæn, hæd, hæt, kæd, kæb, dʌn, nʌn

Allophonic and Dialect Variations

Unlike the velars and bilabials, the alveolars [t] and [d] show considerable variation depending on context (Davenport & Hannahs, 1998). Examples such as *bad boy* [bæbɔɪ] and *sad man* [sæmæn] demonstrate that the closure for the [d] is not alveolar but is at the place of articulation of the following segment: the [b] in *bad boy* and the [m] in *sad man*. These are examples of influences of other consonant sounds.

The alveolar stops also show variation between vowels in a number of varieties, including the phenomenon of flapping found in many North American accents of English. The term *flapping* is used to indicate that the distinction between [t] and [d] is lost because their differences are neutralized between vowels. For example, in United States English pronunciation the words *Adam* and *atom* become homophones, that is, they sound identical, with both words having the flap for the intervocalic [t] and [d]. Davenport and Hannahs (1998) point out that one exception occurs when the stop begins a stressed syllable, as in *attend* [ətɛnd], where the second syllable is stressed.

The varieties of allophones within the [d] sound are a result of the place of tongue contact, which may range from a dental to a palatal location (Carrell & Tiffany, 1960; Edwards, 1997). For example:

1. The point of contact of the tongue tends to extend beyond the alveolar ridge to the top teeth to become a dentalized [d] when the [d] is followed by an interdental, as in *width* [wɪdΘ].

2. A bilateral or palatalized tongue release position occurs when [d] is followed by an [l], as in *candelabra* and *dog* or *heard*, where the [d] is followed or preceded by a sound produced toward the palatal area.

3. Further weakening of the [d] sound can produce an affrication quality or lingua-alveolar fricative, as in [dʒreɪn] for *drain* [dreɪn].

4. A nasal release may occur when [d] is followed by a syllabic nasal, as when *Rodney* [rɑdni] becomes [rɑdni].

5. The [d] may be unreleased in the final position, as when *land* [lænd] becomes [læn].

6. The [d] sound may be lengthened when an arresting [d] is followed by a releasing [d], as in *defend Dan* [difɛd:æn].

7. Omission of the [d] sound may occur when it is preceded or followed by a sound that has a similar articulatory position, as in *friendly*, where the [n] and the [d] are both lingua-alveolar. The [d] may be deleted and an [nd] context would be pronounced [frenli].

Native American English speakers exhibit different degrees of aspiration and placement of aspiration in the production of the [d] sound. Ordinarily, these changes do not present significant problems in the intelligibility of the utterance but could be noticed as different. For example, there are speakers in New York City and other regions who tend to dentalize the alveolar [d], and its effect is audible to the listener.

African Americans may devoice the [d] sound in the final position and lengthen the preceding vowel, as in *good* [gʊ:t] and *said* [sɛ:t]. Or they may delete the [d] when followed by a consonant, as in *could be* [kʊl:bi] (Edwards, 1997). Also, an omission of a final consonant blend could be spoken, as in *played* [pleɪ].

Normal and Deviant Development of the [d] Sound

The [d] sound is usually acquired by the age of 4 years (Sander, 1972) and is one of the most frequently occurring consonant sounds in United States English speech (Calvert, 1986). The [d] sound is often misarticulated (Calvert, 1986).

Nonnative Speaker Pronunciation

The allophonic [d] sound occurs in many sound systems worldwide. In some languages, plosives such as the [d] are not produced with the blade of the tongue against the alveolar ridge as in English (MacKay, 1987). Rather, the tip of the tongue is against the upper teeth. This apicodental (tip or apex of the tongue against the teeth) is characteristic of the Spanish pronunciation of [t] and [d]. This change in position can produce some minor or major changes in the way a native Spanish speaker pronounces the [d] when speaking United States English.

The [d] is often produced without sufficient strength, especially in stressed syllables. In such contexts, Edwards (1997) explains that it may be replaced by the voiced interdental fricative, the *th* [ð]. The word *day* [deɪ] is pronounced [ðeɪ]. Nonnative speakers also have a tendency to devoice [d] in the final position and replace it with its voiceless cognate [t], as when *bed* [bɛd] becomes [bɛt]. Generally speaking, voicing may be a major problem in some foreign dialects of English that results in confusion as to whether the sound is a [d] or a [t].

Strong release of the [d] as the final consonant in a word may result in the addition of an extra syllable (Tiffany & Carrell, 1977). In many foreign dialects of United States English, the speaker is accustomed to adding a vowel sound to the end of certain words because words in many other languages end in vowels. For example, nonnative speakers will add a vowel sound to the word *stand* in the phrase "Stand by me," as in [stændə bai mi].

The [d] sound, with its allophonic variations, is present in the 15 other sound systems of languages predominantly spoken in the United States. These sound systems are Spanish, French, German, Italian, Chinese, Tagalog, Polish, Korean, Portuguese, Japanese, Greek, Vietnamese, Arabic, Hindi (Urdu), and Russian.

Summary

The [d] sound is one of the three voiced stop consonants ([b], [d], [g]), and its voiceless cognate is the [t] sound. In addition to the [t], it is homorganic (linguavelar) with the [s], [z], [l], [n], and with the first sounds in the affricatives [tʃ] and [dʒ]. The letter *d* appears in about the same number of contexts in which it is pronounced as a [d] or as a different sound such as the *ed*

in *picked* or the *dg* in *judge*. The [d] sound is mastered by children at approximately 4 years of age, which is the same age for acquisition of the [k] and [g] sounds. Dialect differences occur in the degree and placement of aspiration, and this sound may be dentalized. Some nonnative speakers tend to dentalize the [d] sound or produce it without sufficient strength. A substitution of the voiced fricative [ð] may occur. Individuals with impaired velopharyngeal closure or other oral neuromuscular impairments may experience difficulty in the production (precision and strength) and maintenance (endurance) of the stop/release phases of the [d] sound, and a portion of the aspiration may escape through the nasal passageway and exhibit other weakened production.

[d] +

Write out the words using orthographic spelling and phonetic symbols. Refer to the Key at the end upon completion.

		Orthographic	Phonetic
1.	[d] + 2 sounds: moisture on ground	_____	[_ ju]
2.	[d] + 1 sound: something we all will do	_____	[_ aɪ]
3.	[d] + 2 sounds: opposite of shallow	_____	[_ i _]
4.	[e] + 3 sounds: girls like to go on them	_____	[_ eɪ _ _]
5.	[d] + 1 sound: slang for money	_____	[_ oʊ]
6.	[d] + 9 sounds: a type of government	_____	[_ ɛ _ ʌ _ _ æ _ ɪ _]
7.	[d] + 7 sounds: a person on insulin	_____	[_ aɪə _ ɛ _ ɪ _]
8.	[d] + 10 sounds: to make distinction	_____	[_ ɪ _ _ _ ɪ _ ə _ e _]
9.	[d] + 7 sounds: a sleuth	_____	[_ i _ ɛ _ _ ɪ _]
10.	[d] + 9 sounds: to show	_____	[_ ɛ _ ə _ _ _ _ e _]

Key: 1. dew [dju]; 2. die [daɪ]; 3. deep [dip]; 4. dates [deɪts]; 5. dough [doʊ]; 6. democratic [dɛmʌkrætɪk]; 7. diabetic [daɪəbɛtɪk]; 8. discriminate [dɪskrɪmənet]; 9. detective [ditɛktɪv]; 10. demonstrate [dɛmənstret]

PHONETIC SYMBOL [k]

EXHIBIT 13-5	Phonetic Symbol [k]

Phonetic Symbol	[k]	[k]
Grapheme Symbols	k, c, ch, ck, cc, kh, x, q	
Diacritic Symbol	k	
Phonic Symbol	K	
Cognate	[g]	
Homorganic	Lingua-Alveolar [g], [h], [ʍ], [w], [ŋ]	
Sound Class	Consonant	
Basic Phonetic Features	Placement: Lingua-Velar Manner: Stop/Plosive Voicing: Minus Voice	
IPA (1999)	[k] #109 Voiceless, Velar, Plosive	

How the Sound Is Produced

The [k] sound is produced in two phases. First the stop phase occurs as the back of the tongue (lingua) closes against the front of the velum (velar) or back portion of the palate as the airflow from the lungs is held (implosion-stop) and compressed in the back of the oral cavity and in the oropharynx. The second phase involving aspiration (explosion) occurs when the compressed air in the oral cavity and oropharynx is released suddenly (plosive) as an audible noise between the tongue and roof of the mouth. The [k] sound is produced with the velopharyngeal port closed and the vocal folds opened, thus it is a voiceless sound. The voiced cognate is the [g] sound, and it is produced with less aspiration than the [k] sound. See **Figure 13-5**.

Different Spellings for the [k] Sound

Transcribe the following words and note the different letters that represent the [k] sound. Refer to the Key at the right upon completion.

Different Spellings				*Key*
k	king _____	kayak _____		kɪŋ, kaɪjæk
	keep _____	baker _____		kip, beɪkɚ
c	copper _____	zinc _____		kɑpɚ, zɪŋk
	tic _____	chic _____		tɪk, ʃɪk
ch	echo _____	chrome _____	ache _____	ɛkoʊ, kroʊm, eɪk
ck	tick _____	luck _____		tɪk, lʌk

cc	access _____	accurate _____		æksɛs, æk3ɪt
	occur _____			oʊkɚ
kh	khaki _____	Khan _____		kæki, kɑn
x (ks)	excess _____	box _____		ɛksɛs, bɑks
cq (kw)	acquittal _____	acquire _____		əkwɪtl, əkwaɪr
	acquit _____			əkwɪt
q	inquire _____	liquid _____		ɪnkwaɪr, lɪkwɪd
	liquor _____			lɪkɚ
que	technique _____	baroque _____		tɛknik, b3oʊk
	Basque _____			bæsk

Different Sounds for the Letter *k*

Transcribe the following words. Refer to the Key at the right upon completion.

					Key
k [k]	king _____				kɪŋ
k (silent)	knee _____	knight _____	knead _____		ni, naɪt, nid

Rules for Spelling and Pronunciation of the [k] Sound

1. The written *k* is pronounced [k], as in *king, tickle*, and *pink*, and when it appears between two vowels within a word, as in *locket, blockade*.

2. The letter *k* and [k] sound are quite dependable in their sound/symbol relationship except when the *k* is silent.

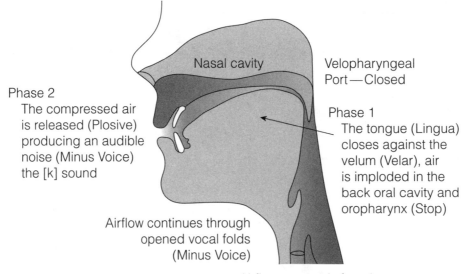

Nasal cavity

Velopharyngeal
Port—Closed

Phase 2
The compressed air
is released (Plosive)
producing an audible
noise (Minus Voice)
the [k] sound

Phase 1
The tongue (Lingua)
closes against the
velum (Velar), air
is imploded in the
back oral cavity and
oropharynx (Stop)

Airflow continues through
opened vocal folds
(Minus Voice)

Airflow proceeds from lungs
and continues through
trachea to larynx

Figure 13-5 [k] pronunciation.

3. The *k* is not pronounced when followed by the letter *n*, as in *knight, knew, knowledge, knuckle,* and *knock.*

4. The *ca, co, cl, cr,* and *cu* spellings become a [k] sound in words such as *can, could, crow,* and *biscuit.*

5. Notice that in a word such as *circle,* the first *c* is pronounced as an [s] and the second *c* as a [k].

6. The consonant blend *ch* represents the [k] sound in some contexts such as *chloroform, technique, ache, echo,* and *chlorinate.* However, the *ch* is pronounced as a [tʃ] in *chime, cheer,* and *chimney* or [ʃ] as in *chalet.*

7. *Tick* and *luck* have four written letters but only three sounds because *ck* is pronounced as a [k] only. The *ck* is always pronounced [k], as in *black, neck,* and *back.*

8. Two adjacent *c* letters (*cc*) may be pronounced as a single [k], as in *acclaim* and when preceding the letter *u* in *occur,* *o* in *accommodation,* and *a* in *staccato.*

9. The consonant blend *kh* in *Khan* and the Hindi word *khaki* is an unusual spelling context for the [k] sound in the initial position.

10. The letter *x* is pronounced as a combination of the [k] and [s] sounds, as in *x-ray, fox, box,* and *exercise.* This rule generally applies when the [k] sound is in the stressed syllable. It is also common for the *x* to be pronounced as a [z] sound when it occurs at the beginning of a word, as in *xebec, xylem,* and *xylophone.*

11. The letter *q* is pronounced as a combination of the [k] and [w] sounds, as in *queen, quiet,* and *quick.* Also the *q* in *appliqué* and *technique* is a [k] sound.

12. The [k] sound is usually spelled with a *k* before the letters *e* and *I*, as in *kind, blanket, kettle,* and it is spelled with a *c* before the letters *a, o,* and *u,* as in *come, cage,* and *cunning.*

13. An intruded [k] sound, not included in spelling, may occur in the *–ngth* context between [ŋ] and [Θ], as in *length* [lɛŋkΘ] and *strength* [strɛŋkΘ].

Words That Include the [k] Sound

Transcribe the following words. Note the position of the [k] sound. Refer to the Key at the right upon completion.

Initial Consonant			*Key*
kit ____	curb ____	kind ____	kɪt, kɚb, kɪnd
coin ____	quit ____	quote ____	kɔɪn, kwɪt, kwoʊt

Unstressed Syllable (Less Aspiration)

Medial Consonant

taken ___			teɪkən
vacant ___	bobcat ___	broken ___	veɪkənt, bɔbkæt, broʊkən
liquor ___	making ___	bacon ___	lɪkɚ, meɪkɪŋ, beɪkən

Stressed Syllable (More Aspiration)

Medial Consonant

become ___   bɪkəm

request ___ include ___ cotton ___   rikwɛst, ɪnklud, kɔtn̩

cupboard ___ keep ___ actor ___   kʌbɝd, kip, æktɚ

Final Consonant

irk ___ bake ___ metric ___   ɝk, beɪk, mɛtrɪk

lyric ___ magic ___ rhythmic ___   lɪrɪk, mædʒɪk, rɪðmɪk

Initial and Final Consonants (More/Less Aspiration)

kick ___ cake ___ coke ___   kɪk, keɪk, koʊk

Kodak ___ click ___ kayak ___   koʊdæk, klɪk, kaɪjæk

clock ___ crook ___   klɑk, krʊk

Initial Blends

<u>sk</u> school ___ sky ___ <u>kr</u> crow ___   skul, skaɪ, kroʊ

crime ___ <u>kl</u> climb ___ clip ___   kraɪm, klaɪm, klɪp

<u>kw</u> quick ___ quite ___   kwɪk, kwaɪt

<u>skr</u> scream ___ screen ___   skrim, skrin

<u>sk(w)</u> squash ___   skwæʃ

Medial Blends

<u>kl</u> chuckle ___ decline ___   tʃʌkl̩, diklaɪn

sparkle ___ <u>lk</u> bulky ___ silky ___   spɑrkl̩, bʊlki, sɪlki

welcome ___ <u>kr</u> increase ___   wɛlkəm, ɪnkris

cockroach ___ recruit ___   kɔkrotʃ, rikrut

<u>rk</u> arcade ___ market ___ turkey ___   ɑrkeɪd, mɑrkɪt, tɝki

<u>ks</u> oxen ___ Jackson ___   ɔksən, dʒæksən

Final Blends

<u>ks</u> picks ___ mix ___   pɪks, mɪks

<u>ked</u> [k] [t] cooked ___ asked ___   kʊkt, æskt

<u>nk</u> [ŋk] sink ___ spank ___   sɪŋk, speɪŋk

<u>sk</u> task ___ risk ___   tæsk, rɪsk

<u>rk</u> pork ___ bark ___   pɔrk, bɑrk

Clusters

<u>rkt</u> jerked ___ <u>exp</u> (ksp) expect ___   dʒɝkt, ɛkspɛkt

<u>kst</u> sixty ___ <u>ngk</u> [ŋk] anchor ___   sɪksti, eɪŋkɚ

drink ___ donkey ___   drɪŋk, dɔŋki

<u>nks</u> [ŋks] pranks ___ thanks ___   præŋks, Θæŋks

<u>nkt</u> [ŋkt] thanked ___ linked ___   Θæŋkt, lɪŋkt

<u>rked</u> [rkt] sparked ___ marked ___   spɑrkt, mɑrkt

Auditory Discrimination

Transcribe the following words. Note the slight difference in pronunciation of the pairs of words. Refer to the Key at the right upon completion.

Cognate Pairs   *Other Minimal Pairs*

[k] (–Voice)	[g] (+Voice)	[k]	[t]	Key
Kay ___	gay ___	key ___	tea ___	keɪ, geɪ, ki, ti
cap ___	gap ___	back ___	bat ___	kæp, gæp, bæk, bæt
came ___	game ___	cake ___	take ___	keɪm, geɪm, keɪk, teɪk
Kate ___	gate ___	scare ___	stare ___	keɪt, geɪt, skɛr, stɛr
curl ___	girl ___	stark ___	start ___	kɝl, gɝl, stɑrk, stɑrt
come ___	gum ___	cry ___	try ___	kʌm, gʌm, kraɪ, traɪ
sink ___	sing ___	cone ___	tone ___	sɪŋk, sɪŋ, koɪn, toɪn
back ___	bag ___	lick ___	lit ___	bæk, bæg, lɪk, lɪt
lock ___	log ___	neck ___	net ___	lɔk, lɔg, nɛk, nɛt
pick ___	pig ___	pick ___	pit ___	pɪk, pɪg, pɪk, pɪt
rack ___	rag ___	knock ___	not ___	ræk, ræg, nɔk, nɔt

[k]	[p]	[k]	[tʃ]	Key
can ___	pan ___	back ___	batch ___	kæn, pæn, bæk, bætʃ
cart ___	part ___	pack ___	patch ___	kɑrt, pɑrt, pæk, pætʃ
keep ___	peek ___	cat ___	chat ___	kip, pik, kæt, tʃæt
ache ___	ape ___	pick ___	pitch ___	eɪk, eɪp, pɪk, pɪtʃ

Allophonic and Dialect Variations

The [k] is a phoneme that contains a large number of sounds principally because the exact point of articulation is strongly influenced by the character of the sounds that precede and follow (Carrell & Tiffany, 1960). Small (1999) states that the different articulatory gestures common for the production of the [k] demonstrate the process of coarticulation during speech production. Keep in mind that a phoneme's identity can be constantly altered by the other phonemes that precede or follow it. In ordinary connected speech when oral stops such as the [k] are produced, the closing stage and/or the release stage may be missing because of the influence of neighboring sounds (Davenport & Hannahs, 1998). Ball and Rahilly (1999) extend the influence beyond the adjacent sounds and state that it can be found that a particular phonetic feature can spread across a series of segments and need not be restricted to influence between neighboring segments. A whole word or string of words can be affected. They use the term *allophonic feature spread* when only the segment (sound) is altered allophonically. On the other hand, if the result is a series of changed phonemes, this falls into the category normally termed *consonant* or *vowel harmony*. Consonant harmony is a process that primarily affects place of articulation (Khan, 1985). Some include other types of assimilation in this category. For example, when *kiss* [kɪs] becomes [sɪs], not only has the [k] been pulled toward the alveolar [s], it has also taken on the characteristics of **stridency**.

In several contexts, the [k] may be released with variable degrees of aspiration. The [k] is released with strong aspiration in these phonemic contexts:

1. In the initial position of a word, as in *choir, key, came, chrome*

2. In the final position when preceded by the [ŋ] sound, as in *thank, zinc, sank*

The [k] is released with moderate aspiration in these phonemic contexts:

1. In the final position, as in *luck, tic, ache, sick, technique*. However, notice the difference in aspiration of the initial [k] sound and final [k] sound in *kick, cake, kayak*. Which [k] sound has the greater amount of aspiration?

2. In the medial position, as in *occur, acquire, rocket, liquid*. Note that the [k] sound occurs in the unstressed syllable.

The [k] is released without audible aspiration in these phonemic contexts:

1. In the final position of a syllable that is followed by a syllable or word that begins with a voiced consonant, as in compound words, *blackmail, jackknifed, breakdown, bike ride, economic news*.

2. In the medial or final position of a syllable or word that is followed by a voiceless consonant, the [k] sound release occurs more with that voiceless consonant, as in [kt] *picked, baked, pink tights, backpack*.

3. In a consonant blend beginning with *s*, as in *score, sky, scream, skin, squirt*.

Carrell and Tiffany (1960) and Ball and Rahilly (1999) observe that if [k] is followed by a front vowel, as in *keep* [kip], *key* [ki], or *keen* [kin], the contact that stops the breath is quite far forward (fronted velar), perhaps even on the hard palate rather than on the velum. In contrast, when words like *car* [kɑr] or *cook* [kʊk] are pronounced, the contact is much farther back because the vowel placement is in the back-vowel position. In contrast to the unrounded lip position of the [k] sound, the lips become rounded in the [kw] context, as in *queen, inquire*. The nasal influence is present in such contexts as [k] plus a nasal [ŋ], as in *bank*. A more lateral plosive occurs when the [k] is followed by an [l] sound, as in *knuckle, pickle, crackle*.

When two adjacent *k* letters (*kk*) occur and the first [k] sound is prolonged [k:] so that the second [k] is not distinctly heard, the results may be somewhat confusing to the listener. For example, *black cat* [blæk:æt] may be heard as "black hat," and *like king* [laɪk:ɪŋ] may be heard as the word *liking* (Carrell & Tiffany, 1960).

The following allophonic variations of the [k] sound (see **Table 13-1**) are indicated utilizing the diacritic

TABLE 13-1	**Allophonic Variation of [k] Sound**	
Allophone	**Example**	**Description**
[k:]	bake cake [ˈbeɪk:eɪk˺]	Lengthening, arresting [k] is followed by a releasing [k]
[ˌʔ]	token [toʊʔ:n]	Glottal stop
[k̃]	weaken [wikn]	Nasalized, before a syllabic nasal
[k]	school [sk ʊl]	Unaspirated release in consonant cluster
[kʰ]	kinder [kʰaɪdɚ]	Aspirated release in initial, stressed
[k˺]	static [stætɪk˺]	Unreleased in final position
[kʷ]	inquire [ɪnkʷwaɪr]	Rounded before a rounded [w] sound
[k]	classic [klæsɪk]	Lateralized release in [kl] blend

marks for phonetic transcription provided by Shriberg and Kent (1995).

Allophonic differences occur among many speakers of United States English. These differences are not usually significant, except in cases of extreme or diminished aspiration. In conversational speech, the context carries the meaning and the production of the [k] sound does not interfere with the comprehension of what is spoken.

Deletion of final consonant *sk* blend, as in [tæs] for *task*, [dɪs] for *disk*, and [æstɚɪs] *asterisk*, is present in the African American dialect.

Normal and Deviant Development of the [k] Sound

Children usually acquire the [k] sound by 4 years of age (Sander, 1972). For reasons that are not entirely clear, the [k] sound seems to be among the English sounds that are relatively difficult to learn (Carrell & Tiffany, 1960). Many children are quite late in learning this sound. The relative age when 90% of children have mastery in at least two positions is 4.0 years (Edwards, 1997), and it appears that the [k] sound in the final position takes the longest to master of the three positions.

1. The substitution of the [t] for [k] as in [tut] for *suit* or [tip] for *keep* result in a fronting substitution error because the [t] and [s] are positioned in the front (lingua-alveolar) and the [k] is positioned in the back (lingua-velar) of the mouth.

2. Edwards (1997) notes that prevocalic, the [t] or [d], and sometimes the [g], may substitute for the [k] sound, as in *cake* [teɪk] or [deɪk] or [geɪk] and [gʌp] for *cup* [kʌp]. Postvocalically, the [t], omission in cake [keɪ] for [keɪk] or glottal [ʔ] replacement as in *talk* [tɔʔ] for [tɔk] may be observed.

3. Certain combinations of [k] may be difficult or awkward to pronounce, such as the [ks] in the word *accept*, which may be pronounced [æsɛpt] with a deletion (omission) of the [k] as a result of fronting because the sounds that follow are all front-positioned sounds. Another example is [sk] as in *ask* [æsk], which may exhibit a fronting substitution as in [æst].

4. There is one context in which stops, including [k], are frequently deleted that occurs uniquely in children with delayed speech—word-final stops (Shriberg & Kent, 1995). Note the final sound deletion in "cake:ca" or "cheek:chee."

5. A phonological backing error may occur, as when the [k] sound is added at the end of a word, as in *knife* [naɪk] for [naɪf].

6. Deletion of initial consonant: *cake* [eɪk] for [keɪk].

7. Cluster reduction: *squirrel* [skɝ] for [skwɝl].

8. Hodson and Paden (1983) report the use of a [w] to initiate final syllables in multisyllabic words, as in *basket* [bæwət] for [bæskət] and *blanket* [bleɪwət] for [bleɪkət].

A speaker with a cleft palate (Carrell & Tiffany, 1960) or other inadequate velopharyngeal closure may produce a weak or distorted [k] sound with a perceptible nasal plosion or a glottal or pharyngeal-type sound.

Nonnative Speaker Pronunciation

The allophonic [k] sound occurs in many sound systems worldwide. When the letter *k* is written, it usually is pronounced as a [k] sound with the exception of when the *k* is silent, as in *knee* [nee] or [ni] and *know* [now] or [noʊ]. Imagine the confusion a nonnative speaker may encounter with the compound word *jackknife*! The *c* is neither an [s] nor a [k] but silent, the first *k* is pronounced [k], and the second *k* is silent because it precedes a letter *n*. Small (1999) notes that of all the stop consonants, the [k] sound has the most variant spellings. No doubt, this also adds to the difficulties of nonnative speakers.

Edwards (1997) indicates that nonnative speakers tend to underaspirate the [k], especially when it occurs as the initial sound in a word. This tendency is more likely to occur among those speakers whose native language is less similar to the production of the United States English [k] sound.

Carrell and Tiffany (1960) indicate that some German speakers may conspicuously overaspirate the [k] sound whereas others may substitute a palatal or velar that loosely resembles the [k] sound. Both French and Scandinavian speakers may give [k] somewhat less aspiration than would the normal English speaker. Scandinavians may produce a lax sound, but this is not true of the French.

The [k] sound, with its allophonic variations, is present in the 15 other sound systems of languages predominantly spoken in the United States. These sound systems are Spanish, French, German, Italian, Chinese, Tagalog, Polish, Korean, Portuguese, Japanese, Greek, Vietnamese, Arabic, Hindi (Urdu), and Russian.

Summary

The [k] sound is the voiceless cognate to the [g] sound and is one of the three ([k], [t], [p]) voiceless stop/plosive consonants. The [k] sound is represented by a wide variety of different orthographic letter symbols, including the unlikely *x, q,* and *c.* The *c* is particularly confusing because it can also be pronounced as an [s] sound. In addition, the [k] in the *kn* context is one of the few sounds that is silent. The amount of aspiration varies somewhat depending on where the [k] sound appears in a word or utterance, but the difference in aspiration does not present any significant barriers to the understanding of native and nonnative speakers. It is one of the later sounds to be mastered by young children and can present some problems in speech production, particularly among those individuals with insufficient velopharyngeal closure.

[k] +

Write out the words using both the orthographic spelling and phonetic symbols. Refer to the Key at the end of the section upon completion.

	Orthographic	Phonetic
1. [k] + 2 sounds: blackbird	_____	[_ _ oʊ]
2. [k] + 1 sound: unlocks	_____	[_ i]
3. [k] + 2 sounds: something done with yarns and needles	_____	[_ ɪ _]
4. [k] + 2 sounds: dessert	_____	[_ eɪ _]
5. [k] + 2 sounds: fly on a windy day	_____	[_ aɪ _]
6. [k] + 7 sounds: a pickle	_____	[_ ju _ ʌ _ _ ɚ]
7. [k] + 7 sounds: a high school course	_____	[_ ɛ _ ɪ _ _ _ i]
8. [k] + 7 sounds: a premature butterfly	_____	[_ æ _ ʌ _ ɪ _ ɚ]
9. [k] + 6 sounds: electricity	_____	[_ ɪ _ ə _ ɑ _]
10. [k] + 6 sounds: unwillingly taken	_____	[_ ɪ _ _ æ _ _]

Key: 1. crow [kroʊ]; 2. key [ki]; 3. knit [nɪt]; 4. cake [keɪk]; 5. kite [kaɪt]; 6. cucumber [kjukʌmbɚ]; 7. chemistry [kɛmɪstri]; 8. caterpillar [kætʌpɪlɚ]; 9. kilowatt [kɪləwɑt]; 10. kidnapped [kɪdnæpt]

PHONETIC SYMBOL [g]

EXHIBIT 13-6	Phonetic Symbol [g]
Phonetic Symbol	[g]
Grapheme Symbols	g, x, c
Diacritic Symbol	g
Phonic Symbol	g
Cognate	[k]
Homorganic	Lingua-Alveolar [k], [h], [ʍ], [w], [ŋ]
Sound Class	Consonant
Basic Phonetic Features	Placement: Lingua-Velar Manner: Stop/Plosive Voicing: Plus Voice
IPA (1999)	[g] #110 Voiced, Velar, Plosive

[g]

How the Sound Is Produced

The [g] sound is produced in two phases. First is the stop (stop) phase as the back of the tongue (lingua) closes against the front of the velum (velar) or back portion of the palate. The incoming air is held (implosion) and compressed in the back of the oral cavity and in the oropharynx. The second phase involving explosion (plosive) occurs when the compressed air in the oral cavity and oropharynx is released suddenly (plosive) as an audible sound (voiced) between the tongue and roof of the mouth. The [g] sound is produced with the velopharyngeal port closed and the vocal folds vibrating to produce the voiced [g] sound. The [g] sound tends to have less force of air than its unvoiced cognate [k]. Usually, the [g] sound does not have any perceptible aspiration. See **Figure 13-6**.

Different Spellings for the [g] Sound

Transcribe the following words. Note the different alphabet letters used for the [g] sound. Refer to the Key at the right upon completion.

Different Spellings			*Key*
g	good ____ gold ____ dignity ____		gʊd, goʊld, dɪgnɪti
	log ____ ghost ____ finger ____		lɔg, goʊst, fɪŋgɚ
gg	trigger ____	bigger ____	trɪgɚ, bɪgɚ
x	example ____		ɛgzæmpl̩

gue	rogue ____	vague ____	roʊg, veɪg
	intrigue ____		ɪntrɪg
gu	guess ____	guard ____	gɛs, gɑrd
	guarantee ____		gɛrænti
c	eczema ____		ɛgzimə

Different Sounds for the Letter g

Transcribe the following words. Note the different sounds that the letter *g* represents. Refer to the Key at the right upon completion.

					Key
gn	(Silent)	gnat ____	gnaw ____		næt, nɔ
	sign ____	though ____	daughter ____		saɪn, ðoʊ, dɔtɚ
gh	[f]	rough ____	laugh ____		rʌf, læf
ng	[ŋ]	ring ____	lung ____		rɪŋ, lʌŋ
	wrong ____	long ____	along ____		rɔŋ, lɔŋ, əlɔŋ
dg	[dʒ]	fudge ____	fridge ____		fʌdʒ, frɪdʒ
	badge ____	lodge ____	pledge ____		bædʒ, lɔdʒ, plɛdʒ
ge	[ʒ]	garage ____			gɚɔʒ
	collage ____	prestige ____			kʌlɑʒ, prɛstiʒ
gh	[p]	hiccough ____			hɪkəp

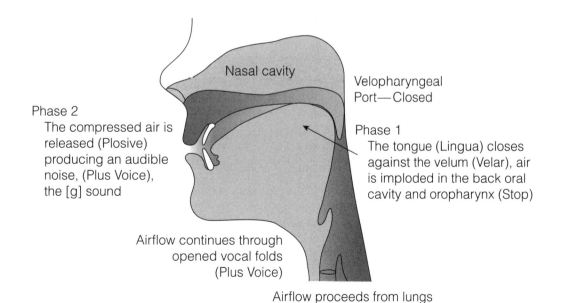

Phase 2
The compressed air is released (Plosive) producing an audible noise, (Plus Voice), the [g] sound

Nasal cavity

Velopharyngeal Port—Closed

Phase 1
The tongue (Lingua) closes against the velum (Velar), air is imploded in the back oral cavity and oropharynx (Stop)

Airflow continues through opened vocal folds (Plus Voice)

Airflow proceeds from lungs and continues through trachea to larynx

Figure 13-6 [g] pronunciation.

Rules for Spelling and Pronunciation of the [g] Sound

1. The written *g* is pronounced [g] when followed by the letters *a*, as in *gave, o*, as in *wagon, u*, as in *gum, l*, as in *glad*, and *r*, as in *grab*.

2. The written *g* is pronounced [g] at the end of words, as in *plug, big, flag, bug, beg*, and *fig*.

3. The written *g* is pronounced as a [dʒ] when followed by the letters *e*, as in *gentle, vegetable, fudge; i*, as in *ginger, region*; and *y*, as in *gypsy*.

4. Two adjacent *g* letters (*gg*) are usually pronounced as one [g] sound, as in *egg, beggar, bigger*, and *trigger*. The word *suggest* is an exception. The first *g* is pronounced [g] and the second *g* is pronounced [dʒ] as in [sʌgdʒɛst].

5. The *gh* combination when preceded by a vowel, as in *tough* and *laughter*, becomes an [f] sound. This is not always the rule and there are several exceptions. Consider the final *gh* in *hiccough* (hiccup), which is actually the [p] sound.

6. The *gh* is silent in *though, night, daughter*, and *weigh* because the *gh* is preceded by a vowel.

7. Only the [g] sound is produced in the word *ghastly, ghetto*, and *ghost*. When *gh* is followed by a vowel or is the first two letters of the word, the *h* is silent.

8. The *x* in *exam, exact* may be pronounced as [gz] when it precedes a vowel and stressed syllable. In other words such as *excite* and *except*, the voiceless consonant follows the *x*, resulting in a [ks] sound combination.

9. The final sound in the word *vague* [gue] and *intrigue* is [g].

10. The word *guess* and other *gu* words are pronounced without the *u*. In the word *language*, the *gu* is pronounced as [gw]: [læŋwɪdʒ].

11. The *g* in the *ng* combination is pronounced as a single sound [ŋ], as in *sing, bring*, and *hanger* but not in *finger, linger*, and *hunger*. Both the [ŋ] and [g] are pronounced, as in *finger* [fɪŋgɚ].

12. The *g* is silent when the letters *gn* begin or end a word, as in *gnat, gnaw*, and *sign*.

13. Both letters in the *gn* combination are pronounced when they appear in the middle of words, as in *signal* and *dignity*.

14. In words such as *beige* and *mirage*, borrowed from the French, the *g* becomes the [ʒ] sound: [beɪʒ] and [mərɑʒ].

Words That Include the [g] Sound

Transcribe the following words. Note the position of the [g] sound in the words. Refer to the Key at the right upon completion.

Initial Consonant			*Key*
give ＿＿	get ＿＿	good ＿＿	gɪv, gɛt, gʊd
gain ＿＿			geɪn

Unstressed Syllable

Medial Consonant

finger ＿＿	legal ＿＿		fɪŋgɚ, ligəl
magnify ＿＿	biggest ＿＿		mægnɪfaɪ, bɪgɛst

Stressed Syllable

Medial Consonant

forget ＿＿	begin ＿＿		fɔrgɛt, bigɪn
cognate ＿＿	suggest ＿＿	regret ＿＿	kɑgnet, sʌdʒgɛst, rigrɛt

Final Consonant

colleague ＿＿	catalog ＿＿	kɑlig, kætələg
twig ＿＿	bug ＿＿	twɪg, bʌg

Initial and Final Consonant

Greg ＿＿	gag ＿＿	gig ＿＿	greɪg, gæg, gɪg

Initial Blends

gl glass ＿＿	glow ＿＿	glove ＿＿	glæs, gloʊ, glʌv
gr grant ＿＿	graceful ＿＿	grade ＿＿	grænt, greɪsfʊl, greɪd
gu [gw] Guam ＿＿	Gwyndolyn ＿＿		gwɑm, gwɪndɔlɪn
guava ＿＿	guacamole ＿＿		gwɔvə, gwɔkʌmoli

Medial Blends

gl angler ＿＿	English ＿＿		eɪŋglɚ, ɪŋglɪʃ
igloo ＿＿	neglect ＿＿	gr fragrant ＿＿	ɪglu, nɛglɛkt, freɪgrənt
hunger ＿＿	agree ＿＿	rg bargain ＿＿	hʌŋgɚ, əgri, bɑrgən
forge ＿＿	target ＿＿		fɔrdʒ, tɑrgɛt
gu [gw] lingua ＿＿	penguin ＿＿		lɪngwə, pɛngwɪn
jaguar ＿＿	gz exact ＿＿		dʒægwɚ, ɛgzækt
examine ＿＿	exotic ＿＿		ɛgzæmɛn, ɛgzɔtɪk,
exhibit ＿＿			ɛgzɪbɪt

Final Blends

gl eagle	___ struggle ___		igḷ, strʌgḷ
rg morgue	___ iceberg ___		mɔrg, aɪsbɝg
gs [gz] bags	___ tugs	___dogs ___	bægz, tʌgz, dɔgz
gd [gd] clogged	___ hugged ___		klɔgd, hʌgd

Clusters

ngl [ŋl] jungle _____	single _____	dʒʌŋgḷ, sɪŋgḷ
triangle _____		traɪŋgḷ

Auditory Discrimination

Transcribe the following words. Note the slight difference in the sounds of the words. Refer to the Key at the right upon completion.

Cognate Pairs		*Other Minimal Pairs*		
[g] (+)	*[k]* (–)	*[g]*	*[ŋ]*	*Key*
ghost ___	coast ___	hug ___	hung ___	goʊst, koʊst, hʌg, hʌŋ
girl ___	curl ___	log ___	long ___	gɝl, kɝl, lɔg, lɔŋ
gum ___	come ___	bag ___	bang ___	gʌm, kʌm, bæg, bæŋ
gab ___	cab ___	wig ___	wing ___	gæb, kæb, wɪg, wɪŋ
good ___	could ___	rug ___	rung ___	gʊd, kʊd, rʌg, rʌŋ
gap ___	cap ___	gag ___	gang ___	gæp, kæp, gæg, geɪŋ
gall ___	call ___	big ___	bing ___	gɔl, kɔl, bɪg, bɪŋ
guild ___	killed ___	slug ___	sling ___	gɪld, kɪld, slʌg, slɪŋ

[g]	*[d]*	*[g]*	*[dʒ]*	*Key*
goes ___	doze ___	egg ___	edge ___	goʊz, doʊz, eɪg, eɪdʒ
gun ___	done ___	go ___	Joe ___	gʌn, dʌn, goʊ, dʒoʊ
go ___	doe ___	gust ___	just ___	goʊ, doʊ, gʌst, dʒʌst
gag ___	dad ___	log ___	lodge ___	gæg, dæg, lɔg, lɔdʒ
big ___	dig ___	slug ___	sludge ___	bɪg, dɪg, slʌg, slʌdʒ
leg ___	led ___	gig ___	jig ___	leɪg, lɛd, gɪg, dʒɪg
goal ___	dole ___	gain ___	Jane ___	goʊl, doʊl, geɪn, dʒeɪn
grain ___	drain ___	bag ___	badge ___	greɪn, dreɪn, bæg, bædʒ

Allophonic and Dialect Variations

During the hold (implosion) phase, there is normally very little voicing. It begins only just before the release. The exact place of articulation varies (Tiffany & Carrell, 1977) from a distinctively forward position, as in the word *geese* [gis] where the front vowel [i] leads the tongue to a forward position, and the word *gong* [gɑŋ] in which the [g] is followed by a lowback vowel.

The release mechanisms for [g] vary from lateral plosion [gl], as in *bugle, eagle, juggle*, to nasal plosion [gn] when *gn* appears in words such as *magnate, stagnate*, and *ignite*; aspirate, affricate, and unreleased forms are also common.

Calvert (1986) reports that as the initial sound, as in *girl*, or immediately following a sibilant consonant (*this girl*), voicing begins with the lingua-velar closure and the [g] is released into the following voiced sound. Between two voiced sounds (*again*) the [g] is a brief closure and release with continued voicing. Before a voiceless consonant (*big coat*), the [g] is closed but not released with voicing. As a final sound (*big*), the [g] is closed and released lightly.

The following allophonic variations of the [g] sound (**Table 13-2**) are shown using the diacritic marks for phonetic transcription provided by Shriberg and Kent (1995).

In individual speech, the [g] sound is pronounced differently depending on the neighboring sounds (Davenport & Hannahs, 1998; MacKay, 1987).

Native English speakers exhibit different degrees of aspiration and placement of that aspiration to the point of either under- or overpronunciation of the [g] sound, but it is not viewed as a significant variance and does not usually call attention to itself in conversational speech.

Edwards (1997) indicates that in the African American dialect speakers tend to devoice [g] to [k] with vowel lengthening in the final position, as in the word *fig* [fɪːk] where the [g] becomes a [k] sound.

Normal and Deviant Development of the [g] Sound

The [g] sound is often observed in the early "goings" of infants, but may not appear as a consistent speech sound until age 3 years (Edwards, 1997). Calvert (1986) states that the [g] sound is mastered by children at about age 4 and is seldom misarticulated. The observations of Carrell and Tiffany (1960) are quite different. They note that in addition to the spelling–pronunciation pitfalls, the [g] sound is frequently involved in "infantile" speech errors, and the typical substitution of [d] for [g] is usually heard among children who also substitute [t] for [k]. Edwards (1997) notes that the most common sound substitution for [g] before vowels is [d] and sometimes [t] or [k]. After vowels or in the final position of a word, [t] or [k]

| TABLE 13-2 | Allophonic Variations of the [g] Sound |

Allophone	Example	Description
[gː]	big girl [bɪgːɚl]	Lengthening, when an arresting [g] is followed by a releasing [g]
[g]	leg [leig]	Unreleased in final position
[gl]	glue [glu]	Lateralized release in [g] blend
[g]	wagon [wægn̩]	Nasalized, before a syllabic nasal
[gʷ]	goat [gʷoʊt]	Rounded before a rounded sound
[ʔ]	forgot [fɔr.ɑt]	Glottal stop
[gʰ]	garden [gʰɑrdn̩]	Aspirated release in initial, stressed
[g]	England [ɪŋg lənd]	Unaspirated release in consonant cluster

occur or the sound may be omitted. A speaker with a cleft palate or other inadequate velopharyngeal closure may produce a weak or distorted [g] sound with a perceptible nasal plosion or a glottal or pharyngeal-type sound (Tiffany & Carrell, 1977).

Nonnative Speaker Pronunciation

The allophonic [g] sound occurs in many sound systems worldwide. One of the dialectal influences on the [g] sound by nonnative speakers occurs in the pronunciation of words such as *sing* [sɪn] in which the [g] sound is added at the end to become [sɪŋg]. Voicing may be diminished or absent, particularly with a Germanic influence where the [g] may be partially or wholly without voice. Such words as *pig* and *hog* may be heard as [pɪk] or [hɑk]. Native Spanish speakers may produce more of a fricative sound that resembles the Spanish [g] than a stop/plosive.

The [g] sound, with its allophonic variations, is present in the 15 other sound systems of languages predominantly spoken in the United States. These sound systems are Spanish, French, German, Italian, Chinese, Tagalog, Polish, Korean, Vietnamese, Portuguese, Japanese, Greek, Arabic, Hindi (Urdu), and Russian.

Summary

The [g] sound is the voiced cognate to the [k] sound and is one of the three ([g], [d], [b]) voiced stop/plosive consonants. The [g] sound is represented by a wide variety of different orthographic letter symbols, including the unlikely *c* and *x*. The [g] sound represents the

g letter consistently with the exception of when it is silent, as in the *gn* digraph. The *gn*, like the *kn*, is silent, as in *gnat, gnaw, sign*. It is present in the initial, medial, and final positions in words. The amount of aspiration varies depending on where the [g] sound appears in a word or utterance, but the difference does not interfere with the listener's ability to understand what is spoken and may be dependent somewhat on contextual cues. It is usually acquired by age 3 and can present speech problems for individuals who exhibit limited velopharyngeal closure such as those with cleft palate.

[g] +

Transcribe the following words. Refer to the Key at the end of the section upon completion.

		Orthographic	Phonetic
1.	[g] + 2 sounds: horse gallop	_____	[_ eɪ _]
2.	[g] + 2 sounds: molecule	_____	[_ i _]
3.	[g] + 3 sounds: the Olympic ____	_____	[_ eɪ _ _]
4.	[g] + 2 sounds: opposite of *gander*	_____	[_ u _]
5.	[g] + 3 sounds: an underground rodent	_____	[_ oʊ _ ɚ]
6.	[g] + 8 sounds: a Texas town	_____	[_ aʊ _ _ ɛ _ _ ə _]

7. [g] + 8 sounds: _____ [_ ə _ ɝ _ _ ə _ _]
   political
   organization

8. [g] + 4 sounds: _____ [_ aɪ _ ɚ _]
   Yellowstone
   attractions

9. [g] + 4 sounds: _____ [_ ɪ _ _ i]
   not innocent

10. [g] + 5 sounds: _____ [_ ɑ _ _ ə _]
    a drinking glass

Key: 1. gait [geɪt]; 2. gene [gɪn]; 3. games [geɪmz]; 4. goose [gus]; 5. gofer [goʊfɚ]; 6. Galveston [gaʊvɛstən]; 7. government [gəvɝnmənt]; 8. geysers [gaɪzɚz]; 9. guilty [gɪlti]; 10. goblet [gɑblət]

SUMMARY

There are three cognate sets of stop consonant phonemes in United States English. Each set has a different anatomic placement. The [p] voiceless and [b] voiced set are bilabial. The [t] voiceless and [d] voiced set are lingua-alveolar, and the [k] voiceless and [g] voiced are lingua-velar. The degree of energy exerted to produce the aspiration (plosive) effect of each sound contributes to their allophonic differences. Where the sound occurs in a word (initial, medial, or final position) predicts the variation in aspiration. Also, the voiced stops have less aspiration than their voiceless counterparts.

There are exceptions and inconsistencies in the orthographic representation of the alphabet symbols and their relationship to the actual sounds produced. For example, the letter *c* may represent either the [k] or [s] sound. In some instances, the symbol is not pronounced at all, such as the [g] in *gnat*. These variations in the rules present confusion both to the native speaker who is acquiring the sounds and to the nonnative speaker who learns the rules only to discover that there are significant exceptions.

Dialect differences are present as evidenced by a shift in placement, such as forward in the dentalization of a [t] or [d] sound to a glottal stop for a [k] or [g] sound. Because the implosion of air in the oral cavity is so critical to the production of the stop consonants, any anatomic abnormality or structural weakness may reduce the effectiveness in the pronunciation of the sound.

TRANSCRIPTION EXERCISE

Complete the matching sets by writing in a word in which the alphabet letters produce a different sound.

Example: t = [t] as in *yacht* but not in *whistle* (silent *t*).

1. p = [p] as in *map* but not in _____.

2. t = [t] as in *stone* but not in _____.

3. d = [d] as in *could* but not in _____.

4. k = [k] as in *echo* but not in _____.

5. g = [g] as in *log* but not in _____.

6. b = [b] as in *baby* but not in _____.

7. p = [p] as in *help* but not in _____.

8. t = [t] as in *Thomas* but not in _____.

9. d = [d] as in *deed* but not in _____.

10. k = [k] as in *occur* but not in _____.

Transcription Exercise

Transcribe the following words. The words contain only those sounds and IPA symbols that have been presented so far. Include the vowel and diphthong symbols where appropriate. Also identify the total number of sounds and syllables. Even though a sound may appear more than once in a word, the total count should include *all* of the sounds. For example, *baby* has four sounds (consonant, diphthong, consonant, vowel).

Examples: guests = [gɛsts] 5 Sounds/1 Syllable

  baby = [beɪbi] 4 Sounds/2 Syllables

Word	Number of Sounds	Number of Syllables	Transcription
1. temple	_____	_____	_____
2. taught	_____	_____	_____
3. reporter	_____	_____	_____
4. phonetics	_____	_____	_____
5. peanuts	_____	_____	_____
6. comb	_____	_____	_____
7. often	_____	_____	_____
8. liberty	_____	_____	_____
9. orient	_____	_____	_____
10. prevent	_____	_____	_____
11. quaint	_____	_____	_____
12. tonight	_____	_____	_____
13. today	_____	_____	_____
14. tough	_____	_____	_____
15. script	_____	_____	_____

True or False

Mark each statement with a T or an F to indicate whether it is true or false.

_____ 1. The [t] and [k] are both lingua-velar sounds.

_____ 2. The velopharyngeal port needs to be closed for all of the stop/plosive sounds.

_____ 3. North United States English has a nonrhotic flap that occurs as a variety of [t] or [d] in such words as *batter* and *hetting*.

_____ 4. The [p] sound occurs in each of the following words: *phone, shepherd, plant*.

_____ 5. The [t] sound occurs in each of the following words: *fished, mopped, buzzed*.

_____ 6. The [d] sound does not occur in each of the following words: *edge, waited, soldier*.

_____ 7. The stop/plosive sounds are present in most of the major sound systems worldwide.

_____ 8. Because the two [d] sounds in the word *deed* have different degrees of aspiration, the last [d] sound is considered a distortion error of the [d] sound.

_____ 9. The voiced stop/plosive sounds have more aspiration than their voiceless cognates.

_____ 10. Coronal (+) is one of the distinctive features of the [k] and [g] sounds.

REFERENCES

Ball, M. J. (1993). *Phonetics for speech pathology*. London, England: Whurr Publishers.

Ball, M. J., & Rahilly, J. (1999). *Phonetics: The science of sound*. London, England: Whurr Publishers.

Calvert, D. R. (1986). *Descriptive phonetics*. New York: Thieme Medical Publishers.

Carrell, J., & Tiffany, W. (1960). *Phonetics: Theory and application to speech improvement*. New York: McGraw-Hill.

Cheng, L. L. (1993). Asian-American Cultures. In D. Battle (Ed.), *Communication disorders in multicultural populations* (pp. 38–77), Boston, MA: Andover Medical Publishers.

Davenport, M., & Hannahs, S. J. (1998). *Introducing phonetics and phonology*. Oxford, England: Oxford University Press.

Edwards, H. T. (1997). *Applied phonetics* (2nd ed.). San Diego, CA: College-Hill Press.

Hodson, B., & Paden, E. (1983). *Targeting intelligible speech: A phonological approach to remediation*. San Diego, CA: College Hill Press.

House, L. (1998). *Introductory phonetics and phonology*. Mahwah, NJ: Lawrence Erlbaum.

Hull, M. A., & Fox, B. J. (1998). *Phonetics for the teacher of reading* (7th ed.). Upper Saddle River, NJ: Merrill.

International Phonetic Association. (1999). *Handbook of the International Phonetic Association*. Cambridge, England: Cambridge: University Press.

Kahn, L. (1985). *Basics of phonological analysis—a programmed learning text*. New York: Little, Brown.

Kayser, H. (1993). Hispanic cultures. In D. Battle (Ed.), *Communication disorders in multicultural populations* (pp. 114–157), Boston, MA: Andover Medical Publishers.

Ladefoged, P. (1993). *A course in phonetics* (3rd ed.). Fort Worth, TX: Harcourt Brace College Publishers.

MacKay, I. R. A. (1987). *Phonetics: The science of speech production*. Boston, MA: Allyn & Bacon.

Sander, E. (1972). When are speech sounds learned? *Journal of Speech and Hearing Disorders, 7*, 55–63.

Shriberg, L., & Kent, R. (1995). *Clinical phonetics* (3rd ed.). Boston, MA: Allyn & Bacon.

Small, L. H. (1999). *Fundamentals of phonetics* (3rd ed.). Boston, MA: Allyn & Bacon.

Tiffany, W. R., & Carrell, J. (1977). *Phonetics: Theory and application*. New York: McGraw-Hill.

Zemlin, W. R. (1998). *Speech and hearing science: Anatomy and physiology* (4th ed.). Upper Saddle River, NJ: Prentice Hall.

Chapter 14

Familiar Phonetic Symbols: Fricative Consonants Analysis and Transcription

PURPOSE

To provide you with the information about fricative sounds that are symbolized with phonetic symbols and alphabet letters that are the same.

OBJECTIVES

This chapter will provide you with information regarding:

1. The identification and description of how the United States English fricative consonants are produced

2. Different spellings for each fricative sound and different sounds for each of the corresponding orthographic (alphabet) letters

3. Rules for spelling and pronunciation of each sound

4. Various contexts in which each sound occurs

5. Examples of cognates and other minimal pairs for auditory discrimination

6. Examples of allophonic variations

7. Normal development and disordered production of each fricative sound

8. Dialect differences and nonnative speaker difficulties

9. Phonetic transcription exercises

IDENTIFICATION OF FRICATIVE CONSONANTS

There are 10 fricative consonant phonemes in United States English speech. As a group, the fricatives form the largest set of consonants in United States English (Edwards, 1997). The fricatives consist of nine standard consonants, comprising four pairs of cognates (plus or minus voice) and [h]. A 10th fricative [ʍ] or [hw] is considered, but few speakers, according to Edwards (1997) and others (see the discussion on the [ʍ] sound), consistently differentiate in their speaking between such words as *where* and *wear*. **Table 14-1** lists the fricatives.

A fricative is defined as a sound that is produced with a narrow constriction through which air escapes with a continuous noise (Shriberg & Kent, 1995).

TABLE 14-1	Fricative Cognate Pairs	
Voiceless	**Voiced**	**Placement**
[f]	[v]	Labiodental
[Ɵ]	[ð]	Linguadental
[ʃ]	[ʒ]	Linguapalatal
[s]	[z]	Lingua-alveolar or linguadental Others
[h]	None	Linguapalatal and lingua-velar or glottal
[ʍ] or [hw]	None	Lingua-velar, bilabial

This "noise" is aperiodic in nature (MacKay, 1987). Aperiodic sounds have no regular period, but contain individual cycles having many different periods. The fricative consonants of United States English are sometimes called *spirates* because of the required turbulence heard as audible friction (Calvert, 1986). Some turbulence occurs as air flows through the glottis and pharynx. However, Calvert (1986) indicates that the primary sources of audible friction for consonants are the structures of the oral cavity: the lips, teeth, tongue, alveolar ridge, palate, and velum. These articulators do not close completely during fricative production but converge to form a slit to create the channel necessary for production of each fricative phoneme (Small, 1999). Audible frication accompanies both the voiceless and voiced fricatives: the voiceless [h], [ʍ], [f], [Ɵ], [s], and [ʃ] and the voiced [v], [ð], [z], and [ʒ]. The voicing feature adds power to the sound that is not present when friction alone is relied on for production (Edwards, 1997). Therefore, more muscular tension and breath pressure are required for the voiceless fricatives than for their voiced cognates. The velopharyngeal port is closed to allow the constricted air stream to exit through the oral cavity and out of the mouth.

Fricative articulation is accomplished by forcing a voiceless or voiced breath stream through a relatively narrow constriction in the vocal tract (Tiffany & Carrell, 1977). The resulting breath stream is either a diffuse friction noise generated as the air stream passes along soft and hard surfaces at the point of constriction, as with [f], or it may be a sound of more strident quality created by directing a concentrated jet of air against the hard palate and dental surfaces, as with the [s] sound. The shape of the constriction is also relevant

and plays a role in the sound produced (MacKay, 1987); hence the slit fricatives such as [Ɵ] and [ð], which are produced with a relatively flat tongue and the space through which air is forced is a wide thin slit as opposed to the rounder grooved posture of the tongue such as for [s] and [z]. Some phoneticians refer to the [s], [z], [ʃ], and [ʒ] sounds as *sibilants* because of their increased strident quality. The sibilants form a major subset of fricatives (Edwards, 1997). They are produced by directing the airflow along a more or less grooved tongue to a hard surface such as the front teeth.

The movement sequence for fricatives includes (1) a foreglide, (2) a hold, and (3) a release. Fricatives, like stops, are considered to be *obstruents* because their production involves an obstruction of the air stream in the vocal tract (Small, 1999). The hold phase is likely to be of relatively greater duration than the other two phases. Tiffany and Carrell (1977) offer some insight into the physiologic aspects of the production of fricatives. They state that the length of the constriction area in the vocal tract varies considerably. Fricatives such as [f] and [Ɵ] have a broad but limited point of constriction formed by the lower lip [f] and teeth and the [Ɵ] is formed by the tongue and teeth. Sounds that are produced with a more open broad channel along a greater length of constriction such as the [ʃ], formed between the tongue and palate, are described as *distributed*. *Concentrated* is the term occasionally used with the sounds like [s] because the jet of air is forced through a relatively narrow channel. Shriberg and Kent (1995) agree that the intensity of the noise varies with place of articulation. The lingua-alveolar fricatives [s] and [z] are among the most intense. An air pressure chamber is created behind the constriction and then released through the narrow constriction or passageway. Noise energy is generated as air escapes through the passage.

The acoustic properties of fricatives as compared with the vowels and other consonants are notable. The [Ɵ] is the weakest of all the sounds and several of the other fricatives such as [f] and [ʃ] may be difficult for the normal listener to discriminate because of their high frequency. Voiced fricatives are somewhat easier to discriminate because of their resonant quality. The acoustic output is subject to modification as a result of resonance within the oral cavity (MacKay, 1987).

Children may develop articulation errors because of their inability to discriminate and may substitute other fricatives such as *fin* for *thin*. Individuals with mild to severe hearing losses may develop confusion in conversations, particularly when the context is unfamiliar or vague. Failure to form a groove is responsible for certain types of lisp (MacKay, 1987). If the front teeth are missing, the air cannot be shaped and a less sibilant fricative sound is produced. In such cases, an attempt to articulate [s] produces a [Ɵ]-like sound, which is identified as a lisp.

The 10 fricative consonants are discussed in sequence of cognate pairs: [s], [z]; [f], [v]; and [h], which are familiar alphabet letters that represent the phonetic sounds. A comprehensive description of each sound and its features is presented. A self-test is included in this chapter. The remaining fricatives are symbolized with relatively less familiar phonetic symbols: [Ɵ], [ð], [ʃ], [ʒ] and [ʍ] and [hw].

PHONETIC SYMBOL [s]

EXHIBIT 14-1	Phonetic Symbol [s]

Phonetic Symbol	[s]	**[s]**
Grapheme Symbols	s, ss, c, sc, sw, st,ps, ce, z, zz, x,scj, tz	
Diacritic Symbol	s	
Phonic Symbol	s	
Cognate	[z]	
Homorganic	Lingua-Alveolar [z], [t], [d], [l], [n]	
Sound Class	Consonant	
Phonetic Features	Placement: Lingua-Alveolar or Lingua (lower) Dental Manner: Fricative or Sibilant Voicing: Minus Voice	
IPA (1999)	[s] #132 Voiceless, Alveolar, Fricative Distinctive Feature Analysis (Chomsky & Halle, 1968) Plus (+): Consonantal, Coronal, Anterior, High, Continuant, Strident Minus (−): Vocalic, Sonorant, Low, Back, Rounded, Distributed, Nasal, Lateral, Tense, Voice	

How the Sound Is Produced

The articulators used to produce the [s] sound may be of the following two pair: (1) the tongue (lingua) and the alveolar ridge (alveolar), or (2) the tongue (lingua) and the lower front teeth (dental). Whatever the preference of the individual, the sound can be made acoustically acceptable with either method of production. See **Figure 14-1**.

In the first position, lingua-alveolar, the sides of the tongue (lingua) are in contact with the upper molars and the alveolar ridge (alveolar) laterally, with the tip of the tongue narrowly grooved and approximating

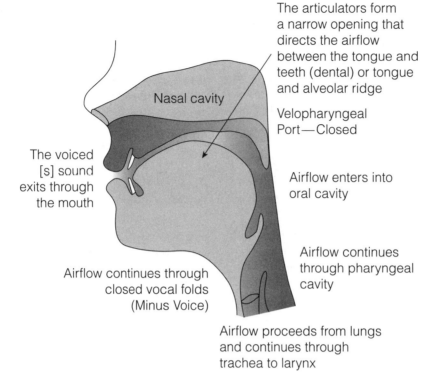

The articulators form
a narrow opening that
directs the airflow
between the tongue and
teeth (dental) or tongue
and alveolar ridge

Velopharyngeal
Port—Closed

Airflow enters into
oral cavity

Airflow continues
through pharyngeal
cavity

Airflow proceeds from lungs
and continues through
trachea to larynx

Airflow continues through
closed vocal folds
(Minus Voice)

The voiced
[s] sound
exits through
the mouth

Nasal cavity

Figure 14-1 [s] pronunciation.

the alveolar ridge just behind the upper incisors. This position provides a narrow airflow channel at the midline of the tongue between the tongue and the anterior portion of the hard palate, the alveolar ridge, and the teeth. The [s] sound is made as the airflow is continuously directed through the narrow channel between the blade of the tongue and the roof of the mouth (hard palate). The audible friction (fricative) of the airflow produces the [s] sound. The upper and lower teeth are slightly apart and the velopharyngeal port is closed.

In the second position, linguadental, the sides (lateral) of the tongue are against the upper molars, the tip of the tongue makes contact behind the lower incisors (dental) near the alveolar ridge (alveolar) and forms a narrow opening through which the airflow is continuously directed against the front teeth. This airflow process causes an audible friction (fricative) noise, resulting in the voiced production of the [s] sound. The [s] sound is made with more force than its cognate, the [z] sound, is.

Different Spellings for the [s] Sound

Transcribe the following words. Refer to the Key at the right upon completion.

Different Spellings			*Key*
s safe ___	lesson ___	this ___	seIf, lɛsən, ðIs
ss class ___	cross ___		klæs, krɔs
accessible ___			ækɛsəbḷ
c city ___	bicycle ___		sIti, baIsIkḷ
lettuce ___			lɛtəs
sc scene ___	science ___		sin, saIəns
scent ___	ascend ___		sɛnt, əsɛnd
sw sword ___			sɔrd
st listen ___	hasten ___		lIsən, hæsən
Christmas ___			krIsməs
ps psalm ___	psychology ___		sɑm, saIkɔlədʒi

ce	race ___	embrace ___		reɪs, ɛmbreɪs
	face ___			feɪs
z	waltz ___	quartz ___		wɑlts, kwɔrts
zz	pizza ___			pitsə
x	six ___	taxi ___	box ___	sɪks, tæksi, bɑks
sch	schism ___			sɪzm or sɪzəm
tz	ritz ___	pretzel ___		rɪts, prɛtsəl

Different Sounds of the Letters That Produce the [s] Sound

Transcribe the following words. Refer to the Key at the right upon completion.

Alphabet Letter	Different Sounds			Key
s	[s]	safe	___	seɪf
	[z]	dogs	___	dɔgz
c	[s]	city	___	sɪti
	[k]	cat	___	kæt
ps	[s]	psalm	___	sɑm
	[ps]	cups	___	kʌps
z	[s]	quartz	___	kwɔrts
	[z]	zoo	___	zu
zz	[s]	pizza	___	pitsə
	[z]	jazz	___	ʤæz
x	[s]	six	___	sɪks
	[k]	extra	___	ɛkstrə

Rules for Spelling and Pronunciation of the [s] Sound

1. The written *s* is pronounced [s], as in *salad, bison, base.*

2. Two adjacent *s* letters (*ss*) are usually pronounced as one [s] sound, as in *access, recess, less.*

3. The *c* is pronounced as [s] in such words as *cite, acid, face, cycle, cent* (*c* before *i, e,* or *y*) but not in words such as *cake* and *county* where the *c* is a [k] sound.

4. The *sc* in the *i, e, y* context, as in *scissors, scenic, scythe,* and *schism,* is pronounced with only the [s] sound. In other contexts, such as *school* or *scone,* the *c* is a [k] sound.

5. The unique *sw* spelling appears in the word *sword* in which the *w* is silent.

6. In the *st* medial position of such words as *listen, hasten,* and *Christmas,* the *t* is silent. Also, the *p* is silent in *psychology* and other words with the *psycho* prefix.

7. Words ending in *ce,* such as *advice, voice, office,* are pronounced with the [s] sound.

8. A few words such as *waltz* and *quartz* that end in the letter *z* are pronounced with an [s] ending. The *zz* in *pizza* is pronounced as [t] [s].

9. The letter *x* is a combination of [k] and [s] or [g] and [z] depending on the context. The [s] is pronounced after the [k] sound as in *axe.*

Words That Include the [s] Sound

The [s] sound appears in all three positions, initial, medial, and final. Transcribe the following words. Refer to the Key at the right upon completion.

Initial Consonant			Key
sample ___	service ___		sæmpl̩, sɝvɪs
sidewalk ___			saɪdwɑk

Unstressed Syllable

Medial Consonant

sedative ___	security ___	sɛdətɪv, səkɝɪti

Stressed Syllable

Medial Consonant

celebrate ___		sɛlʌbreɪt
concern ___	instead ___	kɔnsɚn, ɪnstɛd

Final Consonant

use ___	case ___	ice ___	jus, keɪs, aɪs
analysis ___			ænaʊlɪsɪs

Initial and Final Consonants

spouse ___	spice ___	spaʊs, spaɪs
source ___	suitcase ___	sɔrs, sutkeɪs

Initial Blends

<u>sf</u> sphere ___	sphinx ___			sfɛr, sfɪŋks
sphincter ___	peaceful ___			sfɪŋktɚ, pisfʊl
<u>sk</u> scar ___	skin ___	scout ___		skɑr, skɪn, skaʊt
<u>sl</u> slow ___	slang ___	<u>sm</u> smell ___		sloʊ, sleɪŋ, smɛl
smooth ___	smart ___	<u>sn</u> snack ___		smuð, smɑrt, snæk
sniff ___	snow ___	<u>sp</u> spare ___		snɪf, snoʊ, spɛr
spout ___	spy ___	<u>st</u> staff ___		spoʊt, spaɪ, stæf
stone ___	stop ___	<u>sw</u> swift ___		stoʊn, stɑp, swɪft
swan ___	suede ___			swɑn, sweɪd

Medial Blends

<u>sf</u> forceful ___	asphalt ___			fɔrsfʊl, æsfɔlt
transfer ___	<u>fs</u> lifesaving ___			trænsfɚ, laɪfseɪvɪŋ
<u>sk</u> skin ___	husky ___	mascot ___		skɪn, hʌski, mæskɔt
<u>ks</u> axle ___	expense ___	dextrose ___		æksl̩, ɛkspɛns, dɛkstros
<u>sl</u> asleep ___	priceless ___	nicely ___		əslip, praɪslɛs, naɪsli
<u>ls</u> hillside ___	ulcer ___	also ___		hɪlsaɪd, ɔlsɚ, ɔlsoʊ
<u>sm</u> basement ___	dismiss ___			beɪsmənt, dɪsmɪs
transmit ___	<u>ns</u> insist ___	unseen ___		trænsmɪt, ɪnsɪst, ənsin
principle ___	<u>sp</u> grasping ___			prɪnsəpl̩, ɡræspɪŋ
whisper ___	response ___			ʍɪspɚ, rɪspɔns
<u>ps</u> keepsake ___	chopsticks ___	upset ___		kipseɪk, tʃɑpstɪks, ʌpsɛt
<u>rs</u> herself ___	pursuit ___	horse ___		hɝsɛlf, pɚsut, hɔrs
<u>st</u> constant ___	costume ___			kɑnstɔnt, kɑstum
instead ___	<u>ts</u> outsider ___			ɪnstɛd, aʊtsaɪdɚ
schizophrenic ___	pizzeria ___			skɪtsoʊfrɛnɪk, pitsɚ·iə

Final Blends

<u>fs</u> photographs ___	cliffs ___			foʊtəɡræfs, klɪfs
coughs ___	<u>ks</u> fix ___	rocks ___		kɔfs, fɪks, rɔks
jokes ___	physics ___	<u>sl</u> utensil ___		dʒoʊks, fɪzɪks, jutɛnsɪl
rehearsal ___	carousel ___			rihɝsəl, kɛrʌsɛl
<u>ls</u> false ___	impulse ___	else ___		fɔls, ɪmpɔls, ɛls
<u>ns</u> ounce ___	tense ___	rinse ___		aʊns, tɛns, rɪns
<u>sp</u> clasp ___	lisp ___	wasp ___		klæsp, lɪsp, wɔsp
<u>ps</u> lips ___	slips ___	keeps ___		lɪps, slɪps, kips
<u>rs</u> course ___	sparse ___	endorse ___		kɔrs, spɑrs, ɛndɔrs
<u>st</u> moist ___	wrist ___	test ___		moɪst, rɪst, tɛst
<u>ts</u> dates ___	knits ___	skates ___		deɪts, nɪts, skeɪts
<u>ths</u> wreaths ___	growths ___			riθs, groʊθs

Clusters

<u>rst</u> burst ___	thirst ___	rehearsed ___		bɝst, θɝst, rihɝst
<u>skr</u> scream ___	script ___			skrim, skrɪpt
prescription ___	<u>sks</u> desks ___			pɝskrɪpʃən, dɛsks
masks ___	<u>skw</u> squint ___			mæsks, skwɪnt
squadron ___	<u>spl</u> splash ___			skwɔdrən, splæʃ
splinter ___	split ___	<u>spr</u> sprain ___		splɪntɚ, splɪt, spreɪn
spruce ___	bedspread ___	<u>str</u> street ___		sprus, bɛdsprɛd, strit
strategy ___	stranger ___			strætədʒi, streɪndʒɚ
<u>sts</u> posts ___	wrists ___	digests ___		poʊsts, rɪsts, daɪdʒɛsts
<u>mps</u> bumps ___	stamps ___			bʌmps, stæmps

Adjoining Clusters

<u>kskl/ks</u> exclaim ___	extreme ___			ɛkskleɪm, ɛkstrim
<u>kspr</u> express ___	expensive ___			ɛksprɛs, ɛkspɛnsɪv
<u>kskl</u> exclamation ___				ɛksklʌmeʃən

Auditory Discrimination

Transcribe the following words. Refer to the Key at the right upon completion.

Cognate Pairs   *Other Minimal Pairs*

[s] (−)	[z] (+)	[s]	[θ]	Key
sink ___	zinc ___	sin ___	thin ___	sɪŋk, zɪŋk, sɪn, θɪn
seal ___	zeal ___	face ___	faith ___	sɛl, zɛl, feɪs, feɪθ
race ___	rays ___	saw ___	thaw ___	reɪs, reɪz, sɑ, θɑ
Sue ___	zoo ___	seem ___	theme ___	su, zu, sim, θim
racer ___	razor ___	moss ___	moth ___	reɪsɚ, reɪzɚ, mɑs, mɑθ
price ___	prize ___	lass ___	lath ___	praɪs, praɪz, læs, læθ
bus ___	buzz ___	gross ___	growth ___	bʌs, bʌz, groʊs, groʊθ
lice ___	lies ___	sank ___	thank ___	laɪs, laɪz, seɪŋk, θeɪŋk

[s]	[ʃ]	[s]	[t]	Key
mass ___	mash ___	race ___	rate ___	mæs, mæʃ, reɪs, reɪt
seep ___	sheep ___	pass ___	pat ___	sip, ʃip, pæs, pæt
see ___	she ___	lice ___	light ___	si, ʃi, laɪs, laɪt
class ___	clash ___	base ___	bait ___	klæs, klæʃ, beɪs, beɪt
sock ___	shock ___	see ___	T ___	sɔk, ʃɔk, si, ti
cast ___	cashed ___	rice ___	right ___	kæst, kæʃt, raɪs, raɪt
Swiss ___	swish ___	sick ___	tick ___	swɪs, swɪʃ, sɪk, tɪk
sore ___	shore ___	same ___	tame ___	sɔr, ʃɔr, seɪm, teɪm
gas ___	gash ___	sew ___	tow ___	ɡæs, ɡæʃ, soʊ, toʊ

Allophonic and Dialect Variations

Many varieties of [s] are possible, depending on dentition, mandibular positioning, posture of the tongue tip and blade, and differences in tongue grooving (Edwards, 1997; Tiffany & Carrell, 1977). One example is the palatalization before the [j] sound in which the [s] in *kiss you* becomes more of an [ʃ] sound, as in [kɪʃju]. The anatomic structures play a role in the allophonic differences as does the context in which the sound occurs, including the features of the surrounding vowels or consonant blends and clusters and the position of the sound in the initial, medial, or final segment of the word or utterance.

The [s] and [z] sounds appear differently in words such as *houses* [haʊsəs] or [haʊzəz] and *horses* where there may be two [s] sounds, an [s] and then a [z] sound, or two [z] sounds. Some speakers use the phoneme [z] in the pronunciation of words such as *resource* [risɔrs], which becomes [rizɔrs], *greasy* [grisi], which becomes [grizi], and *absurd* [əbsɝd], which becomes [ɔbzɝd] (Small, 1999).

Normal and Deviant Development of the [s] Sound

The [s] sound is one of the most frequently occurring consonants in the United States English speech (Calvert, 1986). The [s] sound and its cognate [z] are two sounds that span the longest range of different ages at which they are acquired (Sander, 1972). Some children acquire these sounds as early as 3 or 4 years of age; however, the normal range extends to 8 years of age.

The standard [s] production places special demands on the speech production system, and consequently that is probably why it is so frequently misarticulated (Tiffany & Carrell, 1977). Its production includes the following requirements: (1) the tongue must be properly placed and adequately grooved, (2) the air stream must be placed under proper pressure, and (3) the air stream must be directed over the appropriate turbulence-producing obstructions. Tiffany and Carrell (1977) indicate that it is especially important that the hearing mechanism of the speaker be capable of receiving the very high frequencies typical of [s], 4,000 to 7,000 Hertz (Hz). Absence of this feedback can seriously impair the acquisition of this sound.

As mentioned, the [s] is among the most frequently misarticulated consonants, produced variously toward [ɵ] lisping or toward [ʃ] (Calvert, 1986). Abnormal dentition of the teeth may interfere with the directed released of the airflow. Any deformity that disturbs the dentition may make it difficult for the speaker to produce the sound: an over- or underbite, irregular teeth, or an abnormal

opening in the bite are common conditions (Tiffany & Carrell, 1977). The [s] sound is one of the first sounds affected by hearing loss. The most common substitution is [t] followed by [d] (Edwards, 1997). When tongue protrusion is present, a frontal voiceless lisp is produced that resembles the [ɵ] sound. Other errors include [ʃ] and [f], common in *sw* clusters (*swing*) that become [fɪŋ].

Defective [s] sounds are usually classified as one of the following: (1) weak [s] that is appropriate but of low energy; (2) "hishy" or [ʃ]-like sound that is produced by retracted placement of the tongue, a too broad channel of air emission, improper air pressure, or some combination of these; (3) an interdental lisp that sounds more like a [ɵ] substitution; (4) a lateral lisp in which the air emission is directed laterally and escapes over the sides of the tongue; (5) a whistle caused by missing teeth or the effect of dentures; (6) an affricative [ts] particularly produced by hard-of-hearing speakers; (7) a nasal-oral-fricative combination typical of cleft palate speech; and (8) a strident or overly "hissed" [s] (Tiffany & Carrell, 1977).

Nonnative Speaker Pronunciation

Nonnative speaker voicing errors are predominately omissions or failure to pronounce the ends of words (Edwards, 1997). Foreign speakers of United States English may have some problems with [s] although alveolar fricatives are common in the languages of the world (Tiffany & Carrell, 1977). A more anterior and strongly aspirated [s] is spoken by speakers whose native language is German or French, and other speakers may produce a variety of [s] sounds that may sound strange when transferred to United States English diction. Voicing or weakening of the sound so that it may approximate the [z] sound also occurs.

The [s] sound with some variation occurs in Spanish, French, German, Chinese, Korean, Portuguese, Japanese, Arabic, and Hindu (Urdu) (International Phonetic Association, 1999).

Summary

The [s] sound is one of the 10 fricative consonants, and its voiced cognate is the [z] sound. In addition to the [z] sound, it is homorganic (lingua-alveolar) with the [t], [d], [l], and [n] sounds. In addition to its lingua-alveolar placement, with the tongue tip in an upward position, the [s] sound is produced by many speakers with the tip of the tongue downward and pressing against the lower front teeth (dental) position. The [s] sound has a variety of letters and letter combinations that represent its sound and other sounds such as the *c* in *city* and *cat*. Allophonic variations occur as a result of individual differences in the anatomic structures associated with the [s] sound and the context in which the sound occurs. It occurs quite frequently in United States English, and the normal age range for mastery extends from age 4 to 8 years, making it one of the later sounds to be developed. A variation of the [s] sound occurs in many of the sound systems of languages worldwide. Speech production errors include substitutions, deletion, and lisping. The [s] sound may be particularly difficult to acquire for those with a hearing loss or moderate to severe dentition problems.

[s] +

Write the orthographic and phonetic spellings of the following words. Refer to the Key at the bottom of the section upon completion.

	Orthographic	Phonetic
1. [s] + 4 sounds: skin on top of head	_____	[_ _ æ _ _]
2. [s] + 4 sounds: name of fish	_____	[_ æ _ ə _]
3. [s] + 3 sounds: a place of learning	_____	[_ _ u _]

4. [s] + 4 sounds: a loud shout — _____ [_ _ _ i _]

5. [s] + 8 sounds: a study of word sounds — _____ [_ ə _ æ _ _ ɪ _ _]

6. [s] + 7 sounds: bony frame — _____ [_ _ ɛ _ ɪ _ ə _]

7. [s] + 7 sounds: communicable disease — _____ [_ _ ɑ _ _ ɔ _ _]

8. [s] + 4 sounds: girls and boys clubs — _____ [_ _ aʊ _ _]

9. [s] + 6 sounds: a member of a country — _____ [_ ɪ _ ɪ _ ə _]

10. [s] + 7 sounds: movement of blood in body — _____ [_ ɚ _ ju _ e _]

Key: 1. scalp [skælp]; 2. salmon [sæmən]; 3. school [skul]; 4. scream [skrim]; 5. semantics [səmæntɪks]; 6. skeleton [skɛlɪtən]; 7. smallpox [smɑlpɔks]; 8. scouts [skaʊts]; 9. citizen [sɪtɪzən]; 10. circulate [sɚkjulet]

PHONETIC SYMBOL [z]

EXHIBIT 14-2	Phonetic Symbol [z]	
Phonetic Symbol	[z]	**[z]**
Grapheme Symbols	z, zz, s, sth, x, se,ws, ss, ze, cz, ys, sce, sc, si	
Diacritic Symbol	z	
Phonic Symbol	z	
Cognate	[s]	
Homorganic	Lingua-Alveolar {s], [t], [d], [l], [n]	
Sound Class	Consonant	
Basic Phonetic Features	Placement: Lingua-Alveolar orLingua (lower) Dental Manner: Fricative or Sibilant Voicing: Plus Voice	
IPA (1999)	[z] #133 Voiced, Alveolar, Fricative Distinctive Feature Analysis (Chomsky & Halle, 1968) <u>Plus (+):</u> Consonantal, Coronal, Anterior, High, Continuant, Voiced, Strident <u>Minus (–):</u> Vocalic, Sonorant, Low, Back, Rounded, Distributed, Nasal, Lateral, Tense	

How the Sound Is Produced

The articulators used to produce the [z] sound may be one of the following two: (1) the tongue (lingua) and the alveolar ridge (alveolar) or (2) the tongue (lingua) and the lower front teeth (dental). Whatever the preference of the individual, the sound can be made acoustically acceptable with either method of articulation. See **Figure 14-2**.

In the first position, lingua-alveolar, the sides of the tongue (lingua) are in contact with the upper molars and the alveolar ridge (alveolar) laterally, with the tip of the tongue narrowly grooved and approximating the alveolar ridge just behind the upper incisors. This position provides a narrow airflow channel at the midline of the tongue between the tongue and the anterior portion of the hard palate, the alveolar ridge, and the teeth. The [z] sound is made as the voiced (voice) airflow is continuously directed through the narrow channel between the blade of the tongue and the roof of the mouth (hard palate). The audible friction (fricative) of the airflow produces the [z] sound. The upper and lower teeth are slightly apart and the velopharyngeal port is closed.

In the second position, linguadental, the sides (lateral) of the tongue are against the upper molars, and the tip of the tongue makes contact behind the lower incisors (dental) near the alveolar ridge (alveolar) and forms a narrow opening through which the airflow is continuously directed against the front teeth. This airflow process causes an audible friction (fricative) noise, resulting in the voiced production of the [z] sound. The [z] sound is made with less force than its cognate, the [s] sound, is.

Different Spellings for the [z] Sound

Transcribe the following words. Refer to the Key at the right upon completion.

Different Spellings					*Key*
z	zipper ___	zinc ___	zebra ___		zɪpɚ, zɪŋk, zibrə
	daze ___	freeze ___			deɪz, friz
zz	jazz ___	puzzle ___			ʤæz, pʌz̩
	dazzle ___	muzzle ___			dæz̩, mʌz̩
s	has ___	was ___	dogs ___		hæz, wɔz, dɔgz
es	matches ___	washes ___			mætʃəz, wɔʃəz
	mixes ___				mɪksɪz
sth	asthma ___				æzmə
x	xylophone ___				zaɪləfon

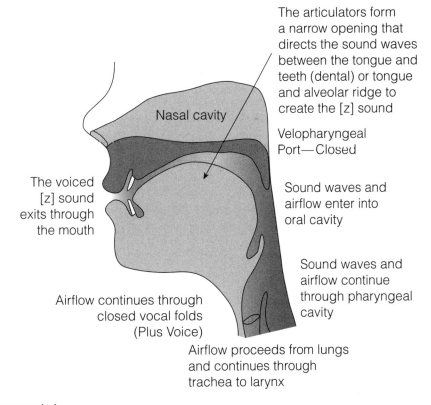

The articulators form a narrow opening that directs the sound waves between the tongue and teeth (dental) or tongue and alveolar ridge to create the [z] sound

Velopharyngeal Port—Closed

Sound waves and airflow enter into oral cavity

Sound waves and airflow continue through pharyngeal cavity

Nasal cavity

The voiced [z] sound exits through the mouth

Airflow continues through closed vocal folds (Plus Voice)

Airflow proceeds from lungs and continues through trachea to larynx

Figure 14-2 [z] pronunciation.

	exit	___ examine ___		ɛgzɪt, ɛgzæmən
se	rose	___ lose ___ bruise ___		roʊz, luz, bruz
ws	news	___ crews ___		nuz, kruz
ss	scissors	___ dessert ___		sɪzɚz, dɪzɚt
ze	sneeze	___ haze ___		sniz, haɪz
cz	czar	___		zɑr
ys	days	___		deɪz
sce	discern	___		dɪzɚn
si	music	___		mjuzɪk

Different Sounds for the Letter z

There are no other sounds that the letter *z* makes. Note, however, that the letter *x* in the initial position of a word, although usually pronounced as a [z] sound as in *Xerox*, is pronounced as an [s] in the word *x-ray* wherein the initial sound is a vowel, as in [ɛks-reɪ]. The *z* is silent in words of French origin, as in *rendezvous*.

Rules for Spelling and Pronunciation of the [z] Sound

1. The written *z* is pronounced [z], as in *zebra, hazy*.
2. Two adjacent *z* letters (*zz*) are usually pronounced as one [z] sound, as in *dizzy, puzzle, jazz*.
3. The final *s* after a vowel or voiced consonant is pronounced as a [z], as in *halves, abides, rivers*.
4. The final *s* in words ending in *es* as in *matches, catches, teaches* is pronounced as a [z] sound.
5. In the word *asthma*, the *s* becomes a [z] sound and the *th* is silent.
6. The *x* at the beginning of a word is pronounced [z], and in words such as *example*, the first consonant is the [g] sound followed by the [z]. This occurs primarily because the [g] sound is voiced.
7. Words spelled with an *se* at the end as in *rose, cruise* have an [s] sound ending.
8. Words that end in *ws* such as *knows, news, crews* end with the [z] sound.
9. Because of the (voiced) vowel that precedes the *ss* letters in *scissors* and *dessert*, the medial sound becomes a [z].
10. The *ze* combination at the end of words as in *sneeze* and *haze* results in the [z] as the last sound.
11. The [z] sound replaces the [s] sound in plural forms, past tense, and possessives after vowels as in *trees* and voiced consonants as in *logs*.
12. The [z] sound is the initial sound in the unique word *czar*.

Words That Include the [z] Sound

The [z] sound appears in the prevocalic, intervocalic, and postvocalic positions and in all three positions, initial, medial, and final. Transcribe the following words. Refer to the Key at the right upon completion.

Initial Consonant   *Key*

zoom _____   zenith _____   zoo _____   zum, zinɪθ, zu

Unstressed Syllable

Medial Consonant

easy _____   pleasant _____   izi, plɛzənt

blazer _____   bleɪzɚ

Stressed Syllable

Medial Consonant

embezzle _____   amusing _____   ɛmbɛzl̩, əmuzɪŋ

incisor _____   ɪnsaɪzɚ

Final Consonant

ribs _____   sneeze _____   rɪbz, sniz

eyes _____   is _____   aɪz, ɪz

Medial Blends

gz exempt	_____ exile	_____	ɛgzɛmpt, ɛgzaɪl
zigzag	_____ mz doomsday	_____	zɪgzæg, dumzdeɪ
groomsman	_____		grumzmən
nz frenzy	_____ Wednesday	_____	frɛnzi, wɛnzdeɪ
Kansas	_____ vs eavesdrop	_____	kænzəs, ivzdrɔp

Final Blends

bz bibs ___ clubs ___			bɪbz, klʌbz
Bob's ___ cobwebs ___			bɔbz, kɔbwɛbz
dz kids ___ crowds ___ sheds ___			kɪdz, kraʊdz, ʃɛdz
mz beams ___ chimes ___			bimz, ʧaɪmz
crumbs ___ nz fines ___ gains ___			krʌmz, faɪnz, geɪnz
retains ___ rz oars ___ dinners ___			riteɪnz, ɔrz, dɪnɚz
cheers ___ thz bathes ___ breathes ___			ʧɪrz, beɪðz, briðz
truths ___ truðz			
vz strives ___ shaves ___			straɪvz, ʃeɪvz
wives ___ zl chisel ___ easel ___			waɪvz, ʧɪzəl, izəl
arousal ___ refusal ___			əraʊzəl, rifjuzʊl

Clusters

ldz builds ___ yields ___ holds ___   bɪldz, jɪldz, hɔldz

ndz kinds ___ sands ___ glands ___   kaɪndz, sændz, glændz

<u>ŋgz</u> bangs ___ songs ___ things ___ bæɪŋz, sɑŋz, Θɪŋz

<u>rdz</u> swords ___ yards ___ sɔrdz, jɑrdz

chords ___ cards ___ kɔrdz, kɑrdz

Auditory Discrimination

Transcribe the following words. Refer to the Key at the right upon completion.

Cognates

[z] (+)		[s] (–)		Key
zip	_____	sip	_____	zɪp, sɪp
zoo	_____	sue	_____	zu, su
zeal	_____	seal	_____	zɪl, sɪl
Z	_____	see	_____	zi, si
zinc	_____	sink	_____	zɪŋk, sɪŋk
hers	_____	hearse	_____	hɝz, hɝs
trays	_____	trace	_____	treɪz, treɪs
maize	_____	mace	_____	meɪz, meɪs

Other Minimal Pairs

[z]		[ʒ]		[z]		[ð]		Key
reason	__	lesion	__	breeze	__	breathe	__	rizən, liʒən, briz, brið
Caesar	__	seizure	__	lays	__	lathe	__	sisɚ, siʒɚ, leɪz, leɪð
bays	__	beige	__	close	__	clothe	__	beɪz, beɪʒ, kloʊz, kloʊð
tease	__	prestige	__	tease	__	teethe	__	tiz, prɛstɪʒ, tiz, tið
hazard	__	azure	__	ties	__	tithe	__	hæzɚd, æʒɚ, taɪz, taɪð

Allophonic and Dialect Variations

Some speakers tend to unvoice [z], particularly in initial and final positions (Tiffany & Carrell, 1977). In the final position, the voicing may disappear shortly after the friction noise begins. Such devoicing may occur in words such as *keys* and also in the medial position in selected words such as *absorb* (Edwards, 1997). The [z] may also become palatalized in connected speech and the [ʒ] sound may be substituted as in *as you* [æʒju].

Related more to a grammatical feature rather than a sound feature is the deletion of the final consonant in African American English that marks plurality as in "There be two dog." This is not to be considered as an omission error of the [z] in [dɑgz]. The [z] sound usually maintains its uniqueness with some acceptable variations that are subtle to the listener. Some speakers produce the [z] sound with the tip of the tongue pressed against the lower front teeth (linguadental) and others pronounce the sound with the tip at various levels between the linguadental position and behind the alveolar ridge.

Normal and Deviant Development of the [z] Sound

The [z] sound is usually acquired by age 8 years (Sander, 1972) and may be frequently misarticulated until mastered. The [z] sound and its cognate, the [s] sound, are some of the last consonants mastered by children and are among the most frequently misarticulated consonants (Calvert, 1986; Edwards, 1997). Edwards (1997) notes that in severe cases, [d] is substituted, followed by [t], or the sound may be omitted. Milder cases may be characterized by a degree of stridency or higher-frequency noise, resulting in a lisping characteristic. Such a lisp may approximate a [ʒ] or a [ð] sound and is often produced with central and lateral airflow. Shriberg and Kent (1995) indicate that distortion of the [z] sound occurs when the tongue gets too close to or actually abuts the alveolar ridge or teeth, which results in a dentalization of the [z] and its cognate [s] sound.

Abnormal dentition (malocclusions) and other pathologic conditions such as those associated with birth defects and neuromuscular development may interfere with the pronunciation of the [z] sound.

Nonnative Speaker Pronunciation

Omissions may result from grammatical deficiencies (plural, possessive, etc.) or from a failure to pronounce the ends of words (Edwards, 1997). Some Europeans, particularly Spanish and Swedish speakers, may substitute the [s] sound regularly (Calvert, 1986). Those who have a strong German accent may devoice the [z] and substitute the [s] sound for the [z] sound, as when the word *nose* [noʊz] becomes [noʊs] (Tiffany & Carrell, 1977). Dentalization (forwarding of the tongue from the alveolar ridge onto the top front teeth) may be present to one degree or another.

Summary

The [z] sound is one of the 10 fricative consonants, and its voiceless cognate is the [s] sound. In addition to the [s] sound, it is homorganic (lingua-alveolar) with the [t], [d], [l], and [n] sounds. In addition to its lingua-alveolar placement, with the tongue tip in an upward position, the [z] sound is produced by many speakers with the tip of the tongue downward and pressing against the lower front teeth (dental) position. The letter *z* is consistent in representing the [z] sound, but the sound can also be represented by the letter *s* and by other letters in peculiar words such as *exit* and *czar* where the [z] is the first sound in the word. The [z] and [s] sounds are among the last to be mastered by children and are frequently misarticulated. A grammatical feature of African American English is the deletion of the final consonant marker on nouns such as *dog* for *dogs*. This is not to be considered a phonological error. Nonnative speakers tend to devoice the [z] sound and substitute the [s] sound, and there is also confusion caused by the use of the *s* spelling for many of the words that are pronounced with a [z] sound.

[z] +

Write the orthographic and phonetic spellings for the following words. Refer to the Key at the bottom of the section upon completion.

	Orthographic	*Phonetic*
1. z + 3 sounds: minus one (1)	_____	[_ i _ o]
2. z + 4 sounds: a black and white striped animal	_____	[_ i _ _ ə]
3. z + 3 sounds: used to fasten two pieces of material	_____	[_ ɪ _ ɚ]
4. z + 3 sounds: behavior of a clown	_____	[_ eɪ _ i]
5. z + 1 sound: place with caged animals	_____	[_ u]
6. z + 4 sounds: signs used in astrology	_____	[_ o _ i æ _]
7. z + 5 sounds: a series of short, sharp angles	_____	[_ ɪ _ _ æ _]
8. z + 4 sounds: enthusiastic about something	_____	[_ ɛ _ ə _]
9. z + 6 sounds: an airborne vehicle	_____	[_ ɛ _ _ ɪ _]
10. z + 5 sounds: a branch of biology	_____	[_ o _ o ʤ i]

Key: 1. zero [ziro]; 2. zebra [zibrə]; 3. zipper [zɪpɚ]; 4. zany [zeɪni]; 5. zoo [zu]; 6. zodiac [zodiæk]; 7. zigzag [zɪgzæg]; 8. zealous [zɛləs]; 9. zeppelin [zɛplɪn]; 10. zoology [zoloʤi]

PHONETIC SYMBOL [f]

EXHIBIT 14-3	Phonetic Symbol [f]

[f]

Phonetic Symbol	[f]
Grapheme Symbols	v, f, ph, vv, zv
Diacritic Symbol	f
Phonic Symbol	f
Cognate	[v]
Homorganic	[v]
Sound Class	Consonant
Basic Phonetic Features	Placement: Linguadental Manner: Fricative Voicing: Minus Voice
IPA (1999)	[f] #128 Voiceless, Linguadental, Fricative Distinctive Feature Analysis (Chomsky & Halle, 1968) Plus (+): Consonantal, Anterior, Continuant, Voiceless, Strident Minus (–): Vocalic, Sonorant, Coronal, High, Back, Low, Rounded, Distributed, Nasal, Lateral, Tense

How the Sound Is Produced

The [f] sound is produced by contact between the lower lip (labio) and the upper front teeth (dental). The airflow from the lungs passes through the open vocal folds (voiceless). The velopharyngeal port is closed, directing the airflow into the oral cavity, and the voiceless [f] is continuously emitted between the teeth and with sufficient force to create audible friction without voicing. The [f] is longer in duration and usually produced with more force than its cognate, the [v] sound. See **Figure 14-3**.

Different Spellings for the [f] Sound

Transcribe the following. Refer to the Key at the right upon completion.

Different Spellings			*Key*
f	fun	_____	fʌn
ph	phone	_____	fon
ff	huff	_____	hʌf
gh	laugh	_____	læf

Different Sounds for the Letter *f*

There are no different sounds for the letter *f*.

Rules for Spelling and Pronunciation of the [f] Sound

1. The *gh* has the sound of [f] when *au* has the sound of short ǎ [æ].

2. The *gh* has the sound of [f] when *ou* has the sound of ô [ɔ], as in *awful, cough,* and *trough*.

3. The letter *f* is never silent in a word. However, it is pronounced as *v* in the word *of* [ʌv] or [ɔv].

4. The *ph* in *phonetics, diphthong, gopher* is pronounced with the [f] sound.

5. Words spelled with the *lf* such as *calf* and *half* omit the [l] sound but such words as *elf, shelf,* and *golf* do not.

6. *F* and *l* are combined to form a consonant blend, as in *fly, flew, flip, flea, float,* and *floor*.

7. *F* is also found in consonant clusters with *r* as in the words *fry, front,* and *from*.

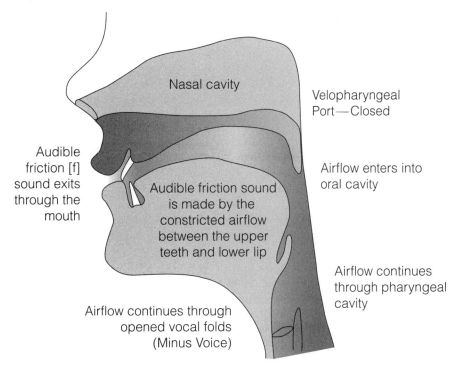

Figure 14-3 [f] pronunciation.

Words That Include the [f] Sound

The [f] sound occurs in all three positions, initial, medial, and final. Transcribe the following words. Refer to the Key at the right upon completion.

Initial Consonant

			Key
field ____	fast ____	five ____	fɪld, fæst, faɪv
fire ____	fork ____	free ____	faɪr, fɔrk, fri
fine ____	phone ____		faɪn, foʊn

Unstressed Syllable

Medial Consonant

taffy ____	offer ____	tæfi, ɔfɚ
coffee ____	notify ____	kɔfi, noʊtɪfaɪ,
edify ____		ɛdɪfaɪ
elephant ____		ɛlʌfənt

Stressed Syllable

Medial Consonant

conform ____	perform ____	kʌnfɔrm, pɝfɔrm
refuse ____	infamous ____	rifjuz, ɪnfʌməs
infinite ____		ɪnfɪnɪt or ɪnfʌnət

Final Consonant

knife ____	life ____	reef ____	naɪf, laɪf, rif
off ____	rough ____	chief ____	ɔf, rʌf, ʧif

Initial and Final Consonants

fife ____	fluff ____	faɪf, flʌf
photograph ____		foʊtoɡræf

Initial Blends

fl fly ____	fled ____	flower ____	flaɪ, flɛd, flaʊɚ
phlegm ____			flɛm
fr fry ____	friend ____	from ____	fraɪ, frɛnd, frɔm

Medial Blends

fl muffler ____	reflect ____	mʌflɚ, riflɛkt
pamphlet ____	lf alfalfa ____	pæmflɛt, aʊlfaʊfə
alphabet ____	skillful ____	aulfʌbɛt, skɪfʊl
fr confront ____	refresh ____	kʌnfrənt, rifrɛʃ
affricate ____		æfrɪkət
rf orphan ____	careful ____	ɔrfən, kɛrfʊl
morphology ____	sf asphalt ____	mɔrfɔloʤi, æsfɔlt
graceful ____	transfer ____	ɡreɪsfʊl, trænsfɚ
ft fifty ____	thrifty ____	fɪfti, θrɪfti

Final Blends

ft laughed ____	left ____	læft, lɛft
fs laughs ____	cliffs ____	læfs, klɪfs
lf gulf ____	yourself ____	ɡɔlf, jɔrsɛlf
Ralph ____	rf scarf ____	rælf, skɑrf
wharf ____	turf ____	wɔrf, tɝf

Auditory Discrimination

Transcribe the following. Refer to the Key at the right upon completion.

Cognates

[f] (–) Voice	*[v] (+) Voice*	*Key*
face ____	vase ____	feɪs, veɪs
surf ____	serve ____	sɝf, sɝv
fat ____	vat ____	fæt, væt
file ____	vile ____	faɪl, vaɪl
few ____	view ____	fu, vu
feel ____	veal ____	fɛl, vɛl

Other Minimal Pairs

[f]	*[θ]*	*[f]*	*[p]*	*Key*
fin ____	thin ____	far ____	par ____	fɪn, θɪn, fɑr, pɑr
offer ____	author ____	leaf ____	leap ____	ɔfɚ, ɔθɚ, lif, lip
free ____	three ____	fry ____	pry ____	fri, θri, fraɪ, praɪ
fought ____	thought ____	fool ____	pool ____	fɔt, θɔt, ful, pul
first ____	thirst ____	fast ____	past ____	fɝst, θɝst, fæst, pæst
fret ____	threat ____	flee ____	plea ____	frɛt, θrɛt, fli, pli

[f]	*[s]*	*Key*
feel ____	seal ____	fɛl, sɛl
fine ____	sign ____	faɪn, saɪn
fed ____	said ____	fɛd, sɛd

fame _____	same _____	feɪm, seɪm
feet _____	seat _____	fit, sit
fun _____	sun _____	fʌn, sʌn

Allophonic and Dialect Variations

The allophonic variations occur as a result of three factors: (1) the position of the [f] sound within the word or utterance, initial, medial, or final; (2) whether it appears in the stressed or unstressed portion of the word; and (3) the influence of the consonant blend or vowel context because the [f] sound is somewhat "preprogrammed" by these other sound features. The strength, duration, and loudness (noise) of this fricative consonant may change depending on these factors, but, in general, any altered allophonic production of the [f] sound does not interfere with speaker and listener understanding of meaning. For example, when the [f] sound occurs after a labial such as in *comfort*, the [f] sound is weaker and may be more of a labial fricative rather than a labial dental. The initial position in *foot* has a different allophonic element than in the word *off*.

The [f] sound depends on the nature of a constricted airflow and its resultant turbulence for the precise quality of its "noise" element (Tiffany & Carrell, 1977). There is relatively little variation of this sound in native speech. When the sound is deliberately pronounced in isolation, the teeth may be in contact with a point fairly well out on the carmine border of the lip. In connected speech, the teeth often touch the upper part of the inner surface of the lower lip, presumably because this involves less contrast with the positions of the articulators for preceding and following sounds.

Native speakers rarely have any conspicuous errors of pronunciation and/or articulation involving the [f] sound, presumably because the articulatory pattern for the sound is relatively simple, and there are good visual and tactile cues (Edwards, 1997; Tiffany & Carrell, 1977). Edwards (1997) states that there is no significant dialect variations for the [f] sound, but some speakers may substitute the [Θ] for the [f] sound at the end of words such as *trough* [trɑf]: [trɑΘ].

Normal and Deviant Development of the [f] Sound

The [f] sound is generally acquired by age 4 years. Edwards (1997) states that prevocalic substitutions include [b] and [p]. In the postvocalic position, the [p] is substituted or the sound may be omitted. Because of a dental malocclusion, some children may find it difficult to make the necessary labiodental contact. Tiffany and Carrell (1977) report that children are more likely to choose [f] as a substitute for another sound such as the voiceless *th* [Θ]. The [f] sound is mastered between the ages of 2 and 4 years.

Nonnative Speaker Pronunciation

Among foreign speakers, failure to produce an acceptable approximation of United States English [f] is not usually a problem, although the bilabial fricative is not uncommon (Tiffany & Carrell, 1977). German speakers may produce the [f] somewhat weaker than a native speaker does. Japanese and Korean are two languages that do not have the [f] sound. The other predominant languages spoken in the United States do include the [f] in their sound systems.

Summary

The [f] sound is one of the 10 fricative consonants, and its voiced cognate is the [v] sound. It is homorganic (labiodental) with the [v] sound. The [f] sound is represented by several different alphabet letters and is usually mastered by age 4 years. Allophonic variations are the result of differences in the fricative noise as determined by the context of the sound. Native speakers produce this sound with ease most of the time. The [f] sound or its variations appear in many of the sound systems of languages worldwide; however, it is absent in many Pacific Rim or Asian languages. Structural abnormalities such as dental malocclusions and limitations to the lower lip and/or other neuromuscular weaknesses may interfere with an acceptable production of the [f] sound. Generally, the correction of the [f] sound is enhanced as a result of its visual and tactile features.

[f]+

Write the orthographic and phonetic spellings of the following words. Refer to the Key at the bottom of the section upon completion.

	Orthographic	Phonetic
1. [f] + 3 sounds: domestic animals live here	_____	[_ ɑ _ _]
2. [f] + 5 sounds: to say goodbye	_____	[_ ɑ _ _ ɛ _]
3. [f] + 8 sounds: superlative for great	_____	[_ æ _ _ æ _ _ ɪ _]

4. [f] + 3 sounds: _____   [_ i _ _]
   a meal with a lot
   of food

5. [f] + 4 sounds: _____   [_ imɛ _]
   opposite of male

6. [f] + 3 sounds: _____   [_ ɪ _ _]
   a type of violin

7. [f] + 3 sounds: _____   [_ ɝ _ _]
   opposite of last

8. [f] + 3 sounds: _____   [_ _ æ _]
   each nation has one

9. [f] + 7 sounds: _____   [_ _ ɛ _ _ ə _ _]
   the characteristic
   of being bendable

10. [f] + 3 sounds: _____   [_ oʊ _ i]
    not real

Key: 1. farm [fɑrm]; 2. farewell [fɛrwɛl]; 3. fantastic [fæntæstɪk]; 4. feast [fist]; 5. female [fimɛl]; 6. fiddle [fɪdl̩]; 7. first [fɝst]; 8. flag [flæg]; 9. flexible [flɛksəbl̩]; 10. phony [foʊni]

PHONETIC SYMBOL [v]

EXHIBIT 14-4   Phonetic Symbol [v]

[v]

Phonetic Symbol	[v]
Grapheme Symbols	v, f, ph, vv, zv
Diacritic Symbol	v̰
Phonic Symbol	V̰
Cognate	[f]
Homorganic	[f]
Sound Class	Consonant
Basic Phonetic Features	Placement: Linguadental Manner: Fricative Voicing: Plus Voice
IPA (1999)	[v] #129 Voiced, Linguadental, Fricative Distinctive Feature Analysis (Chomsky & Halle, 1968) Plus (+): Consonantal, Anterior, Continuant, Voiced, Strident Minus (−): Vocalic, Sonorant, Coronal, High, Back, Low, Rounded, Distributed, Nasal, Lateral, Tense

How the Sound Is Produced

The [v] sound is produced by contact between the lower lip (labio) and the upper front teeth (dental). The airflow from the lungs activates the vocal folds to vibrate (voicing). The velopharyngeal port is closed, directing the airflow into the oral cavity, and voiced [v] is continuously emitted between the teeth and with sufficient force to create audible friction with voicing. The [v] is shorter in duration and usually produced with less force than its cognate, the [f] sound, is. See **Figure 14-4.**

Different Spellings for the [v] Sound

Transcribe the following. Refer to the Key at the right upon completion.

Different Spellings		*Key*
v	vegetable	vɛdʒətəbl̩
f	of	ʌv
ph	Stephen	stivən
vv	navvy (slang for navigator)	nævi

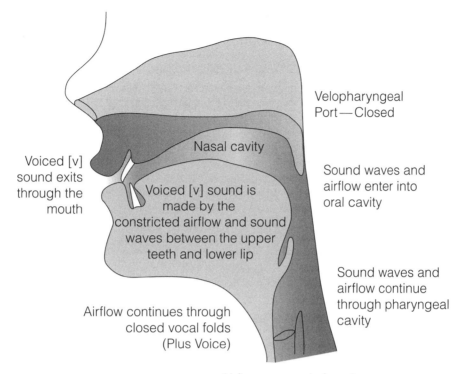

Velopharyngeal Port—Closed

Nasal cavity

Voiced [v] sound exits through the mouth

Sound waves and airflow enter into oral cavity

Voiced [v] sound is made by the constricted airflow and sound waves between the upper teeth and lower lip

Sound waves and airflow continue through pharyngeal cavity

Airflow continues through closed vocal folds (Plus Voice)

Airflow proceeds from lungs and continues through trachea to larynx

Figure 14-4 [v] pronunciation.

	flivver (old, cheap car)	flɪvɚ
zv	rendezvous	rɑndəvu

Different Sounds for the Letter v

None: the letter *v* is quite reliable in representing the [v] sound.

Rules for Spelling the [v] Sound

1. The *v* in most spelling contexts is written *v*.
2. Two adjacent *v* letters (*vv*) may be pronounced as a single [v].
3. The [f] sound in *of* is replaced with the voiced cognate [v]: [ʌv].
4. The *ph* in the word *Ste__ph__en* when pronounced as *Ste__v__en* is replaced with the [v] sound.

Words That Include the [v] Sound

The [v] sound occurs in all three positions, initial, medial, and final. Transcribe the following. Refer to the Key at the right upon completion.

Initial Consonant   *Key*

very _____ vase _____ vote _____   vɛri, veɪs, voʊt

valley _____ victory _____   væli, vɪktɔri

Medial Consonant

sliver _____ nervous _____   slɪvɚ, nɝvəs

travel _____ paving _____ even _____   trævəl, peɪvɪŋ, ivən

Final Consonant

believe _____ glove _____   bilive, glʌv

five _____ love _____ of _____   faɪv, lʌv, ʌv

Stressed Syllable

convex _____ convey _____   kɑnvɛks, kɑnveɪ

review _____ revolt _____ veto _____   rivu, rivɔlt, vɛto

Unstressed Syllable

given _____ having _____   gɪvən, hævɪŋ

river _____ clover _____ devote _____   rɪvɚ, kloʊvɚ, divoʊt

Blends

vd starved _____   vz waves _____   stɑrvd̩, weɪvz

lv silver _____   involve _____   sɪlvɚ, ɪnvɑlv

vl carnival _____   lvd solved _____   cɑrnəvl, sɔlvd̩

lvz evolves _____   ivɑlvz

Initial and Final Consonant

valve _____   visive _____   vælv, vɪsɪv

votive _____   voʊtɪv

Audible Discrimination

Cognates

Transcribe the following words. Refer to the Key at the right upon completion.

[v] (+) Voice		[f] (−) Voice		Key
vine	_____	fine	_____	vɑɪn, fɑɪn
live	_____	life	_____	laɪv, laɪf
vile	_____	file	_____	vaɪl, faɪl
vault	_____	fault	_____	vɔlt, fɔlt
versed	_____	first	_____	vɝst, fɝst
save	_____	safe	_____	seɪv, seɪf

Other Minimal Pairs

[v]	[z]	[v]	[ð]	Key
have __	has __	ever __	whether __	hæv, hæz, ɛvɚ, wɛðɚ
pave __	pays __	vine __	thine __	pæv, pæz, vaɪn, ðaɪn
grave __	graze __	cave __	scathe __	greɪv, greɪz, keɪv, skeɪð
clove __	close __	vat __	that __	kloʊv, kloʊz, væt, ðæt
veal __	zeal __	van __	than __	vɛl, zɛl, væn, ðæn
rove __	rose __	vie __	thy __	roʊv, roʊz, vaɪ, ðaɪ

Allophonic and Dialect Variations

Because fricatives depend on the nature of a constricted airflow and its resultant turbulence for the precise quality of their "noise" element, wide variations are encountered in their production (Tiffany & Carrell, 1977). However, there is relatively little variation with the [f] and [v] sounds in native language. Tiffany and Carrell (1977) further explain that there is no special tongue position for [v] and coarticulation is strongly influenced by the surrounding vowels that influence the exact position of dental-lip contact, as in the words *veal* and *vote*.

When [v] follows a bilabial sound, as in *subversive*, the [v] may become more like a bilabial fricative. In the final

position, as in *half*, and when it is followed by a voiceless consonant in conversational speech *I have time now*, the [v] may become an [f] sound: [aɪ hæf taɪm noʊ]. Also, there is an allophonic difference in the production of the [v] sound when it occurs in a stressed or unstressed syllable. Consider the difference in such words as *reverse* [rɪvɝs] (stressed syllable) and *given* [gɪvən] (unstressed syllable).

Speakers of African American English substitute the [b] for the [v] in all positions in words (Edwards, 1997) and substitute the [v] for the [ð] (voiced *th*) in the medial *feather* [fɛðɚ:fɛvɚ] and final *smooth* [smuð:smuv] (Calvert, 1986). General American and Southern American speakers may substitute the [b] for the [v] in the medial and final positions. In informal speech, there may be a tendency to substitute the [b] sound in the medial position, as in *seven* [sɛbən]. Hawaiians substitute a labiodental fricative [v] for the intervocalic [w], as in *Ewa* and *Hawaii* (Calvert, 1986).

Normal and Deviant Development of the [v] Sound

The [v] sound is usually acquired between ages 4 and 8 years (Sander, 1972). The [v] is mastered by age 8, which is much later than age of acquisition of its voiceless cognate, the [f] sound, which is mastered by age 4 (Sander, 1972). The [v] sound is misarticulated rather frequently (Calvert, 1986). The most common prevocalic substitution is [b] (Edwards, 1997). At the end of an utterance, [f] is common or the sound may be omitted.

Nonnative Speaker Pronunciation

Nonnative speakers tend to substitute the [w] or [b] for the [v], and the [v] tends to become devoiced, especially in the final position in a word. Spanish speakers may substitute [b] for initial [v] and produce a voiced bilabial fricative in the medial position (Calvert, 1986).

Summary

The [v] sound is one of the 10 fricative consonants, and its voiceless cognate is the [f] sound. It is only homorganic (labiodental) with the [f] sound. The letter *v* is consistent in representing the [v] sound, and the sound is also produced using the letters *of, Stephen*, and is omitted in words such as *rendezvous*. The [v] sound may not be mastered until age 8 years, which is a later age of acquisition than for most of the other sounds. Consequently, it is misarticulated frequently. Dialect and nonnative speaker errors consist of the substitution of the [b] and for the [v] to become devoiced with the [f] substitution.

[v] +

Write the orthographic and phonetic spellings of the following words. Refer to the Key at the bottom of the section upon completion.

Orthographic Phonetic

1. [v] + 7 sounds: _____ [_ æ _ _ ɪ _ e _]
to inoculate

2. [v] + 4 sounds: _____ [_ ɪ _ ə _]
the Roman
goddess; a
planet

3. [v] + 5 sounds: _____ [_ eɪ _ ə _ _]
not occupied

4. [v] + 12 sounds: _____ [_ ɛ _ _ _ ɪ _ə _ _ ɪ _ _]
an entertainer

5. [v] + 6 sounds: _____ [_ ɚ _ ɪ _ ə _]
opposite of
horizontal

6. [v] + 5 sounds: _____ [_ aɪ _ _ e _]
to shake

7. [v] + 9 sounds: _____ [_ ɪ _ io _ ə _ ɛ _]
a case containing
a video tape

8. [v] + 8 sounds: _____ [_ iɛ _ _ ɑ _ i _]
a native of
Vietnam

9. [v] + 6 sounds: _____ [_ aɪ _ ə _ ɛ _]
a dietary
supplement

10. [v] + 6 sounds: _____ [_ oʊi _ _ ɛ _]
an [s] is a v_
sound

Key: 1. vaccinate [væksɪnet]; 2. Venus [vɪnəs]; 3. vacant [veɪkənt]; 4. ventriloquist [vɛntrɪləkwɪst]; 5. vertical [vɚtɪkəl]; 6. vibrate [vaɪbret]; 7. videocassette [vɪdiokəsɛt]; 8. Vietnamese [viɛtnɑmiz]; 9. vitamin [vaɪtəmɛn]; 10. voiceless [voʊislɛs]

PHONETIC SYMBOL [h]

EXHIBIT 14-5	Phonetic Symbol [h]

		[h]
Phonetic Symbol	[h]	
Grapheme Symbols	h, j	
Diacritic Symbol	h	
Phonic Symbol	h	
Cognate	None	
Homorganic	Lingua-Velar [k], [g], [ŋ], [w], [ʍ] Linguapalatal [ʃ], [ʒ], [r], [j]	
Sound Class	Consonant	
Basic Phonetic Features	Placement: Lingua-Velar, Linguapalatal Manner: Fricative Voicing: Minus Voice	
IPA (1999)	[h] #146 Voiceless, Glottal, Fricative Distinctive Feature Analysis (Chomsky & Halle, 1968) Plus (+): Low, Continuant Minus (−): Vocalic, Consonantal, Sonorant, Coronal, Anterior, High, Back, Rounded, Distributed, Nasal, Lateral, Tense, Voiced, Strident	

How the Sound Is Produced

The airflow from the lungs progresses through the slightly constricted vocal folds (voiceless). This physical condition creates a soft, diffused friction (fricative) sound as the airflow is expelled through the glottis (glottal). The velopharyngeal port is closed to permit the airflow to make contact with the soft (velar) and hard palate (palatal) areas to enhance the friction quality of the voiceless [h] sound. Unlike many other sounds that are produced with rather distinct and consistent postures, there is no given placement of the tongue and lips critical to the production of the [h] sound. Rather, it appears that the oral cavity and the articulators assume the configuration for the next anticipated sound when the [h] is spoken in context. Because of its short duration, the [h] may be considered a glide. The airflow is emitted with greater turbulence in comparison with other fricatives. This is necessary to make the [h] audible. See **Figure 14-5**.

The constriction involved in the production of the [h] sound is at the glottis and this sound is sometimes considered to be a voiceless *glottal* fricative (Edwards, 1986; International Phonetic Association, 1999).

Different Spellings for the [h] Sound

Transcribe the following words. Refer to the Key at the right upon completion.

Different Spellings				Key
h	he ____	perhaps ____	have ____	hi, pɚhæps, hæv
j	Navajo ____			nævəhoʊ

Different Sounds of the Letters That Produce the [h] Sound

Transcribe the following words. Refer to the Key at the right upon completion.

Different Sounds			Key
h [h]	he ____		hi
wh [ʍ]	what ____	when ____	ʍɑt, ʍɛn
	where ____	which ____	ʍɛr, ʍɪtʃ
sh [ʃ]	shoe ____	wish ____	ʃu, wɪʃ
	washer ____		wɔʃɚ

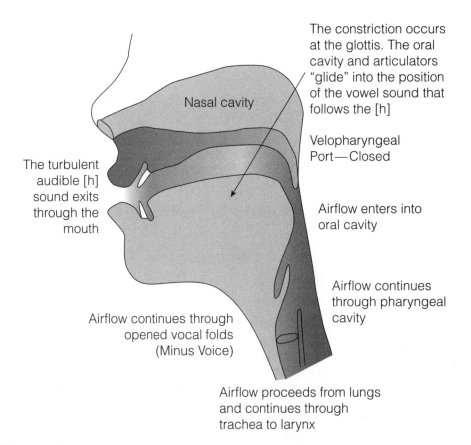

The constriction occurs at the glottis. The oral cavity and articulators "glide" into the position of the vowel sound that follows the [h]

Velopharyngeal Port—Closed

Airflow enters into oral cavity

Airflow continues through pharyngeal cavity

Nasal cavity

The turbulent audible [h] sound exits through the mouth

Airflow continues through opened vocal folds (Minus Voice)

Airflow proceeds from lungs and continues through trachea to larynx

Figure 14-5 [h] pronunciation.

ph [f]	phony	———		foʊni
	telephone	———		tɛləfon
	triumph	———		traɪəmf
ch [ʧ]	change	———		ʧeɪnʤ
	cherry	——— chin ———		ʧɛri, ʧɪn
gh [f]	enough	———		inʌf
	tough	——— rough ———		tʌf, rʌf
h [h]	he			hi
h (silent)	honor	——— herb ———		ɑnɚ, ɝb
	honorary	——— heir ———		ɑnɚɛri, ɛɪr
	hour	———		aʊɚ
h (silent)	oh	——— ah ———night ———		oʊ, ɑ, naɪt
gh (silent)	though	——— Hugh ———		ðoʊ, hju
	thought	——— ghost ———		Ɵɔt, goʊst
kh (silent)	khaki	———		kæki
rh (silent)	rhetoric	———		rɛtɔrɪk

Rules for Spelling and Pronunciation of the [h] Sound

1. The letter *h* is pronounced as [h], as in *here, hurry, inhalation, behavior,* and *uphill.*

2. In the *wh* context, as in *which, whenever, why,* and *whether,* the *wh* is pronounced as a voiceless [ʍ] (hw) fricative sound.

3. In the *sh* context, both the *s* and *h* form an entirely different sound, the [ʃ] as in *should, show, dishwasher,* and *brush.*

4. When the *h* appears in the *ph* context, as in *phonology, morphology,* and *photograph,* the *ph* is pronounced as the [f] sound.

5. The *h* in *honor, heir,* and *herb* is not pronounced, so the *h* is silent. However, the [h] sound is pronounced in *Herb.*

6. The *h* is silent in the pronunciation of exclamations such as *Oh!* and *Ah!*

7. In the *gh* context, as in *ghost* and *ghastly,* the *h* is silent, and both of the letters *gh* are silent as in *though, thought, Hugh,* and *thigh.*

8. The *h* is silent when it follows the consonants [k], as in *khaki,* and [r], as in *rhetoric.*

9. In the preferential spelling of the word *Navajo* versus *Navaho,* the letter *j* has the [h] sound.

Words That Include the [h] Sound

The [h] sound occurs in the prevocalic (initial) and intervocalic (medial) positions but not in the final position. Transcribe the following words. Refer to the Key at the right upon completion.

Initial Consonant		*Key*
hurry ———	Henry ———	hɝɪ, hɛnri
hemisphere ———	harmonize———	hɛmɪsfɛr, hɑrmənaɪz
hamburger ———	Hawaii ———	hæmbɚgɚ, həwaɪi

Unstressed Syllable

Medial Consonant

vehicle ————	mohair ————	vihɪkl̩, mohɛɪr
forehead ————	cowhide ————	fɔrhɛd, kɑʊhaɪd

Stressed Syllable

Medial Consonant

ahoy ———	behave ———	əhɔɪ, biheɪv
behind ———	perhaps ———	bihaɪnd, pɚhæps
inherit ———	rehearsal———	ɪnhɛrɪt, rihɝsəl

Final Consonant

[None]

Auditory Discrimination
Contrast Minimal Pairs

[h] +	*[h] –*	*[h]*	*[ʍ]*	*Key*
hat	——at	——hen	——when	hæt, æt, hɛn, wɛn
hand ——	and ——	high ——	why ——	hænd, ænd, haɪ, waɪ
high ——	eye ——	heat ——	wheat ——	haɪ, aɪ, hit, wit
his	——is	——height ——	white	hɪz, ɪz, haɪt, waɪt
hold ——	old ——	hitch ——	which ——	hoʊld, oʊld, hɪʧ, wɪʧ
hair ——	air ——	heel ——	wheel ——	hɛɪr, ɛɪr, hɛl, wɛl
had ——	ad ——	hay ——	whey ——	hæd, æd, heɪ, weɪ
Herb ——	herb ——			hɝb, ɝb
here	——ear ———			hɛr, ɛr

[h]	*[f]*	*[h]*	*[Θ]*	*Key*
hill __	fill __	high __	thigh __	hɪl, fɪl, haɪ, Θaɪ
he __	fee __	hick __	thick __	hi, fi, hɪk, Θɪk
hit __	fit __	heard __	third __	hɪt, fɪt, hɜ˞d, Θɜ˞d
her __	fur __	Hank __	thank __	hɜ˞, fɜ˞, heɪŋk, Θeɪŋk
head __	fed __	hum __	thumb __	hɛd, fɛd, hʌm, Θʌm
hair __	fair __	heft __	theft __	hɛɪr, fɛɪr, hɛft, Θɛft
hold __	fold __	horn __	thorn __	hoʊld, foʊld, hɔrn, Θɔrn

[h]		*[s]*		*Key*
halt _____		salt _____		hɔlt, sɔlt
hat _____		sat _____		hæt, sæt
hand _____		sand _____		hænd, sænd
he _____		see _____		hi, si
had _____		sad _____		hæd, sæd
her _____		sir _____		hɜ˞, sɜ˞
head _____		said _____		hɛd, sɛd

Allophonic and Dialect Variations

Some speakers omit the [h] before [ju], as in *humor, human*, and *humid* [hjumɪd], and for some speakers, part of the turbulence contributing to audible friction for [h] may occur at the glottis rather than at the velum and palate above and the surface of the tongue below (Calvert, 1986). The voiceless [h] may become voiced when presented between two vowels, as in *treehouse* [trihaʊs] (Edwards, 1997). This may also occur after a nasal resonant, as in *downhill* [daʊnhɪl], and the [h] becomes more voiced than voiceless. The [h] may be omitted when it occurs in the unstressed position, as when *forehead* [fɔrhɛd] becomes [fɔrɛd]. Some speakers substitute a glottal stop, as in *hello* [hʌlo] or [hɛlo] when the initial [h] is omitted and a glottal stop is substituted, as in [ʔʌlo].

The [h] sound may be considerably weakened or even lost in connected speech (House, 1998; Tiffany & Carrell, 1977). Initial sounds are quite commonly obliterated in conversational speech when they occur in unstressed positions in words and phrases, such as *It's to his credit* [ɪts tu ɪz krɛdət], when spoken in a natural manner. Pronunciation changes under the influence of stress. For example, when speakers emphasize a specific intent *I have none?* [aɪ hæv nʌn], then the [h] sound is present.

Subtle allophonic variations occur depending on contact of the articulators and surrounding context.

When the articulators that influence the constricted airflow (manner) are predominantly at the tongue–palate or glottal contact is made, the [h] sound is affected. The context is determined by the distinctive features of the surrounding vowels and consonant sounds. For example, during the production of [h], the articulators take on the shape of the vowel that follows, as in *hoop* [hʊp] (rounded, back vowel) and *heap* [hip] (unrounded, front vowel) (House, 1998; Small, 1999). The speaker's lips take on the posture of the vowel even before the [h] sound is produced.

No significant dialect variation has been reported for the [h] sound in United States English (Edwards, 1997), and native speakers are not likely to have difficulty from misarticulation of this sound (Tiffany & Carrell, 1977). Speakers of certain English dialects tend to delete [h], as in *Here now* [ir naʊ]. Speakers of Southern American speech tend to add the [h], as in *it* [hɪt] for [ɪt], which depicts an earlier English pronunciation of this pronoun. In many accents of English, [h] can occur only before stressed vowels or before the approximant [j], as in *hue* [hju] (Ladefoged, 1993). Some speakers of English also sound [h] before [w] so that they contrast *which* [hwɪtʃ] and *witch* [wɪtʃ]. The [ʍ] symbol is used to express [hw] phonetically, as in *which* [ʍɪtʃ].

Normal and Deviant Development of the [h] Sound

The [h] sound is mastered early by 3 years of age (Calvert, 1986) and is seldom misarticulated. Rarely is the [h] sound a problem, probably because of its vowel-like quality (Edwards, 1997). It may be omitted or replaced with a glottal stop.

Nonnative Speaker Pronunciation

With insufficient airflow, nonnative speakers may substitute a glottal stop for the [h] sound and may produce a voiceless velar fricative if the articulators are not positioned correctly (Edwards, 1997). In foreign dialects, the errors are numerous (Tiffany & Carrell, 1977). In the French dialect, the [h] may be omitted or a non-English variant may be substituted such as the velar fricative of German speakers.

According to the U. S. Census Bureau (1990), in addition to United States English, 15 other languages are spoken prominently in the United States. Those that have an [h] sound similar to United States English are German, Korean, Arabic, and Hindi. Those who do not include the [h] sound are Spanish, French, Chinese, Portuguese, and Japanese.

Summary

The [h] sound is one of the 10 fricative sounds in United States English, and it has no cognate and neither does it appear in the final position in words even though the letter *h* appears there. It is mastered between the ages of 2 and 3 years and is one of the earliest sounds to be acquired, perhaps because of its vowel-like quality. It is seldom misarticulated and is usually deleted in the unstressed position in words and phrases. Allophonic variations occur as a result of differences in the point at which the constriction of airflow makes contact, such as in glottal or palatal positions. A glottal stop may be substituted in some instances. There are minor dialect differences, and nonnative speakers may produce the [h] sound with some variation depending on point of contact between airflow and articulators (glottal, velar, palatal).

REFERENCES

Calvert, D. R. (1986). *Descriptive phonetics*. New York: Thieme Medical Publishers.

Chomsky, N. & Halle, Morris (1968). *The sound pattern of english*. New York: Harper & Row.

Edwards, H. T. (1997). *Applied phonetics* (2nd ed.). San Diego, CA: College-Hill Press.

House, L. (1998). *Introductory phonetics and phonology*. Mahwah, NJ: Lawrence Erlbaum.

International Phonetic Association. (1999). *Handbook of the International Phonetic Association*. Cambridge, England: Cambridge University Press.

Ladefoged, P. (1993). *A course in phonetics* (3rd ed.). Fort Worth, TX: Harcourt Brace College Publishers.

MacKay, I. R. A. (1987). *Phonetics: The science of speech production*. Boston, MA: Allyn & Bacon.

Sander, E. (1972). When are speech sounds learned? *Journal of Speech and Hearing Disorders, 37*, 55–63.

Shriberg, L., & Kent, R. (1995). *Clinical phonetics* (3rd ed.). Boston, MA: Allyn & Bacon.

Small, L. H. (1999). *Fundamentals of phonetics: A practical guide for students* (3rd ed.). Boston, MA: Allyn & Bacon.

Tiffany, W. R., & Carrell, J. (1977). *Phonetics: Theory and application*. New York: McGraw-Hill.

U.S. Census Bureau. (1990). Table 5. Detailed list of languages spoken at home for the population 5 years and over by state: 1990. Retrieved from http://www.census.gov/prod/2010pubs/acs-12.pdf

Chapter 15

Unfamiliar Phonetic Symbols: Fricative Consonants Analysis and Transcription

PURPOSE

To describe the fricative sounds symbolized by unfamiliar phonetic symbols.

OBJECTIVES

This chapter will provide you with information regarding:

1. Characteristics of the cognate fricative consonant pair [Ɵ] and [ð]

2. Characteristics of the cognate fricative consonant pair [ʃ] and [ʒ]

3. Characteristics of the [hw] and [ʍ] sounds

4. Transcription exercises throughout the chapter

The previous chapter discusses the fricative sounds that have familiar symbols that are the same as the alphabet letters. The four fricative consonants presented in this chapter have symbols that are not alphabet letters and that have unusual configurations. They consist of two sets of cognate pairs, the voiceless *th* [Ɵ] and the voiced *th* [ð], and the voiceless *sh* [ʃ] and the voiced [ʒ] that represents the *z* sound in *azure* [æʒɚ]. Remember that the only difference between the two sounds of a cognate pair is voicing. The manner in which the airflow is modified and the placement of the articulators are the same. In addition, the [hw] and [ʍ] are fricatives; they are the same sound. They do not have corresponding sounds such as the other cognates.

PHONETIC SYMBOL [Ө]

EXHIBIT 15-1	**Phonetic Symbol [Ө]**	

		[Ө]
Phonetic Symbol	[Ө]	
Grapheme Symbol	th	
Diacritic Symbols	th, th, Ө	
Phonic Symbol	Th	
Cognate	[ð]	
Homorganic	Linguadental [ð]	
Sound Class	Consonant Fricative	
Basic Traditional Features	Placement: Linguadental Manner: Fricative Voicing: Minus Voice	
International Phonetic Alphabet (IPA) (International Phonetic Association [IPA], 1999)	[Ө] #130 Voiceless Dental Fricative	

How the Sound Is Produced

The airflow from the lungs moves through the opened vocal folds to the oral cavity. A channel for the airflow to continue is formed with the sides of the tongue pressing against the molars. The tongue is flattened and shifted forward, and the tip of the tongue (lingua) approximates the edge or inner surface of the upper front teeth (dental). The airflow is continuously emitted through the constricted channel, and audible friction (fricative) occurs as the airflow is expelled between the upper front teeth and tongue. The bottom teeth usually are in contact with the undersurface of the tongue tip. The lips are apart and in a neutral position. The [Ө] is of longer duration and has more turbulence than its cognate, the voiced [ð]. See **Figure 15-1**.

The [Ө] sound may also be produced by forming a constriction between the apex of the tongue and the posterior portion of the upper central incisors (Small, 1999). The placement is then considered as dental as opposed to interdental where the tongue placement is between the upper and lower front teeth.

Different Spellings for the [Ө] Sound

The [Ө] sound has only one spelling, *th*. It occurs in all positions. Transcribe the following words. Refer to the Key at the right upon completion.

Different Spellings   *Key*

Initial

thin _____   three _____   ӨIn, Өri

Medial

arithmetic _____   author _____   ərIӨmətIk, ɔӨɚ

Final

bath _____   month _____   bæӨ, mʌnӨ

Different Sounds of the Letters That Produce the [Ө] Sound

Transcribe the following words. Refer to the Key at the right upon completion.

              Key

th [Ө] thin _____   th [ð] then _____   ӨIn, ðɛn

th [Ө] thin _____   t [t] tin _____   ӨIn, tIn

Rules for Spelling and Pronunciation of the [Ө] Sound

1. The *th* at the beginning of a word, as in *thirst, thought,* and *thing*, is pronounced with the [Ө] sound.

2. The *th* at the beginning of words that represent pronouns, as in *these, those, thy, their, them,* and other words such as *than*, are not pronounced with the [Ө] sound.

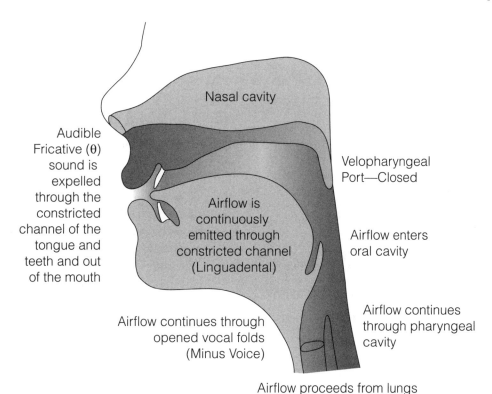

Figure 15-1 [Ɵ] pronunciation.

3. There are also two choices for the pronunciation of the *th* in the medial position in a word. In words such as *diphthong, author*, and *athlete*, the voiceless [Ɵ] is used. In words such as *southern, leather, mother, whether*, the voiced [ð] sound is used.

4. In the context at the end of a word, the voiced [ð] is used, as in *bathe* and *breathe*. The [Ɵ] is used in most other *th* word endings, as in *math, growth, underneath*, and *path*.

5. There are a few exceptions where the *th* is pronounced as a [t], as in *Thomas, Thames*, and *Theresa*.

Words That Include the [Ɵ] Sound

The [Ɵ] sound occurs in all three positions, initial, medial, and final. Transcribe the following words. Refer to the Key at the right upon completion.

Initial Consonant

thought ___ thirsty ___

thunder ___ thankful ___ theme ___

Key

Ɵɔt, Ɵɝsti

Ɵʌndɚ, Ɵeɪŋkfʊl, Ɵim

Unstressed Syllable

Medial Consonant

author _____ healthy _____

anything _____ plaything _____

ɔƟɚ, hɛlƟi

ɛniƟɪŋ, pleɪƟɪŋ

Stressed Syllable

Medial Consonant

faithful ___ withhold ___

athlete ___ truthful ___ ethical ___

feɪƟfʊl, wɪƟhoʊld

æƟlit, truƟfʊl, ɛƟɪk|

Final Consonant

twentieth ___ teeth ___

youth ___ beneath ___ length ___

twɛntiƟ, tiƟ

yuƟ, biniƟ, lɛŋƟ

Initial Blends

thr threw _____ throne _____

thrill _____ thread _____

Ɵru, Ɵroʊn

 Ɵrɪl, Ɵrɛd

Medial Blends

lth healthy _____ wealthy _____

hɛlƟi, wɛlƟi

209

filthiest	_____	<u>nth</u> anther	_____	filθiɛst, ænθɚ
monthly	_____	panther	_____	mʌnθli, pænθɚ
<u>thr</u> bathroom	_____	thread	_____	bæθrum, θrɛd
throw	_____	arthritis	_____	θroʊ, ɑrθraɪtəs
<u>rth</u> birth	_____	north	_____	bɝθ, nɔrθ
worth	_____	orthodox	_____	wɔrθ, ɔrθədɑks

Final Blends

<u>rth</u> forth	_____	north	_____	earth	_____	fɔrθ, nɔrθ, ɝθ
<u>ngth</u> strength	_____	length	_____			strɛŋθ, lɛŋθ
<u>nth</u> eleventh	_____	strengthen	_____			əlɛvɛnθ, strɛŋθən
month	_____	<u>dth</u> width	_____			mʌnθ, wɪdθ
hundredth	_____	<u>lth</u> wealthier	_____			həndɚɛθ, wɛlθiɚ
unhealthy	_____					ənhɛlθi
filth	_____	<u>tbs</u> months	_____			fɪlθ, mʌnθs
Keith's	_____	depths	_____			Kiθs, dɛpθs

Auditory Discrimination

Transcribe the following words. Refer to the Key at the right upon completion.

Contrast Minimal Pairs

[θ] (–)		*[ð] (+)*		*Key*
ether	_____	either	_____	iθɚ, iðɚ
throw	_____	through	_____	θroʊ, ðoʊ
teeth	_____	teethe	_____	tiθ, tið
thin	_____	this	_____	θɪn, ðɪs

Other Minimal Pairs

[θ]		*[f]*		*Key*
three	_____	free	_____	θri, fri
thigh	_____	fie	_____	θaɪ, faɪ
death	_____	deaf	_____	dɛθ, dɛf
author	_____	offer	_____	ɔθɚ, ɔfɚ
threat	_____	fret	_____	θrɛt, frɛt

[θ]	*[s]*	*[θ]*	*[t]*	*Key*
thin _	sin _	three _	tree _	θɪn, sɪn, θri, tri
thigh _	sigh _	thin _	tin _	θaɪ, saɪ, θɪn, tɪn

path _	pass _	thigh _	tie _	pæθ, pæs, θaɪ, taɪ
faith _	face _	thick _	tick _	feɪθ, feɪs, θɪk, tɪk
thing _	sing _	both _	boat _	θɪŋ, sɪŋ, boʊθ, boʊt

Allophonic and Dialect Variations

The [θ] is acoustically one of the weakest speech sounds in the language (Calvert, 1986; Carrell & Tiffany, 1960). It is produced with the least amount of physical energy and is therefore among the most difficult to hear. The [θ] sound takes on a voicing quality in co-articulation with a voiced consonant, as when *with much* [wɪθ mətʃ] becomes [wɪð mətʃ] (Edwards, 1997). The differences between the [θ] and [ð] sounds are often slight, and distinctions in meaning do not often depend on whether one says [θ] or [ð]. There is such a wide variation in the amount of voicing on these sounds that, in conversational speech, it is often nearly impossible to say whether a given sound should be considered voiced or voiceless. For example, the word *with* could be pronounced as [wɛθ] or [wɪð] in *with us* and as [wɪθ] in *with Sam*. Or, more likely, it is acoustically an allophonic variation of either sound and not a distinct [θ] or [ð] sound.

In the typical New York City dialect, the [θ] becomes dentalized when it occurs before or between vowels, as when *think* [θɪŋk] becomes [tɪŋk] (Edwards, 1997). In African American speech, the [θ] becomes a [t] when it precedes a vowel, as when *thought* [θɔt] or [θɑt] becomes [tɔt] or [tɑt]. When it occurs intervocalic, in the final position, or when followed by an *r*, an [f] is substituted, as in [nʌfən] for *nothing*, [wɪf] for *with*, and [foʊt] for *throat* (House, 1998; VanRiper, 1979).

Normal and Deviant Development of the [θ] Sound

The [θ] sound is one of the last sounds to be mastered by children (Calvert, 1986) and is acquired between the ages of 4 and 7 years (Sander, 1972). It is one of the most difficult United States English sounds to perceive because it is one of the weakest sounds acoustically (House, 1998).

The [θ] sound is among the most frequently misarticulated consonants, and the [f] is frequently a substitution for it (Calvert, 1986; Carrell & Tiffany, 1960). Presumably, because the [θ] is produced with a relatively reduced amount of energy, a child may have difficulty in perceiving it and that is why it is so frequently misarticulated. Intelligibility may be adequate when [f] or [s] is substituted for the [Ɵ] sound, but it may be reduced when a [t] or [d] substitution occurs or when the [Ɵ] is omitted (Edwards, 1997).

A lingual lisp occurs when a person with such a lisp uses a [Ɵ] in place of the [s] sound, as in [Ɵ] for *see* [si] (VanRiper, 1979).

Nonnative Speaker Pronunciation

The [Ɵ] is very difficult for most foreign-born speakers to learn, and they frequently substitute the [t] or [s] sound (Calvert, 1986). Very few languages use the [Ɵ] sound, and nonnative speakers find it difficult to pronounce and often substitute another phoneme (House, 1998). Among the European languages, this sound appears only in English, Gaelic, Greek, and Spanish. German, Dutch, and Scandinavian language equivalents to the [Ɵ] usually start with the *d* letter (VanRiper, 1979). A dentalized [t] occurs when there is insufficient breath support, and the [f] and [s] may vary because of the differences in the placement of the articulators (Edwards, 1997).

Words that include the *th* sound often present problems to nonnative speakers not only because of the possibility of the lack of appropriate dentalization or voicing, but also because the written *th* represents both the [Ɵ] and [ð] sounds (Carrell & Tiffany, 1960).

According to the U. S. Census Bureau (1990), 15 languages, other than American English, are spoken most prominently in the United States. Those that include the [Ɵ] sound as listed in the *Handbook of the International Phonetic Association* (IPA, 1999) and other sources include Arabic, Spanish, Italian, Greek, and Russian. The sound systems of languages that do not include the [Ɵ] sound are French, German, Chinese, Tagalog, Polish, Korean, Vietnamese, Portuguese, Japanese, and Hindi.

Summary

The [Ɵ] sound is one of the 10 fricative consonants, and its voiced cognate is the [ð] sound. It is only homorganic (linguadental) with its cognate and no other sounds. It is one of the last sounds to be mastered and, acoustically, it is difficult to hear. The [Ɵ] sound is quite consistently spelled with the *th*, although nonnative speakers may be confused because the *th* also represents other sounds. Allophonic variations exist between the pronunciation of the two *th* sounds [Ɵ] and [ð], and it may be difficult within certain contexts to differentiate exactly which sound is actually spoken. Dialect differences occur with the substitution of the [t] or [f]. In addition to those two sounds, nonnative speakers may substitute the [d] or [s]. Only a few languages of the world include the [Ɵ] sound. Children often substitute other sounds, produce a "lisping" sound, or delete the sound.

[Ɵ] +

Complete the following brain teaser to increase your phonetic sound/symbol recognition and transcription skills. Provide the orthographic and phonetic spellings for the clues given.

		Orthographic	Phonetic
1.	[Ɵ] + 2 sounds: the opposite of thin	_____	/ _ɪ _/
2.	[Ɵ] + 5 sounds: holds objects to corkboard	_____	/ _ʌ_ _æ _/
3.	[Ɵ] + 4 sounds: a Master's project	_____	/_i_ə_/
4.	[Ɵ] + 3 sounds: to need liquid	_____	/_ɝ_ _/
5.	[Ɵ] + 4 sounds: robbers	_____	/_i_ə_/
6.	[Ɵ] + 7 sounds: temperature indicator	_____	/_ɚ_æ_ɛ_ɚ/
7.	[Ɵ] + 2 sounds: an idea	_____	/_ɑ_/
8.	[Ɵ] + 3 sounds: a day of the week	_____	/_ɝ_ _eɪ/
9.	[Ɵ] + 4 sounds: unlucky number	_____	/_ɝ_i_/
10.	[Ɵ] + 6 sounds: a breed of horse	_____	/_ɚ_oʊ_ _ɛ_/

Key: 1. thick [Ɵɪk]; 2. thumbtack [Ɵʌmtæk]; 3. thesis [Ɵisəs]; 4. thirst [Ɵɝst]; 5. thieves [Ɵivəz]; 6. thermometer [Ɵɚmɛmɛtɚ]; 7. thought [Ɵɑt]; 8. Thursday [Ɵɝzdeɪ]; 9. thirteen [Ɵɝtin]; 10. thoroughbred [Ɵɚoʊbrɛd]

PHONETIC SYMBOL [ð]

EXHIBIT 15-2	Phonetic Symbol [ð]	
Phonetic Symbol	[ð]	**[ð̃]**
Grapheme Symbol	th	
Diacritic Symbols	th, <u>th</u>, th, Ѳ	
Phonic Symbol	th	
Cognate	[Ѳ]	
Homorganic	Linguadental [Ѳ]	
Sound Class	Consonant Fricative	
Basic Traditional Features	Placement: Linguadental Manner: Fricative Voicing: Plus Voice	
IPA (1999)	[ð] #131 Voiced Dental Fricative	

How the Sound Is Produced

The airflow from the lungs activates the vibration of the vocal folds (voiced). The velopharyngeal port is closed, allowing the airflow to enter the tongue pressing against the molars. The tongue is flattened and shifted forward and the tip of the tongue (lingua) approximates the edge or inner surface of the upper front teeth (dental). The airflow is continuously emitted through the constricted channel, and audible friction (fricative) occurs as the airflow is expelled between the upper front teeth and the tongue. The bottom teeth usually are in contact with the undersurface of the tongue tip. The lips are apart and in a neutral position. The [ð] is of lesser duration and turbulence than its cognate, the voiceless [Ѳ]. An additional dental placement may be used to produce the [ð] sound by forming a constriction between the apex of the tongue and the posterior portion of the upper central incisors (Small, 1999). The production of the [ð] sound may be interdental by placing the tongue between the teeth (Small, 1999). See **Figure 15-2**.

Different Spellings for the [ð] Sound

Transcribe the following words. Refer to the Key at the right upon completion.

Different Spellings			*Key*
th	third ___ ethical ___		ðɝd, ɛðɪkɔl
	python ___ growth ___ depth ___		paɪðɑn, groʊð, dɛpð
the	breathe ___ bathe ___ clothe ___		brið, beɪð, kloʊð

Different Sounds of the Letters That Produce the [ð] Sound

Transcribe the following words. Refer to the Key at the right upon completion.

								Key
th	[ð]	then ___		th	[Ѳ]	thin	___	ðɛn, Ѳɪn
th	[ð]	there ___		th	[t]	Thomas	___	ðɛr, tɑməs

Rules for Spelling and Pronunciation of the [ð]

1. The [ð] sound for the *th* occurs in words such as *this, their (there), them, those,* and *they.*

2. Such words as *smooth* and *with* are produced with the [ð] sound.

3. The *th* in the medial position followed by *er,* as in *neither, father, other,* and *leather,* is pronounced with the [ð] sound.

4. When *ing* follows the *th,* as in *soothing, tithing, clothing,* and *teething,* the *th* is pronounced with the [ð] sound.

5. Words such as *mouth, moth,* and *booth* have the [ð] for the *th.* When these words are in the plural form, as in *mouths, moths,* and *booths,* the *th* is pronounced with the [ð] sound.

6. The voiced [ð] and the voiceless [Ѳ] can be found in similar spelling contexts. This makes it difficult to discern which sound the *th* represents, as in <u>*thatch*</u> voiceless [Ѳ] and <u>*that*</u> voiced [ð].

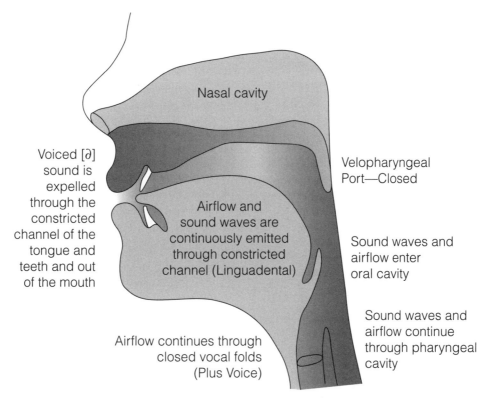

Figure 15-2 [ð] pronunciation.

The [ð] has a long history (House, 1998). The symbol itself originates from the Old English use of the *d*, from the Roman alphabet. In the fifteenth century, the scribes began to use the *y* to replace the *eth*, which introduced words such as *ye* into the language. The [ð] became voiced during the modern period and is now represented by the *th* in spelling.

Words That Include the [ð] Sound

The [ð] sound occurs in all three positions, initial, medial, and final. Transcribe the following words. Refer to the Key at the right upon completion.

Initial Consonant   *Key*

the _____   these _____   ðʌ, ðiz

then _____   thus _____   their _____   ðɛn, ðʌs, ðɛr

Unstressed Syllable

Medial Consonant

breathing _____   brother _____   briðəŋ, brʌðɚ

worthy _____   soothing _____   wɝði, suðɪŋ

Stressed Syllable

Medial Consonant

without _____   therein _____   wɪðaʊt, ðɛrɪn

thyself _____   therefore _____   ðaɪsɛlf, ðɛrfoʊr

themselves _____   ðɛmsɛlvz

Final Consonant

lathe _____   teethe _____   clothe _____   læð, tið, kloʊð

smooth _____   scathe _____   smuð, skeɪð

Final Blends

<u>thd</u> bathed ___   seethed ___   baɪðd, sɪðd

<u>rth</u> further ___   northern ___   farther ___   fɝðɚ, norðrn, fɑrðɚ

<u>ths</u> (z) seethes ___   teethes ___   sɪðz, tiðz

smoothes ___   breathes ___   smuðz, briðz

Auditory Discrimination

Transcribe the following words. Refer to the Key at the right upon completion.

Contrast Minimal Pairs

[ð] (+)	[Ɵ] (−)	Key
though _____	throw _____	ðu, Ɵroʊ
these _____	theme _____	ðiz, Ɵim
this _____	thin _____	ðɪs, Ɵɪn
either _____	ether _____	iðɚ, iƟɚ
booths _____	booth _____	buðz, buƟ

Other Contrast Pairs

[ð]	[v]	Key
that _____	vat _____	ðæt, væt
than _____	van _____	ðæn, væn
either _____	fever _____	iðɚ, fɛvɚ
they'll _____	veil _____	ðeɪl, vɛl
scathe _____	cave _____	skeɪð, keɪv

[ð]	[d]	Key
father _____	fodder _____	fɑðɚ, fɔdɚ
they _____	day _____	ðeɪ, deɪ
bathe _____	bayed _____	baɪð, baid
though _____	dough _____	ðoʊ, doʊ
lather _____	ladder _____	læðɚ, lædɚ

[ð]	[z]	Key
teethe _____	tease _____	tɪð, tiz
tithe _____	ties _____	taɪð, taɪz
seethe _____	sees _____	sɪð, siz
breathe _____	breeze _____	brɪð, briz
thee _____	Z _____	ðɪ, zi

Allophonic and Dialect Variations

The [ð] tends to be dentalized when it is coarticulated with an alveolar phoneme, as in *hit those* [hɪt doz] and *meet them* [mit dəm], so it is pronounced somewhere between a [ð] and a [d] (Edwards, 1997). Remember that an allophone loses its distinction when it becomes more like a different sound rather than a "shading" of the original sound and is then considered a substitution rather than an allophone of a phoneme such as [ð].

A dentalized [d] replaces the [ð] when it is followed by a vowel in the typical New York City dialect (Edwards, 1997). African American speakers may substitute the [d] when [ð] appears prevocalic, as in *they* [deɪ] for [ðeɪ], and in the postvocalic position, the [ð] may become a [v] as when *smooth* [smuð] becomes [smuv]. The word *the* is among the most common words spoken in United States English and quite often is pronounced [dʌ] rather than [ðʌ] in connected speech. Using [diz] for *these* [ðiz] and [doʊz] for *those* [ðoʊz]

is very common. It is almost impossible to speak more than one or two utterances without using these words.

Two other examples of dialect differences in conversational speech include the phrases *is that so* [ɪz ðæt soʊ], which becomes [ɪsætsoʊ], and *was there* [wʌz ðɛr], which becomes [wʌzɛr] (Carrell & Tiffany, 1960).

Normal and Deviant Development of the [ð] Sound

The [ð] sound is mastered rather late between the ages of 5 and 8 years, and its voiceless cognate [Ɵ] is mastered within the same time period (Sander, 1972).

The [ð] sound is one of the last to be mastered by children and is among the most frequently misarticulated consonants (Calvert, 1986). The [ð] sound may be omitted or [v], [z], [d], or [t] may be substituted, as when *mother* [mʌðɚ] becomes [mʌvɚ] and *that* [ðæt] becomes [ʌæt] (Carrell & Tiffany, 1960; Edwards, 1997).

Nonnative Speaker Pronunciation

The [ð] is very difficult for most foreign-born speakers to learn and is present only in English, Spanish, and Danish among European languages (Calvert, 1986). The problems with the sound are similar to those for the [Ɵ] sound (Edwards, 1997). A dentalized [d] occurs when there is not sufficient airflow. Placement difficulties result in a [v] or [z] substitution, and confusion may arise because both the voiced [ð] and voiceless [Ɵ] sounds are identified by the *th* letters. The dentalized affricate [dð] and the alveolar stop that includes the influence of the [d] sound are present in some foreign dialects (Carrell & Tiffany, 1960). Nonnative speakers may also unvoice [ð] to the extent that it sounds like the [Ɵ] sound. This error is quite common among persons with a German or Scandinavian language background.

Of the 15 most prominent languages spoken in the United States other than English, according to the U.S. Census Bureau (1990), those that include the [ð] sound as listed in the *Handbook of the International Phonetic Association* (IPA, 1999) and other sources are Arabic, Spanish, Greek, Italian, and Russian, excluding French, German, Chinese, Tagalog, Polish, Korean, Vietnamese, Portuguese, Japanese, and Hindi (Urdu).

Summary

The [ð] sound is one of the 10 fricative consonants, and its voiceless cognate is the [Ɵ] sound. It is only homorganic (linguadental) with its cognate and no other sounds. It is one of the last sounds to be mastered by children around age 8 years and is quite consistent in its sound/spelling correlation.

Allophonic variations occur when the sound becomes more dentalized, and both native and nonnative speakers of United States English tend to substitute other sounds such as [d], [v], and [z]. It sometimes loses its unique sound characteristics during conversational speaking when substitutions replace the actual sound. Substitution errors among young children include a variety of sounds. The [ð] is one of the least common sounds among the languages of the world.

PHONETIC SYMBOL [ʃ]

EXHIBIT 15-3	Phonetic Symbol [ʃ]	
Phonetic Symbol	[ʃ]	**[ʃ]**
Grapheme Symbols	sh, ch, ss, ce, ci, ti, x, chs, sci, sch, psh, ssi, su, si	
Diacritic Symbol	sh	
Phonic Symbol	Sh	
Cognate	[ʒ]	
Homorganic	Linguapalatal [ʒ] [r] [j] [h] Final sound: [t͡ʃ] [d͡ʒ]	
Sound Class	Consonant	
Basic Phonetic Features	Placement: Lingua-Palatal-Alveolar Manner: Fricative/Sibilant Voicing: Minus Voice	
IPA (1999)	[ʃ] #134 Voiceless Postalveolar Fricative	

How the Sound Is Produced

The airflow from the lungs progresses through the opened vocal folds (voiceless) into the oral cavity because the velopharyngeal port is closed. The sides of the tongue (lingua) are pressed laterally against the molars and/or alveolar ridge (alveolar) to provide a channel for the air to continue to the front of the mouth. The blade and tip of the tongue are raised toward the front part of the palate (palatal) or alveolar ridge, and the airflow creates a turbulent audible (fricative) noise that continues through the channel formed between the tongue and the roof of the mouth. The lips are rounded and may be in a forward position. The front teeth are slightly apart. The more open constriction for [ʃ] is formed by the closely held tongue blade and the hard palate (Small, 1999). This articulation is posterior to the constriction of the alveolar fricatives [s] and [z]. Therefore, [ʃ] is considered by many phoneticians to have a postalveolar articulation (IPA, 1999). The [ʃ] exerts more pressure than its cognate [ʒ]. See **Figure 15-3**.

Different Spellings for the [ʃ] Sound

Transcribe the following words. Refer to the Key at the right upon completion.

Different Spellings

					Key
sh [ʃ]	shoe	___	show	___	ʃu, ʃoʊ
	shocking	___	shoulder	___	ʃɑkɪŋ, ʃoʊldɚ
ch [ʃ]	machine	___	Chicago	___	məʃɪn, ʃəkɑgo
	chef	___	chic	___	ʃɛf, ʃik
ss [ʃ]	issue	___	tissue	___	ɪʃu, tɪʃu
	assure	___	fissure	___	əʃoʊr, fɪʃɚ
ce [ʃ]	ocean	___			oʊʃən
ci [ʃ]	special	___	social	___	spɛʃʊl, soʊʃʊl
	racial	___	associate	___	ræʃʊl, əsoʊʃɛt
	precious	___	licorice	___	prɛʃəs, lɪkɚɪʃ
ti [ʃ]	auction	___	motion	___	ɔkʃən, moʊʃən
	vacation	___	nation	___	vekeɪʃən, neɪʃən
	fractious	___			frækʃəs

Chapter 15

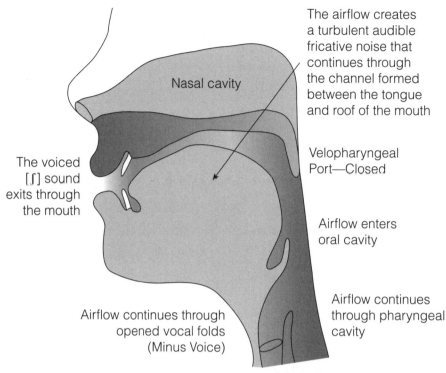

The voiced [ʃ] sound exits through the mouth

Nasal cavity

The airflow creates a turbulent audible fricative noise that continues through the channel formed between the tongue and roof of the mouth

Velopharyngeal Port—Closed

Airflow enters oral cavity

Airflow continues through pharyngeal cavity

Airflow continues through opened vocal folds (Minus Voice)

Airflow proceeds from lungs and continues through trachea to larynx

Figure 15-3 [ʃ] pronunciation.

x [ʃ]	anxious ___	luxury	___	eɪnkʃəs, lʌkɚi	
chs [ʃ]	fuchsia ___			fuʃə	
sci [ʃ]	conscious___	conscience	___	kɑnsʃə, kɑnʃɛns	
sch [ʃ]	schwa ___			ʃwɑ	
psh [ʃ]	pshaw ___			ʃɑw	
ssi [ʃ]	mission ___	passion	___	mɪʃən, pæʃən	
	omission ___	profession	___	omɪʃən, profɛʃən	
su [ʃ]	sure ___	sugar	___	ʃoʊr, ʃɪgɚ	
si [ʃ]	mission ___	transmission___		mɪʃən, trænsmɪʃən	

Different Sounds of the Letters That Produce the [ʃ] Sound

Transcribe the following words. Refer to the Key at the right upon completion.

Key

ch	[ʃ]	chef ___	ch [ʧ]	chin	___	ʃɛf, ʧɪn
su	[ʃ]	sugar ___	su [s]	sun	___	ʃɪgɚ, sʌn
ss	[ʃ]	tissue ___	ss [z]	scissors___		tɪʃu, sɪzɚz
ce	[ʃ]	ocean ___	ce [s]	nice	___	oʃən, naɪs
ci	[ʃ]	social ___	ci [s]	city	___	soʊʃʊl, sɪti
ti	[ʃ]	nation ___	ti [t]	tidy	___	næʃən, taɪdɪ

x	[ʃ]	anxious ___	x [k] extra	___	eɪkʃəs, ɛkstrə
si	[ʃ]	mission ___	si [s] simple	___	mɪʃən, sɪmpl̩

Rules for Spelling and Pronunciation of the [ʃ] Sound

1. The *sh* is always pronounced as [ʃ], as in *shock, fishing, wash*, except when it appears in a compound word such as *grasshopper*.

2. The *ch* as in *chief* and *church* is pronounced as a [ʃ] in *chef, machine*, and *Chevrolet*.

3. In words such as *sugar, insurance*, and *sure*, the *su* context is pronounced as [ʃ] unlike the *su* in *sun* or *subway*.

4. When two adjacent *s* letters (*ss*) occur, as in *tissue, issue*, and *fissure*, the [ʃ] sound is produced.

5. In words with the *ssi* context, the *i* is silent, as in *mission, passion*, and *profession*.

6. Infrequently, such as in the *ce* in *ocean*, such letters become the [ʃ] sound.

7. The *ci* as in *special, precious*, and *associate* is pronounced as the [ʃ] sound.

8. The *i* in the *ti* context as in *auction, motion, vacation* is nonfunctional and the sound produced is the [ʃ].

216

9. The [ʃ] is unique in its pronunciation as the *x* in *anxious*.

10. The *chs* is an uncommon usage of the [ʃ] sound.

11. The *sch* sounds as in *school* and *scholar* are changed to the [ʃ] sound in the word *schwa*.

12. Another unusual use of the [ʃ] sound occurs in the word *pshaw*, which is an expression of irritation or disapproval.

Words That Include the [ʃ] Sound

The [ʃ] occurs in all three positions, initial, medial, and final. Transcribe the following words. Refer to the Key at the right upon completion.

Initial Consonant   *Key*

shop	_____	schwa	_____	ʃɑp, ʃwɑ
sugar	_____	chaperone	_____	ʃɪgɚ, ʃæpɚon
chandelier	_____			ʃændəlɛɪr

Unstressed Syllable

Medial Consonant

vivacious	_____			vaɪveɪʃəs
transition	_____	possession	_____	trænsɪʃən, posɛsʃən
technician	_____			tɛknɪʃən

Stressed Syllable

Medial Consonant

cashier	_____	dishes	_____	kæʃɛɪr, dɪʃəs
ashore	_____	ocean	_____	əʃour, oʃən
marshal	_____			mɑrʃʊl

Final Consonant

cherish	_____	mustache	_____	ʧɛrɪʃ, məstæʃ
crush	_____	afresh	_____ licorice _____	krʌʃ, əfrɛʃ, lɪkɚɪʃ

Initial Blends

<u>shr</u> shrine	_____	shrubbery	_____	ʃraɪn, ʃrʌbɛri
shred	_____	shriek	_____	ʃrɛd, ʃrik

Medial Blends

<u>rs</u> censorship	_____	airship	_____	sɛnsɚʃɪp, ɛɪrʃɪp
partial	_____	portion	_____	pɑrʃʊl, pɔrʃən

Final Blends

<u>shed</u> brushed	_____	washed	_____	brʌʃt, wɑʃt
famished	_____	unleashed	_____	fæmɪʃt, ənliʃt
<u>rsh</u> marsh	_____	harsh	_____	mɑrʃ, hɑrʃ

Auditory Discrimination

Transcribe the following words. Refer to the Key at the right upon completion.

Cognates

[ʃ] (–)		[ʒ] (+)		*Key*
glacier	_____	glazier	_____	gleɪʃɚ, gleɪʒɚ
Aleutian	_____	allusion	_____	əluʃən, əluʒən
Confucian	_____	confusion	_____	kɑnfjuʃən, kɑnfjuʒən
mash	_____	Madge	_____	mæʃ, mæʒ
mesher	_____	measure	_____	ɛʃɚ, meɪʒɚ

Other Minimal Pairs

[ʃ]		[θ]		*Key*
rash	_____	wrath	_____	ræʃ, ræθ
shy	_____	thigh	_____	ʃaɪ, θaɪ
shin	_____	thin	_____	ʃɪn, θɪn
hash	_____	hath	_____	hæʃ, hæθ
sheaf	_____	thief	_____	ʃif, θif
shore	_____	Thor	_____	ʃor, θor

[ʃ]	[ʧ]	[ʃ]	[s]	*Key*
ship _____	chip _____	sheep _____	seep _____	ʃɪp, ʧɪp, ʃip, sip
mash _____	match _____	shock _____	sock _____	mæʃ, mæʧ, ʃok, sɔk
wash _____	watch _____	gash _____	gas _____	wɑʃ, wɑʧ, gæʃ, gæs
shore _____	chore _____	sheet _____	seat _____	ʃor, ʧor, ʃit, sit
wish _____	witch _____	mash _____	mass _____	wɪʃ, wɪʧ, mæʃ, mæs
dishes _____	ditches _____	cashed _____	cast _____	dɪʃəs, dɪʧəs, kæʃt, kæst

Allophonic and Dialect Variations

No significant allophonic variation has been reported for this sound (Edwards, 1997). It may be underpronounced or weakened, but the [ʃ] sound still maintains its identity (Carrell & Tiffany, 1960). As with each of the sounds, there exists some allophonic variations as a result of different variables including context, the influence of the surrounding sounds, and the position of the sound within the word, that is, initial, medial, or final.

The [ʃ] sound is not often involved in dialect errors of native speakers (Carrell & Tiffany, 1960). In Old English, the [ʃ] was called the long *s* (House, 1998). The use of the long *s* [ʃ] as a variation of [s] continued until the 1800s.

Normal and Deviant Development of the [ʃ] Sound

Children master the [ʃ] sound between the ages of 4 and 7 years, and they master its cognate, the [ʒ] sound, between the ages of 6 and 8 years (Sander, 1972). The [ʃ] sound is frequently misarticulated and is highly affected by abnormal dentition (Calvert, 1986; House, 1998). The [ʃ] sound is subject to some of the same kinds of defects as are associated with the [s] sound (Carrell & Tiffany, 1960). The sound may be produced with a lateral feature or may be distorted as a result of severe dental malocclusions. It can be overly weak, partially or completely voiced as in its cognate [ʒ], or may be produced as the affricate [ʧ].

Edwards (1997) indicates that the most frequent severe substitutions for the [ʃ] sound are the [t] followed by the [d] sound. He states that the [ʃ] may also be omitted and that milder errors, judged in terms of their intelligibility, are [s] (depalatalization) and [ʧ] (affrication). Both of these errors result in lisping sounds, which may be different as a result of the placement features of the [s] and [ʧ] sounds.

Nonnative Speaker Pronunciation

Spanish speakers are likely to substitute [ʧ], and some Europeans may make the [ʃ] too far back on the palate or may round and protrude the lips to a greater degree than for the United States English [ʃ] sound (Calvert, 1986).

Of the 15 most prominent languages spoken in the United States other than English, according to the U.S. Census Bureau (1990), those that include the [ʃ] sound listed in the *Handbook of the International Phonetic Association* (IPA, 1999) and other sources are French, German, Italian, Portuguese, Japanese, Arabic, Hindi (Urdu), and Vietnamese. The languages that do not have the [ʃ] sound are Greek, Spanish, Chinese, Korean, Polish, and Russian.

Summary

The [ʃ] sound is one of the 10 fricative consonants, and its voiced cognate is the [ʒ] sound. It is homorganic (linguapalatal) with the [ʒ], [r], [j], [h], and the second sounds in the [ʧ] and [ʤ] cognates. It has multiple spelling symbols that could be confusing to those learning the sound. There appears to be no significant allophonic or dialect variations. Approximately one-half of the other prominent languages spoken in the United States have the [ʃ] sound in their sound system. Some of the speech sound errors include the substitution of the [t], [d], or [s], and distortions may occur as a result of dental malocclusions that produce a lisping.

PHONETIC SYMBOL [ʒ]

EXHIBIT 15-4	Phonetic Symbol [ʒ]
Phonetic Symbol	[ʒ]
Grapheme Symbols	s, z, g, si, ti, ge, zi, zs, ssi
Diacritic Symbol	zh, zh ʒ
Phonic Symbol	zh
Cognate	[ʃ]
Homorganic	Linguapalatal [ʃ] [r] [j] [h] Final Sounds: [ʧ] [ʤ]
Sound Class	Consonant
Basic Phonetic Features	Placement: Lingua-Palatal-Alveolar Manner: Fricative/Sibilant Voicing: Plus Voice
IPA (1999)	[ʒ] #135 Voiced Postalveolar Fricative

[ʒ]

How the Sound Is Produced

The airflow from the lungs progresses through the closed vocal folds (voiced) into the oral cavity because the velopharyngeal port is closed. The sides of the tongue (lingua) are pressed laterally against the molars and/or alveolar ridge (alveolar) to provide a channel for the air to continue to the front of the mouth. The blade and tip of the tongue are raised toward the front part of the palate (palatal) or alveolar ridge, and the airflow creates a tur- bulent audible (fricative) noise that continues through the channel formed between the tongue and the roof of the mouth (palatal). It is also referred to as a postalveolar fricative. The lips are rounded and may be in a forward position. The front teeth are slightly apart. The [ʒ] re- quires less air pressure than its [ʃ] cognate. See **Figure 15-4**.

Different Spellings for the [ʒ] Sound

Transcribe the following words. Refer to the Key at the right upon completion.

Different Spellings				*Key*
s [ʒ]	leisure _____	measure _____		liʒɚ, meɪʒɚ
	treasure _____			trɛʒɚ
z [ʒ]	glazier _____	azure _____		gleɪʒɚ, æʒɚ
g [ʒ]	regime _____			rəʒim
si [ʒ]	occasion _____	fantasia _____		oʊkeɪʒən, fænteɪʒə
	vision _____			vɪʒən
ti [ʒ]	equation _____			ikweɪʒən
ge [ʒ]	rouge _____	garage _____		ruʒ, gərɔʒ
zi [ʒ]	brazier _____			breɪʒiɚ

zs [ʒ]	Zsa Zsa Gabor _____	ʒɔ ʒɔ gʌbor
ssi [ʒ]	scission _____	sɪʒən

Different Sounds of the Letters That Produce the [ʒ] Sound

Transcribe the following words. Refer to the Key at the right upon completion.

							Key
s	[ʒ]	measure _____	s	[s]	sun	_____	meɪʒɚ, sʌn
z	[ʒ]	glazier _____	z	[z]	zoo	_____	gleɪʒɚ, zu
g	[ʒ]	regime _____	g	[g]	gone	_____	rəʒim, gɑn
si	[ʒ]	vision _____	si	[s]	sign	_____	vɪʒən, saɪn
ti	[ʒ]	equation _____	ti	[t]	time	_____	ikweɪʒən, taɪm
ge	[ʒ]	age _____	ge	[g]	get	_____	eɛʒ, gɛt
zi	[ʒ]	brazier _____	zi	[z]	zinc	_____	breɪʒɚ, zɪŋk
ssi	[ʒ]	scission _____	ssi	[ʃ]	mission _____		skɪʒən, mɪʃən

Rules for Spelling and Pronunciation of the [ʒ] Sound

1. The *s* is pronounced as the [ʒ] in *treasure, version, lesion*, and *Persia*.

2. The *z* is pronounced as a [ʒ] in *seizure* and *azure*.

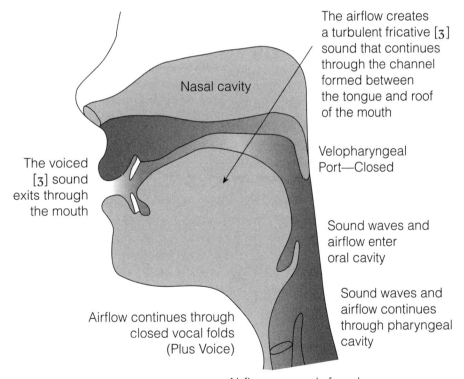

The airflow creates a turbulent fricative [ʒ] sound that continues through the channel formed between the tongue and roof of the mouth

Nasal cavity

Velopharyngeal Port—Closed

The voiced [ʒ] sound exits through the mouth

Sound waves and airflow enter oral cavity

Sound waves and airflow continues through pharyngeal cavity

Airflow continues through closed vocal folds (Plus Voice)

Airflow proceeds from lungs and continues through trachea to larynx

Figure 15-4 [ʒ] pronunciation.

3. The *g* as in *regime*, *bourgeois*, and *negligee* is pronounced as a [ʒ] sound.

4. The *i* in the context of *si* is silent and the *si* is pronounced as a [ʒ], as in *vision, inclusion, revision*.

5. The *ti* is pronounced as a [ʒ] in the word *equation*.

6. In French, in words that end in *ge*, as in *rouge* and *garage*, the final sound is the [ʒ].

7. The *zi* context in the word *brazier* is pronounced as a [ʒ] sound.

8. Zsa Zsa Gabor's name provides an interesting spelling: *zs* for the [ʒ] sound.

9. The *ssi* in the word *scission* (*schism*) is pronounced with the [ʒ] sound.

Words That Include the [ʒ] Sound

The [ʒ] sound occurs in the intervocalic (medial) and postvocalic (final) positions but not in the initial position. Transcribe the following words. Refer to the Key at the right upon completion.

Initial Consonant — *Key*

[None]

Unstressed Syllable

Medial Consonant

supervision _____ — supɚvɪʒən

profusion _____ fantasia _____ — profjuʒən, fænteɪʒə

Stressed Syllable

Medial Consonant

regime _____ Roger _____ — rəʒim, rɑʒɚ

Asiatic _____ casually _____ — eʒiætɪk, kæʒjuli

measurement _____ — meɪʒɚmɛnt

Final Consonant

prestige _____ corsage _____ — prɛstɪʒ, kɔrsɑʒ

massage _____ mirage _____ — mʌsɑʒ, mɪrɔʒ

fuselage _____ — fjusəlɑʒ

Consonant Blend

ged sabotaged _____ — sæbətɔʒd̩

camouflaged _____ garaged _____ — kæməflɑʒd̩, gərɑʒd̩

Auditory Discrimination

Transcribe the following words. Refer to the Key at the right upon completion.

Contrast Minimal Pairs

[ʒ] (+)		[ʃ] (–)		Key
glazier	_____	glacier	_____	gleɪʒɚ, gleɪʃɚ

azure	_____	assure	_____	æʒɚ, əsɔr
allusion	_____	Aleutian	_____	əluʒən, əluʃən
measure	_____	mesher	_____	meɪʒɚ, mɛʃɚ
confusion	_____	Confucian	_____	kɑnfjuʒən, kɑnfjuʃən
pleasure	_____	pressure	_____	plɛʒɚ, prɛsɚ

Other Contrast Pairs

[ʒ]	[ʤ]	[ʒ]	[z]	Key
lesion ____	legion ____	beige ____	bays ____	liʒən, liʤən, beɪʒ, beɪz
pleasure ____	pledger ____	seizure ____	Caesar ____	plɛʒɚ, plɛʤɚ, siʒɚ, sizɚ
rouge ____	huge ____	ruse ____		ruʒ, huʤ, ruz
vision ____	pigeon ____			vɪʒən, pɪʤən

Allophonic and Dialect Variations

The [ʒ] sound is subjected to the same rules of assimilation of context as any other sound, and there are, no doubt, some variations when the sound appears between vowels of different features and as the final postvocalic sound. This sound does not appear in the initial position in United States English speech (House, 1998). Its use began during the Modern English period as a fricative found in French loan words. In certain phonemic environments, the [ʒ] sound may resemble the other sibilant sounds such as [s], [z], and its cognate [ʃ]. It is common for the voicing not to continue through to the termination of the fricative noise in the final consonant position (Carrell & Tiffany, 1960).

Native speakers do not often produce incorrectly the differences in the production of the [ʒ] phoneme (Carrell & Tiffany, 1960), although they may be underpronounced or unvoiced to some degree. The [ʒ] sound has been replaced with [ʤ] by some speakers, as when pronunciation of the word *garage* [gərɑʒ] becomes [gərɑʤ] and *camouflage* [kæməflɑʒ] becomes [kæməflɑʤ]. Some speakers may retain a diphthongized [ju] after [ʒ], as when *azure* [æʒur] becomes [æʒjur] and *closure* [kloʊʒur] becomes [kloʊʒjur], which may sound somewhat pedantic. Edwards (1997) indicates that no significant dialect variation has been reported for this sound.

Normal and Deviant Development of the [ʒ] Sound

The [ʒ] is one of the last consonants that children develop and master, usually between the ages of 6 and 8 years and older (Sander, 1972). It is one of the least frequently occurring sounds in English (Calvert, 1986; House, 1998). As with other sibilants, the most common substitution in severe cases is [d], followed by [t] (Edwards, 1997). Other substitutions include the [z], [dʒ], and [tʃ]. The sound also may be omitted.

The [ʒ] shares with [ʃ] the difficulties resulting from malocclusions and the lateral lisp (Carrell & Tiffany, 1960). Children who have not learned the [ʃ] sound, which is developed earlier, usually fail to acquire the [ʒ] as well and are likely to substitute another fricative, frequently the [z] sound.

As mentioned, Edwards (1997) indicates that the most frequent severe substitutions for the [ʒ] sound are the [t], followed by the [d] sound. He states that the [ʒ] may also be omitted and that milder errors, judged in terms of their intelligibility, are [s] (depalatalization) and [tʃ] (affrication). Both of these errors result in lisping sounds, which may be different as a result of the placement features of the [s] and [tʃ].

Nonnative Speaker Pronunciation

Of the 15 most prominent languages spoken in the United States other than English, according to the U.S. Census Bureau (1990), those that include the [ʒ] sound according to the *Handbook of the International Phonetic Association* (IPA, 1999) and other sources are French, German, and Portuguese. The languages that do not have the [ʒ] sound include Spanish, Chinese, Korean, Japanese, Arabic, and Hindi (Urdu). Also, the [ʒ] is present in Italian, Tagalog, Polish, Vietnamese, Greek, and Russian.

Summary

The [ʒ] sound is one of the 10 fricative consonants, and its voiceless cognate is the [ʃ] sound. It is homorganic (linguapalatal) with the [ʃ], [r], [j], [h], and the second sounds in the [tʃ] and [dʒ] cognates. It is a later sound that children master between ages 6 and 8 years and older. It occurs infrequently in United States English and not at all in the initial position in words. Multiple alphabet letters represent the sound, and these same letters also represent other sounds that may be confusing to first learners. It is not a common sound found in many of the other prominent languages spoken in the United States. Individuals with dental malocclusions may include a lisping sound, and speakers with impairments of the palate may have difficulty producing this sound.

PHONETIC SYMBOLS [hw] OR [ʍ]

EXHIBIT 15-5	Phonetic Symbols [hw] or [ʍ]
Phonetic Symbol	[hw] or [ʍ]
Grapheme Symbol	wh
Diacritic Symbols	hw, wh
Phonic Symbol	wh
Homorganic	Lingua-Velar: [k], [g], [h], [w], [ŋ] Bilabial: [p], [b], [m], [w]
Sound Class	Consonant
Basic Phonetic Features	Placement: Lingua-Velar, Bilabial Manner: Fricative/Glide Voicing: Minus Voice
IPA (1999)	[ʍ] #169 Voiceless Labial-Velar Fricative

[hw] [ʍ]

Note: The [ʍ] has historically been transcribed as [hw] (House, 1998), and both phonemes were pronounced. House indicates that during Middle English, the *hw* spelling disappeared and was replaced by *wh, w,* and *h*. Unofficially, the [hw] is often used (MacKay, 1987) and may present more confusion when handwritten because the [ʍ] symbol resembles the [m] symbol. The reader should be aware that both symbols are still widely used for the same sound.

How the Sound Is Produced

The [hw] sound has some unique characteristics that need to be understood. The [hw] phonetic symbols represent the *wh* orthographic spelling. The reverse positioning [hw], which is an Old English spelling, is more descriptive of how the sound is actually produced. The [hw] starts as an [h] and ends as a rounded glide. It is considered to be a glide because it is always made as a movement and is pronounced with the mouth (articulators) in motion. See **Figure 15-5**.

The lips (bilabial) may be slightly rounded during the friction (fricative) initiation of the [h] portion of this sound. The muscles of the lips tighten during the completion (glide) [w] portion of the sound. The vocal folds are slightly adducted (closed) to create the turbulence of the airflow, but the [hw] sound is still considered voiceless. However, when it appears in the intervocalic position, *no<u>wh</u>ere*, the sound usually becomes a voiced fricative. The back of the tongue (velar) and the velopharyngeal port are closed. The airflow is directed through the oral cavity and through the constricted (fricative) opening of the lips with sufficient force to produce audible friction.

Different Spellings for the [hw] or [ʍ] Sound

Note: Pronounce the *wh* as the [hw]–[ʍ] so that you can get a sense of how it is produced and how it sounds even though your natural tendency may be to use the [w] sound. An obvious "slight breeze" escapes between the lips as the [ʍ] is produced, as in *wheat*. It is absent in [w] in *was*.

Transcribe the following words. Refer to the Key at the right upon completion.

Different Spellings				*Key*
wh	when	___ which ___	wheat ___	ʍɛn, ʍɪʧ, ʍit
w	sway	___ swim ___		sweɪ, swɪm
	switch	___ twirl ___		swɪʧ, twɝl
u	persuade ___	suede ___		pɝsweɪd, sweɪd

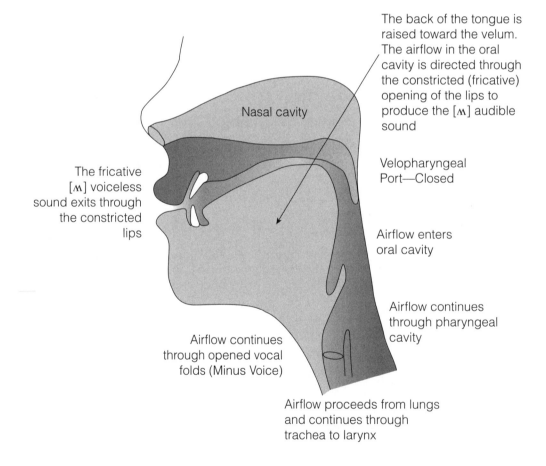

The back of the tongue is raised toward the velum. The airflow in the oral cavity is directed through the constricted (fricative) opening of the lips to produce the [ʍ] audible sound

Nasal cavity

Velopharyngeal Port—Closed

The fricative [ʍ] voiceless sound exits through the constricted lips

Airflow enters oral cavity

Airflow continues through pharyngeal cavity

Airflow continues through opened vocal folds (Minus Voice)

Airflow proceeds from lungs and continues through trachea to larynx

Figure 15-5 [hw] and [ʍ] pronunciation.

Different Sounds of the Letters That Produce the [hw] or [ʍ] Sound

Transcribe the following words. Refer to the Key at the right upon completion.

Key

[ʍ]	swim ___	w	[w]	was ___			swɪm, wɑz
[ʍ]	suede ___	u	[ʌ]	us ___			sweɪd, ʌs
			[ju]	use ___			juz
[ʍ]	when ___	wh	[h]	who ___			ʍɛn, hu

Rules for Spelling and Pronunciation of the [hw] or [ʍ] Sound

1. The written *wh* is pronounced as [hw] or [ʍ], as in *when, white, anywhere.*

2. The written *wh* is pronounced as [h], as in *who, whole,* and *whoop.*

3. The *w* is pronounced as a [hw] or [ʍ], as in *twenty, twin, thwart.*

4. The *u* in *su* combinations is produced as a [hw] or [ʍ] glide, as in *persuade, suede.*

5. The *wh* can occur in initial and middle positions in words but not before other consonants or at the end of words.

Words That Include the [hw] or [ʍ] Sound

The [ʍ] or [hw] sound occurs in the initial and medial positions but not in the final position. Transcribe the following words. Refer to the Key at the right upon completion.

Initial Consonant

Key

whip ___	while ___	ʍɪp, ʍaɪl
wheel ___	whale ___	ʍɪl, ʍeɪl

Unstressed Syllable

Medial Consonant

anywhere ___	ɛniʍɛr
worthwhile ___	wɝθʍaɪl

Stressed Syllable

Medial Consonant

twenty ___	sweet ___	tʍɛnti, sʍit
schwa ___	twinkle ___	ʃʍɔ, tʍɪŋkl̩
suede ___	overwhelm ___	sweɪd, ovɚʍɛlm

Final Consonant

[None]

Auditory Discrimination

Transcribe the following words. Practice pronouncing the [ʍ] sound even though it may not be in your personal dialect.

Contrast Minimal Pairs

[ʍ] (–)		[w] (+)		*Key*
whey ___		way ___		ʍaɪ, waɪ
where ___		wear ___		ʍɛr, wɛr
whether ___		weather ___		ʍɛðɚ, wɛðɚ
which ___		witch ___		ʍɪʧ, wɪʧ
whine ___		wine ___		ʍaɪn, waɪn

Others

[ʍ]	[h]	[ʍ]	[f]	*Key*
wheat ___	heat ___	whig ___	fig ___	ʍit, hit, ʍɪg, fɪg
whale ___	hail ___	wheel ___	feel ___	ʍeɪl, hɛl, ʍɪl, fɛl
whim ___	him ___	whale ___	fail ___	ʍɪm, hɪm, ʍeɪl, feɪl
when ___	hen ___	while ___	file ___	ʍɛn, hɛn, ʍaɪl, faɪl
white ___	height ___	white ___	fight ___	ʍaɪt, haɪt, ʍaɪt, faɪt

Allophonic and Dialect Variations

In the intervocalic position, as in *nowhere*, the [ʍ] usually becomes the [w] voiced fricative (Calvert, 1986). Tiffany and Carrell (1977) indicate that the allophonic variations are somewhat subtle and occur as a result of voicing and the degree of the aspirated release of airflow through the constricted area. Speakers have a tendency to add a degree of voicing that may be a result of the assimilation of the following vowel sound and also reduce the amount of aspirated airflow that produces less energy or noise that is associated with the pronunciation of the [ʍ] sound. Most speakers of United States English do not make a distinction between the voiced and voiceless [w] in their speech habits (Small, 1999); therefore, the [ʍ] sound is not really acknowledged.

In several dialects of United States English, the [hw] or [ʍ] has been replaced with the [w] sound. Carrell and Tiffany (1960) indicate that although words such as *where* and *why* are marked with the [ʍ] in most dictionaries, the aspirate quality and unvoicing may be sharply reduced, or entirely absent, in context. An example is the paired words *wear* and *where* that are usually indistinguishable in informal speech in most United States English dialects. These authors speculate that the [w] and [ʍ] contrast is in the process of being lost. Some United States English speakers habitually omit or reduce the friction and add voicing to the [ʍ] so that it is closer to [w], as in *when* [wɛn] for [ʍɛn] and when *white* [waɪt] becomes [ʍaɪt] (Calvert, 1986).

In some dialects of English, the initial sound of words such as *which* and *when* is produced with the voiceless [ʍ], also written as [hw] (Edwards, 1997). Some phoneticians also use [ʍ] to represent the [w] glide when it follows a voiceless consonant in words such as *twin* and *sweet*. Small (1999) presents one of the most straightforward responses to this issue wherein he adopts only the [w] sound and omits any discussion of the [ʍ] sound because most speakers of United States English do not make a distinction between the voiced and voiceless sounds in their speech habits. House (1998) agrees that the [ʍ] sound is disappearing from common usage and is being replaced by most speakers at the conversational level with the [w]. She adds that historically the [ʍ] was transcribed as [hw] and both phonemes were pronounced. During the Middle English period, the *hw* was replaced by *wh, w,* or *h.* Ladefoged (1993) adds that the contrast between [w] and [ʍ] seems to be disappearing in most forms of English so that in those dialects in which it occurs, [ʍ] is more likely to be found only in the less common words such as *whether* rather than in frequently used words such as *what.* However, the [ʍ] sound does still exist and should be considered a part of the inventory of United States English sounds.

Normal and Deviant Development of the [ʍ] Sound

Children usually master the [ʍ] sound between the ages of 5 and 10 years (Sander, 1972). The [ʍ] is one of the last sounds children master (Calvert, 1986) and is among the most frequently misarticulated consonants.

Rarely does this sound serve as a clinical target (Edwards, 1997). Any acoustical differences that result from the use of the [w] substitution do not present a problem to the listener in the determination of a *wh* word in context. Such words usually closely resemble homonyms. Otherwise, such minimal pairs as *which, witch* and *weigh, whey* require more precision and effort to reduce any ambiguity of their meanings when presented alone or out of context.

Nonnative Speaker Pronunciation

Continental Europeans frequently have difficulty learning the [ʍ] sound (Calvert, 1986). The [v] sound is substituted, as when *when* [vɛn] becomes [ʍɛn] or *white* [vaɪt] becomes [ʍaɪt]. Also, the cognate of [v], the [f] sound, may also be substituted, as when *white* becomes [faɪt], particularly in the German dialect. The [ʍ] sound does not appear as a distinct sound in any of the other 15 major languages spoken in the United States.

Summary

The [ʍ] sound is one of the 10 fricative consonants. It is homorganic with lingua-velar [k], [g], [h], [w], [ŋ], and the bilabial [p], [b], [m], and [w]. Children master the [ʍ] sound at approximately 6 to 9 years old, making it one of the last sounds to be acquired. There is a prevalence among native speakers to substitute the voiced [w] for the voiceless [ʍ], and nonnative speakers may substitute the [b], [f], or [v] sound. A discrepancy between spelling and pronunciation may present some confusion to both native and nonnative speakers, as in *wh* in *who* [hu] and *when* [ʍɛn]. Most listeners accept the substitution of the [w] for the [ʍ], and it is seldom considered a clinical issue, particularly because many phoneticians agree that the [ʍ] sound is being used less frequently and may be nonexistent in many United States English dialects.

SUMMARY

There are four cognate sets of fricative consonants and two other fricatives, the [h] and [hw] or [ʍ]. Each set has a different anatomic placement. The voiceless [f] and the voiced [v] are labiodental. The voiceless *th* [θ] and the voiced *th* [ð] are linguadental (upper front teeth), the voiceless [ʃ] and the voiced [ʒ] are linguapalatal, and the voiceless [s] and voiced [z] are either lingua-alveolar or linguadental (lower front teeth). The voiceless [h] is linguapalatal and lingua-velar or glottal, and the [ʍ] [hw] is bilabial, lingua-velar. The alveolar and palatal fricatives are much more intense than the others and are identified as sibilants or stridents ([s], [z], [ʃ], and [ʒ]). The other fricatives require weaker energy and may, under certain conditions, be difficult to discriminate. However, the fricatives such as [f], [v], [θ], and [ð] have high visibility (cues to the listener) and relatively low frequency of occurrence in United States English.

The fricatives are distinctive in that the velopharyngeal port is closed, and the oral pharyngeal cavities function as chambers to capture the air pressure behind the constriction. The airflow is then channeled by the shaped articulators through a narrow constriction, and a continuous fricative aperiodic noise is generated. Because their production involves an obstruction of the airflow in the vocal tract, fricatives are also labeled as **obstruents**. Fricatives are perceived and discriminated by their voicing, the frequency range of the aperiodic "noise," and their relative loudness.

Developmental acquisition of the fricative sounds varies. Children master the [h] and [f] by age 4 years and master the [ð], [ʒ], and [ʍ] later; these latter sounds may not be stabilized until age 8 years. With the exception of the [h] and [ʍ], the other fricatives occur in the initial, medial, and final positions in words. A wide variety of alphabet letters represents the sounds of the fricatives, and some very unusual relations occur such as the *gh* for the [f] in *laugh*, the *f* for [v] in *of*, the difference in the *th* in *thin* and *then*, the *x* for the [ʃ] in *anxious*, and the *x* for [s] in *taxi*. The high-frequency, weak-energy output may make the perception of these sounds difficult.

Because of the constriction feature of fricatives, abnormalities to the oral-pharyngeal areas that result in weakness, lack of endurance, and imprecise placement of the articulators can result in articulation errors such as substitutions and distortions. The latter results in frontal or lateral lisps.

The 10 fricative sounds represent 40% of the United States English consonant sounds.

MIRROR PUZZLE

Following are words that spell a different word when spelled backward. Watch for different vowel sounds. Phonetically transcribe the words in the spaces provided. For example, but = bʌt and tub = tʌb. The Key is presented after the puzzle.

1.	but	bʌt	tub	tʌb
2.	not	_____	ton	_____
3.	mood	_____	doom	_____
4.	net	_____	ten	_____
5.	draw	_____	ward	_____
6.	reed	_____	deer	_____
7.	gel	_____	leg	_____
8.	strap	_____	parts	_____
9.	tar	_____	rat	_____
10.	stop	_____	pots	_____
11.	step	_____	pets	_____
12.	slap	_____	pals	_____

Key:

1.	but	bʌt	tub	tʌb
2.	not	nɑt	ton	tʌn
3.	mood	mud	doom	dum
4.	net	nɛt	ten	tɛn
5.	draw	drɑw	ward	wɑrd
6.	reed	rid	deer	dɪr
7.	gel	gɛl	leg	leɪg
8.	strap	stræp	parts	pɑrts
9.	tar	tɑr	rat	ræt
10.	stop	stɑp	pots	pɑts
11.	step	stɛp	pets	pɛts
12.	slap	slæp	pals	paɪls

WORDS THAT RHYME

Identify three other words that rhyme with the following words and transcribe each phonetically.

1. <u>rice</u>   2. <u>seat</u>   3. <u>rhyme</u>

_____   _____   _____

_____   _____   _____

_____   _____   _____

4. <u>trail</u>   5. <u>string</u>   6. <u>coast</u>

_____   _____   _____

_____   _____   _____

_____   _____   _____

7. <u>maid</u>   8. <u>small</u>   9. <u>pull</u>

_____   _____   _____

_____   _____   _____

_____   _____   _____

10. <u>trick</u>

_____

_____

_____

REFERENCES

Calvert, D. R. (1986). *Descriptive phonetics*. New York, NY: Thieme Medical Publishers.

Carrell, J., & Tiffany, W. (1960). *Phonetics: Theory and application to speech improvement*. New York, NY: McGraw-Hill.

Edwards, H. T. (1997). *Applied phonetics* (2nd ed.). San Diego, CA: College-Hill Press.

House, L. (1998). *Introductory phonetics and phonology.* Mahwah, NJ: Lawrence Erlbaum.

International Phonetic Association. (1999). *Handbook of the International Phonetic Association.* Cambridge, England: Cambridge University Press.

Ladefoged, P. (1993). *A course in phonetics* (3rd ed.). Fort Worth, TX: Harcourt Brace College Publishers.

MacKay, I. R. A. (1987). *Phonetics: The science of speech production.* Boston, MA: Allyn & Bacon.

Sander, E. (1972). When are speech sounds learned? *Journal of Speech and Hearing Disorders, 37,* 55–63.

Small, L. H. (1999). *Fundamentals of phonetics: A practical guide for students* (3rd ed.). Boston, MA: Allyn & Bacon.

Tiffany, W. R., & Carrell, J. (1977). *Phonetics: Theory and application.* New York, NY: McGraw-Hill.

U.S. Census Bureau. (1990). *Table 5. Detailed list of languages spoken at home for the population 5 years and over by state: 1990.* Retrieved from http://www.census.gov/prod/2010pubs/acs-12.pdf

VanRiper, C. (1979). *An introduction to general American phonetics.* New York, NY: Harper & Row.

Chapter 16

Affricate Consonants: Two Sounds Combine to Make One

PURPOSE

To introduce you to the United States English affricative consonants.

OBJECTIVES

This chapter will provide you with information regarding:

1. The identification and description of how the United States English affricate consonants are produced

2. Different spellings for each stop sound and different sounds for each of the corresponding orthographic letters

3. Rules for spelling and pronunciation of each sound

4. Various contexts in which each sound occurs; examples of cognates and other minimal pairs for auditory discrimination

5. Examples of allophonic variations, dialect differences, and nonnativespeaker difficulties

6. Normal development and disordered production of each sound

7. Phonetic transcription exercises throughout the chapter and self-quiz

Remember the *dialect variations* when referring to the transcription keys. This applies particularly to the [ɑ], [ɔ] and the [i], [ɪ] sounds.

CHARACTERISTICS OF AFFRICATIVES

The inventory of United States English consonants contains two affricates, the [ʧ] in *ch* in and the [ʤ] in *jam*. The question arises whether to consider each of these as one segment or as a sequence of a stop plus a fricative. For example, native speakers have the intuition that each affricate is a single segment, despite the two letters required to symbolize it. Also, English words do not begin with a sequence of stop plus fricative. This suggests that English has a constraint against syllable-initial stop-fricative sequences.

According to Ball and Lowry (2001), an affricate is a combination of a stop and a fricative, and the acoustic characteristics of both sounds can be seen on a spectrographic display. There is a break for the stop followed by the high-frequency noise of the second sound.

Affricatives are considered as a combination of sounds involving a stop (complete closure) [t] or [d] followed by a fricative (noise) segment [ʃ] or [ʒ] (Shriberg & Kent, 2003). These authors explain that air pressure built up during the stop phase is released as a burst of noise, similar in duration to that of fricative sounds, and fricatives are produced only at the palatal place of production.

Small (1999) provides a detailed description, indicating that affricates are obstruents that begin as an alveolar stop in which the tongue tip contacts the posterior alveolar ridge. There is a corresponding increase in intraoral pressure in the oral cavity to create the [t] or [d] component of the affricate. This air pressure is then forced through the constriction formed by the tongue and palate to create a turbulent noise [ʃ] or [ʒ].

Although [tʃ] and [dʒ] are the only English sounds classified as affricates, other sound combinations have affricative characteristics (Carrell & Tiffany, 1960; MacKay, 1987). Examples include the [θ], as in *eighth*, and [ð] as in *outside*. The [ð] voiceless dental or alveolar affricate occurs in German, Italian, Canadian French, and other languages. Other combinations are [dʒ] as in *adds*, and [dr] as in *dream*, both of which have a tendency toward "affrication" because their production involves a glide from a stop to a fricative. Calvert (1986) even suggests that the [kʍ] and [ks] are combined as affricatives. These combinations are considered as individual, distinct, and separate sounds rather than as affricates.

MacKay (1987) offers an explanation as to why the [tʃ] and the [dʒ] are each considered as one sound. An affricate is a speech sound made up of a plosive and a homorganic (same or similar place of articulation) fricative, with the two articulated in one movement and acting together as a single unit. You may ask, "What sets these two sounds apart from the other sounds to constitute affricates?" MacKay states that the difference between an affricate and a simple sequence of plosive and fricative can be based on purely phonetic reasons, but it is more often based on phonemic grounds.

Furthermore, MacKay (1987) states that to meet the phonetic criteria for an affricate, the following characteristics must be present:

1. The plosive and fricative are homorganic.
2. The sounds are closely fused by the most direct transitional movement possible.
3. The total duration is not much greater than the usual duration of either component part.

The phonemic criterion, which is more usual, is that the affricate be produced as if it were a single segment in the sound system of a given language. Examples are words such as *jam* [dʒæm], *judge* [dʒʌdʒ], and *chin* [tʃɪn]. It would be confusing to both the speaker and the listener to pronounce the initial sound in these words as two separate sounds! The phonetic and phonemic definitions can be in conflict, however.

A comprehensive description of the two affricates sounds, the voiceless [tʃ] and voiced [dʒ] cognate pair, and their features is presented.

PHONETIC SYMBOL [tʃ]

EXHIBIT 16-1	Phonetic Symbol [tʃ]

Phonetic Symbol	[tʃ]	**[tʃ]**
Grapheme Symbol	ch	
Diacritic Symbols	ch, ch, tʃ	
Phonic Symbol	ch	
Cognate	[dʒ]	
Homorganic	[dʒ] and Lingua-Alveolar: [t], [d], [s], [z], [l], [n] Linguapalatal: [ʃ], [ʒ], [r], [j], [h]	
Sound Class	Consonant	
Basic Phonetic Features	Placement: Lingua-Alveolar [t] to Linguapalatal [ʃ] Manner: Affricate Voicing: Minus Voice	
International Phonetic Alphabet (IPA) (International Phonetic Association [IPA], 1999)	[tʃ] #213 Voiceless, Postalveolar, Affricative	

How the Sound Is Produced

The airflow from the lungs continues through the opened vocal folds (voiceless). The velopharyngeal port is closed, and the sound is directed into the oral cavity. The sides of the tongue (lingua) are pressed against the upper molars or palate (palatal). The tip of the tongue seals the oral cavity by touching close on or just behind the alveolar ridge (alveolar). This seal results in the stoppage (stop) of the compressed air. The airflow is then released through the broad opening between the alveolar ridge and the front of the tongue, which directs the airflow through and against the slightly opened front teeth (fricative). Its cognate, the voiced [ʤ], is generally produced with less force. See **Figure 16-1**.

The [ʧ] is produced with a single burst of air pressure, although it includes elements of both the [t] (stop) and [ʃ] fricative sounds.

Different Spellings for the [ʧ] Sound

Transcribe the following words. Refer to the Key at the right upon completion.

Different Spellings						Key
c	cello	___				ʧɛloʊ
ch	charm	___	choose	___		ʧɑrm, ʧuz
	teacher	___	match	___	niche ___	tiʧɚ, mæʧ, nɪʧ
t	righteous	___				raɪʧəs
tu	actual	___	obituary	___		æʧuʊl, obiʧjuɛri
	natural	___	adventure	___		næʧɚʊl, ædvɛnʧɚ
	contractual	___				kəntræʧʊl
ture	lecture	___	feature	___		lɛkʧɚ, fiʧɚ
	nature	___	gesture	___		neɪʧɚ, ʤɛʧɚ
tion	question	___	congestion	___		kwɛʧən, kɑnʤɛʃən
	mention	___				mɛnʧən
tch	batch	___	kitchen	___	hitch ___	bæʧ, kɪʧən, hɪʧ
	itch	___	hatchery	___		ɪʧ, hæʧɚi
ntc	tincture	___				tɪnʧɚ
nsion	mansion	___	pension	___		mænʧən, pɛnʧən
	tension	___				tɛnʧən

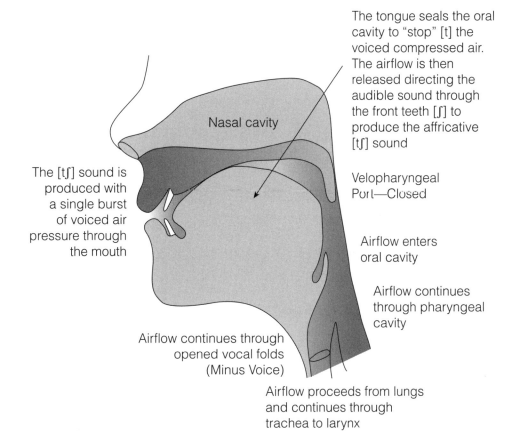

The [tʃ] sound is produced with a single burst of voiced air pressure through the mouth

Nasal cavity

The tongue seals the oral cavity to "stop" [t] the voiced compressed air. The airflow is then released directing the audible sound through the front teeth [ʃ] to produce the affricative [tʃ] sound

Velopharyngeal Port—Closed

Airflow enters oral cavity

Airflow continues through pharyngeal cavity

Airflow continues through opened vocal folds (Minus Voice)

Airflow proceeds from lungs and continues through trachea to larynx

Figure 16-1 [ʧ] pronunciation.

Different Sounds for the [ʧ] Letters

Transcribe the following words. Refer to the Key at the right upon completion.

Key

c	[ʧ]	cello	_____	[s]	city	_____	ʧɛloʊ, sɪti
				[k]	cat	_____	kæt
t	[ʧ]	nature	_____	[t]	tot	_____	neɪʧɚ, tɑt
ch	[ʧ]	charm	_____	[ʃ]	chevron	_____	ʧɑrm, ʃɛvrɑn
				[k]	chemistry	_____	kɛmɪstri
s	[ʧ]	mansion	_____	[s]	sun	_____	mænʧən, sʌn

The Digraph *ch*

The spelling pronunciation problems presented by the digraph *ch* are complicated because word origin plays a major role (Carrell & Tiffany, 1960). You may need to consult a dictionary for the pronunciation of unfamiliar words. In general, however, the initial *ch* in English is more often [ʧ] or [ʃ] than [k], although it may be any one of these three. Those words with predominantly Greek origins such as *chemistry* and *character* begin with the [k] sound. An approximation of the French influence remains in English, as in [ʃ] in *champagne* and *chalet*. Where such original pronunciations are not retained, the sound is [ʧ] as in *chap* [ʧæp] because the word has been anglicized or for other reasons.

Rules for Spelling and Pronunciation of the [ʧ] Sound

1. The *ch* may have the [ʧ] sound as in *charm, kitchen, itch*, but the *ch* also frequently is pronounced as a *sh* sound [ʃ], as in *chevron, machine*, and *nonchalant*. In addition, the *ch* becomes a [k] sound, as in *school, character*, and *chemistry*.

2. The *ch* has an unusual pronunciation in the Italian word *cello*.

3. Another unusual context is the *t* [ʧ] as in *righteous*.

4. In the *tu* context, as in *natural, actual*, and *obituary*, the *tu* is pronounced [ʧ].

5. Similarly, the *ture* context, as in *gesture, forfeiture*, and *immature*, changes the *t* to a [ʧ] sound.

6. The *tion* and *tain* contexts change the *t* to a [ʧ] sound, as in *combustion, digestion*, and *Christian*.

7. The *t* is silent or absorbed in the [ʧ] sound when it precedes the *ch* as in *hatch, itch*, and *kitchen*.

8. An unusual context is *ntc*, as in *tincture*.

9. The *s* is replaced with the [ʧ] sound in *mansion, tension*, and *pension*.

Words That Include the [ʧ] Sound

The [ʧ] occurs in all three positions: initial, medial, and final. Transcribe the following words. Refer to the Key at the right upon completion.

Initial Position   *Key*

cheer _____   charity _____   chili _____   ʧɛr, ʧɛriti, ʧɪli

Unstressed Syllable

Medial Position

adventure _____   ædvɛnʧɚ

literature _____   temperature _____   lɪtɚəʧɚ, tɛmpɚʧɚ

Stressed Syllable

Medial Position

recharge _____   riʧɑrdʒ

unchanged _____   richer _____   ənʧeɪnʒd, riʧɚ

Final Position

advantage _____   much _____   ædvæntɪʧ, mʌʧ

sandwich _____   sændwɪʧ

Initial and Final Positions

church _____   ʧɝʧ

Medial Blends

r̲c̲h̲ archway _____   ɑrʧweɪ

porches _____   fortunate _____   porʧəs, forʧuneɪt

Final Blends

n̲c̲h̲ bench __   branch __   munch __   bɛnʧ, brænʧ, mʌnʧ

Clusters

n̲c̲h̲e̲d̲ lunched _____   pinched _____   lʌnʧt, pɪnʧt

searched _____   sɝʧt

Auditory Discrimination

Transcribe the following words. Refer to the Key at the right upon completion.

Contrast Minimal Pairs

[ʧ] (–)		*[ʤ] (+)*		*Key*
choke	_____	joke	_____	ʧoʊk, ʤoʊk
chip	_____	jip	_____	ʧɪp, ʤɪp
cheap	_____	jeep	_____	ʧip, ʤip
cheer	_____	jeer	_____	ʧɛr, ʤɛr
chain	_____	Jane	_____	ʧeɪn, ʤeɪn
rich	_____	ridge	_____	rɪʧ, rɪʤ
search	_____	surge	_____	sɝʧ, sɝʤ
etch	_____	edge	_____	ɛʧ, ɛʤ
batch	_____	badge	_____	bæʧ, bæʤ
H	_____	age	_____	eɪʧ, eɪʤ

Other Contrast Pairs

[ʧ]	*[ʃ]*	*[ʧ]*	*[t]*	*[ʧ]*	*[k]*
choose ___	shoes ___	chew ___	two ___	cheep ___	keep ___
ditch ___	dish ___	chin ___	tin ___	ditch ___	Dick ___
match ___	mash ___	match ___	mat ___	patch ___	pack ___
cheap ___	sheep ___	catch ___	cat ___	chick ___	kick ___
batch ___	bash ___	chin ___	tin ___	watch ___	walk ___
witch ___	wish ___	chain ___	cane ___		

Key (left to right): ʧuz, ʃuz, ʧu, tu, ʧip, kip, dɪʧ, dɪʃ, ʧɪn, tɪn, dɪʧ, dɪk, mæʧ, mæʃ, mæʧ, mæt, pæʧ, pæk, ʧip, ʃip, kæʧ, kæt, ʧɪk, kɪk, bæʧ, ʧɪn, tɪn, wɑʧ, wɑk, wɪʧ, wɪʃ, ʧeɪn, keɪn

Allophonic and Dialect Variations

Variations among the allophones of the [ʧ] are somewhat prominent (Carrell & Tiffany, 1960). The sounds that precede and follow affect the production of the [ʧ] sound. The position of the vowel, as in *which* (front), leads to a somewhat advanced tongue contact, whereas the tongue assumes a more posterior position as influenced by the [ɑ] back vowel in *wall*. The change in tongue position alters the fricative release posture and produces some subtle variations in the sound. The [ʧ] may become rounded when it precedes a rounded vowel, as in *chalk* [ʧɑl] or [ʧɑk] in contrast to *chin* [ʧɪn] where it is more unrounded (Edwards, 1997).

Certain speakers may still manifest influence of the Early Modern period. For example, the [ʧ] originates from the *tj* in such words as *question* [kwɛsjən] to [kwɛsʧən] and *literature* [lɪtərətjʊr] to [lɪtərətʃʊr] or even with syllable reduction, as in [lɪtrətʧɚ].

Some of the major allophone variants of [ʧ] are (1) alveolar-plus-palatal [ʧ], (2) alveolar-plus-glide [tj], (3) weaker or less distributed palatal (lisping), (4) fricative [ʃ], and (5) alveolar *ts* (Carrell & Tiffany, 1960).

No significant dialect variations have been reported (Edwards, 1997). However, some speakers may substitute the [ʧ] for the *tr* blend, as when *train* [treɪn] becomes [ʧreɪn] and Chicago [ʃəkɑgo] becomes [ʧəkɑo].

Normal and Deviant Development of the [ʧ] Sound

Children master the [ʧ] sound by age 7 years (Sander, 1972). Errors associated with failure to learn [ʧ] are present in children with speech delay (Carrell & Tiffany, 1960). Substitutions occur such as [ʃ] for [ʧ], as when *chicken* [ʧɪkən] becomes [ʃɪkən], and the [ʧ] may be substituted, as when *church* [ʧɝʧ] becomes [ʃɝʃ].

Persons with cleft palate may grossly distort the [ʧ] sound and may produce a glottal or pharyngeal stop followed by a nasal fricative release (Carrell & Tiffany, 1960). Children with delayed speech may (1) delete, (2) stop, (3) voice, and/or (4) distort the [ʧ] affricate sound (Shriberg & Kent, 2003).

Nonnative Speaker Pronunciation

The production of the [ʧ] phoneme is not particularly hard for the foreign speaker to produce, but the spelling rules are frequently misleading (Carrell & Tiffany, 1960). For example, the *ch* digraph in French is uniformly the [ʃ] sound, and there is no palatal or alveolo-palatal plosive in that sound system. Therefore, the [ʧ] and [ʤ] may be pronounced as [ʃ] and [ʒ]. Also, the *ts* may be substituted by some foreign speakers.

In addition to English, the U.S. Census Bureau (1990) identified 15 other languages predominantly spoken in the United States. The following sound systems of these languages contain the [ʧ] sound with some allophonic variations (IPA, 1999). Spanish, French, German, Italian, Chinese, Vietnamese, Japanese, Hindi, and Russian have the [ʧ] or anallophonic variation. Languages that do not include the [ʧ] sound are Tagalog, Polish, Korean, Greek, and Arabic.

Summary

The voiceless [ʧ] and its cognate, the voiced [ʤ], are the two affricatives spoken in United States English. The airflow begins as a stop and completes with a fricative constriction. It is one of the later sounds that children master, by age 7 years. The allophonic variations are a result of the influence of the sounds that surround the [tʃ] sound and of the degree of air pressure during the stop and fricative stages. Nonnative speakers may have difficulty because of the various alphabet letters that represent the [tʃ] sound and the influence of their native language, such as French and German. Children with delayed speech may substitute other stops or fricatives and/or may delete the sound.

PHONETIC SYMBOL [dʒ]

EXHIBIT 16-2	Phonetic Symbol [dʒ]
Phonetic Symbol	[dʒ]
Grapheme Symbols	g, gg, dg, dge, d, ge, di, dj, j
Diacritic Symbols	j, dʒ, g
Phonic Symbol	j
Cognate	[tʃ]
Homorganic	[tʃ] and Lingua-Alveolar: [t], [d], [s], [z], [l], [n] Linguapalatal: [ʃ], [ʒ], [r], [j], [h]
Sound Class	Consonant
Basic Phonetic Features	Placement: Lingua-Alveolar [d] to Linguapalatal [ʒ] Manner: Affricate Voicing: Plus Voice
IPA (1999)	[dʒ] #214 Voiceless, Postalveolar, Affricative

How the Sound Is Produced

The airflow from the lungs activates the vocal folds (voice). The velopharyngeal port is closed and the sound is directed into the oral cavity. The sides of the tongue (lingua) are pressed against the upper molars or palate (palatal). The tip of the tongue seals the oral cavity by touching close on or just behind the alveolar ridge (alveolar). This seal results in the stoppage (stop) of the compressed air. The airflow is then released through the broad opening between the alveolar ridge and front of the tongue, directing the airflow through and against the slightly opened front teeth (fricative). Its cognate, the voiceless [tʃ], is generally produced with more force. The [dʒ] sound is produced with a single burst of air pressure, although it includes elements of both the [d] (stop) and [ʒ] fricative sounds. See **Figure 16-2**.

Different Spellings for the [dʒ] Sound

Transcribe the following words. Refer to the Key at the right upon completion.

Different Spellings				Key
j	jam	___	project ___	dʒæm, prɑjɛct
	adjutant	___	object ___	ædʒutənt, ɑbdʒɛt
	enjoy	___		ɛndʒoɪ
gg	exaggerate	___	suggestion ___	ɛgædʒə·eɪt, sədʒɛstən
	jiggle	___	juggle ___	dʒɪgl̩, dʒʌgl̩
dg	fidget	___	budget ___	fɪdʒɛt, bʌdʒɛt,
	gadget	___		gædʒɛt
dge	ridge	___	fudge ___	rɪdʒ, fʌdʒ,
	edge	___		ɛdʒ
g	tragic	___	imagination ___	trædʒɪk, ɪmædʒɪneɪʃən
	physiology	___	stage ___	fɪzɪɑlədʒi, steɪdʒ
d	gradual	___	graduation ___	grædʒʊl, grædʒueɪʃən
	educator	___		ɛdʒukeɪtə·
dj	adjust	___	adjournment ___	ədʒʌst, ədʒə·nmɛnt

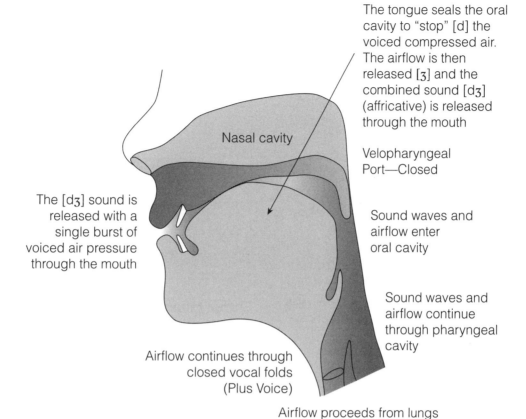

The tongue seals the oral cavity to "stop" [d] the voiced compressed air. The airflow is then released [ʒ] and the combined sound [ʤ] (affricative) is released through the mouth

Nasal cavity

Velopharyngeal Port—Closed

The [ʤ] sound is released with a single burst of voiced air pressure through the mouth

Sound waves and airflow enter oral cavity

Sound waves and airflow continue through pharyngeal cavity

Airflow continues through closed vocal folds (Plus Voice)

Airflow proceeds from lungs and continues through trachea to larynx

Figure 16-2 [ʤ] pronunciation.

adjunct	_____	adjective	_____	æʤənkt, æʤɛtɪv
di	soldier	_____		soʊʤɚ
ge	college	_____	avenge	_____	kɑlɛʤ, əvɛnʤ
	engage	_____	courage	_____	ɛnɡeɪʤ, kɝcɪʤ
	generous	_____			ʤɛnɚəs

Different Sounds of the Letters That Produce the [ʤ] Sound

Transcribe the following words. Refer to the Key at the right upon completion.

Key

j	[ʤ]	jam	___	j [j]	hallelujah	___	ʤæm, hæləlujə
g	[ʤ]	stage	___	g [g]	go	___	steɪʤ, goʊ
gg	[ʤ]	suggest	___	gg [g]	wiggle	___	sʌʤɛst, wɪgl̩
d	[ʤ]	educator	___	d [d]	done	___	ɛʤjukeɪtɚ, dʌn
di	[ʤ]	soldier	___	di [d]	did	___	soʊʤɚ, dɪd

Rules for Spelling and Pronunciation of the [ʤ] Sound

1. The *j* is consistent in representing the [ʤ] sound, as in *jacket, adjust,* and *object.*

2. When two adjacent *g* letters (*gg*) occur, as in *suggestion, juggle,* and *exaggerate,* the [ʤ] sound is pronounced.

3. In the *dg* combination, only the single sound [ʤ] is produced, as in *budget, gadget,* and *fidget.*

4. The [ʤ] sound is pronounced for the letter *g* in the initial or medial position of a word when followed by an *i, e,* or *y,* as in *gin, general, agent, gyrate, gypsum,* and *gypsy.*

5. The *d* in the *du* context, as in *gradual* and *education,* is pronounced as the [ʤ] sound.

6. In the *dj* context, the [ʤ] sound is produced, as in *adjust, adjective.*

7. The *di* in such words as *soldier* is considered as one sound, the [ʤ].

8. In the *ge* context, the *e* is silent and words such as *college, avenge*, and *courage* have [dʒ] as the final sound.

Words That Include the [dʒ] Sound

The [dʒ] sound occurs in all three positions: initial, medial, and final. Transcribe the following words. Refer to the Key at the right upon completion.

Initial Position			Key
jaw ___	gem ___	job ___	dʒɑ, dʒɛm, dʒɑb
giant ___	janitor ___	geologist ___	dʒaɪnt, dʒænətɚ, dʒialodʒɛst

Unstressed Syllable

Medial Position

hydrogen ___	origin ___	haɪdrodʒən, ɑrɪdʒɪn
manager ___	oxygen ___	mænədʒɚ, ɑksidʒən

Stressed Syllable

Medial Position

lodger ___	cages ___	ajar ___	lɑdʒɚ, keɪdʒz, ɑdʒɑr
agile ___	adjustment ___		ædʒʊl, ədʒʌstmɛnt

Final Position

advantage ___	privilege ___	ædvænteɪdʒ, prɪvɪlɛdʒ
edge ___	wage ___	siege ___	ɛdʒ, weɪdʒ, sidʒ

Initial and Final Positions

judge ___	George ___	dʒʌdʒ, dʒordʒ

Medial Blends

ng angel ___	ranger ___	eɪndʒl, reɪnʒɚ
oranges ___	nj injured ___	ɑreɪndʒz, ɪnʒɚd
enjoy ___	injection ___	ɛndʒoɪ, ɪndʒɛkʃən
rg merger ___	converges ___	mɚdʒɚ, kɑnvɚdʒəs
allergy ___	rd cordial ___	ælɚdʒi, kɑrdʒʊl

Final Blends

rg enlarge ___	diverge ___	ɛnlɑrdʒ, divɚdʒ
surge ___	ng avenge ___	sɚdʒ, əvɛndʒ
arrange ___	sponge ___	əreɪndʒ, spʌdʒ
dged judged ___	budged ___	jʌdʒt, bʌdʒt

Auditory Discrimination

Transcribe the following words. Refer to the Key at the right upon completion.

Cognates

[dʒ] (+)		[tʃ] (–)		Key
joke	___	choke	___	dʒoʊk, tʃoʊk
jip	___	chip	___	dʒɪp, tʃɪp
jeep	___	cheap	___	dʒip, tʃip
jeer	___	cheer	___	dʒɛr, tʃɛr
Jane	___	chain	___	dʒeɪn, tʃeɪn
ridge	___	rich	___	rɪdʒ, rɪtʃ
surge	___	search	___	sɚdʒ, sɚtʃ
edge	___	etch	___	ɛdʒ, ɛtʃ
badge	___	batch	___	bædʒ, bætʃ
age	___	H	___	eɪdʒ, eɪtʃ

Other Minimal Pairs

[dʒ]		[dz]		[dʒ]		[j]		[dʒ]		[g]	
rage	___	raids	___	Jack	___	yak	___	edge	___	egg	___
wage	___	wades	___	jail	___	yell	___	ledge	___	leg	___
budge	___	buds	___	jam	___	yam	___	James	___	games	___
hedge	___	heads	___	jet	___	yet	___	Joe	___	go	___
age	___	aids	___	joke	___	yoke	___	ridge	___	rig	___
siege	___	seeds	___	Jell-o	___	yellow	___	budge	___	bug	___
wedge	___	weds	___	Jew	___	you	___	jail	___	gale	___
edge	___	Ed's	___	jeer	___	gear	___	jet	___	get	___
badge	___	bag	___								

Key (left to right): reɪdʒ, reɪdz, dʒæk, jæk, ɛdʒ, ɛg, weɪdʒ, weɪdz, dʒɛl, jɛl, lɛdʒ, lɛg, bʌdʒ, bʌdz, dʒæm, jæm, dʒeɪmz, geɪmz, hɛdʒ, hɛds, dʒɛt, jɛt, dʒoʊ, goʊ, eɪdʒ, eɪdz, dʒoʊk, joʊk, rɪdʒ, rɪg, sidʒ, sidz, dʒɛloʊ, jɛloʊ, bʌdʒ, bʌg, wɛdʒ, wɛdz, dʒu, ju, dʒɛl, gɛl, ɛdʒ, ɛdz, dʒɛr, gɛr, jɛt, gɛt, bædʒ, bæg

Allophonic and Dialect Variations

Edwards (1997) reports that the [dʒ] becomes rounded when it precedes a rounded vowel, as in *juice* [dʒus]. This cognate pair of [tʃ] voiceless and [dʒ] voiced appears rather consistently as substitutes for the voiceless [t] and voiced [d] in such contexts as *want you* [wɑntʃu] and when *did you?* [dɪdju] becomes [dɪdʒu]. Tiffany and Carrell (1977) offer the example of speakers who produce an overly weak allophone of [dʒ] in connected speech, as when *I pledge allegiance* may be pronounced [aɪ pɛʒəlɪʒəs] wherein the [dʒ] sounds more like the [ʒ] sound. Although these are not considered true allophonic variations, because the sounds themselves change, such changes are influenced by the surrounding sounds. Other subtle allophonic variations occur as a result of differences in the production of the distinctive features of stop/plosive and fricative when the airflow release is modified with increased or reduced force.

In more precise conversational speaking, the words *Did you?* are pronounced as [dɪdju], but more often the general pronunciation substitutes the [ʤ] sound, as in [dɪʤu] or [dɪʤə]. Calvert (1986) provides examples of dialect differences in words such as when *medium* [midiəm] becomes [miʤəm] and tedious [tidiəs] becomes [tiʤəs]. He indicates that in Louisiana *Cajuns* [keɪʤənz] is a derivative of the original word *Arcadians* [arkeidiənz]. Because of its affricative characteristics of a combination of two sounds, the [d] and [ʒ], one sound may dominate or demonstrate the influence of similar sounds such as [s], [z], [ʃ], and [ʒ]. For example, the [nʤ] cluster may be pronounced as [nʒ] in which *orange* may be either [arnʤ] or [arnʒ] (Tiffany & Carrell, 1977).

Normal Development of the [ʤ] Sound

Children master the [ʤ] sound between the ages of 4 and 7 years (Sander, 1972). Edwards (1997) reports that the most frequent severe deviations are [d], followed by [t], or omission. In milder cases, [ʒ] (deaffrication with stridency maintained) or [ʤ] (depalatalization) may occur. Simultaneous deaffrication and depalatalization of this sound results in [d] or [z]. An affricated voiced frontal lisp, [ʤ], or an affricated voiced lateral lisp, [lʤ], may also be observed. Among young children, those who have not learned [ʧ] usually cannot produce the [ʤ] sound (Tiffany & Carrell, 1977). Children with delayed speech may (1) delete, (2) stop, (3) voice/devoice, and/or (4) distort the affricate sounds (Shriberg & Kent, 2003). The basic affricate characteristics of the [ʤ] sound lend themselves to a level of complexity in its production. Although voicing remains a constant, the placement shifts from lingua-alveolar to linguapalatal, and the manner in which the airflow is modified requires an adjustment from a stop to a fricative mode. From an orthographic perspective, the letter *j* represents the [ʤ] symbol in words that begin with a *d*. Children have been taught that the *d* represents the initial and final sounds in words such as *did*, and it is difficult to conceptualize the affricative blending of two sounds into one as is required in [ʤ].

Nonnative Speaker Pronunciation

Speakers of foreign languages and dialects most often confuse the [ʤ] sound (VanRiper, 1979). VanRiper indicates that this is probably because there was no letter *j* in the Latin alphabet, which is the basis of western European scripts. Consequently, when the letter *j* was introduced, it was given different values in different languages. For example, in Scandinavia and Germany, the letter *j* is sounded as the United States English [j], as in *yellow* [jɛlo], so *jump* [ʤʌmp] becomes [jʌmp]. In English, it is the [ʤ] sound, and in French it is the [ʒ] sound, as in *just* [ʒʌst] for [ʤʌst]. Those with German accents may also substitute the voiceless cognate [ʧ] for the [ʤ] sound to the extent that *job* [ʤab] may be pronounced [ʧap]. Tiffany and Carrell (1977) offer this example of some German dialects of United States English where the [ʧ] is substituted for the [ʤ] sound in the phrase "I urge you to judge his age": [aɪ ɝʧ ju tə ʧʌʧ hɪz eʧ].

Of the 15 predominant languages spoken in the United States, other than English (U. S. Census Bureau, 1990), the following languages have the [ʤ] sound with some allophonic variations: Spanish, French, Italian, Polish, Japanese, Arabic, Hindi, and Russian. Those that do not include the [ʤ] sound are German, Chinese, Tagalog, Korean, Vietnamese, Portuguese, and Greek.

Summary

The affricate concept is interesting in that there are two sounds [d] and [ʒ] that produce the [ʤ] sound, which is considered one sound. There are only two American English affricates, the [ʤ] and its voiceless cognate [ʧ]. One could compare the affricates to the diphthongs in that both begin with one sound and shift or glide into another while maintaining the definition of one sound. Several of the alphabet letters represent both the [ʤ] sound and other sounds, and there are differences among the sound systems of the world with regard to the pronunciation of the letter *j*, as in *just, jam*, and so forth. Young children master the [ʤ] sound between the ages 4 and 7 years. This sound is rather complex in its production from its initial stop, lingua-alveolar features to its terminal fricative, linguapalatal features.

SUMMARY OF AFFRICATIVE CONSONANTS

The two affricates [ʧ] and [ʤ] are unique in that they comprise four sounds that are considered individual sounds ([t], [ʃ], [d], and [ʒ]), and yet, as affricates, two sounds are united to form one sound: the voiceless [ʧ] and its voiced cognate [ʤ]. What defines them as affricates is their stop-fricative and homorganic characteristics. There are many inconsistencies between spelling and pronunciation of alphabet letters and phonetic symbols, and it seems that for almost every rule there is an exception. Nonnative speakers may experience confusion in translating the printed word to the spoken word because of these exceptions.

Developmentally, the affricatives come later in acquisition, between ages 4 and 7 years, and young children may have some difficulty in pronunciation, resulting in distortions, substitutions, or deletions.

REFERENCES

Ball, M. J., & Lowry, O. (2001). *Methods in clinical phonetics*. London, England: Whurr Publishers.

Calvert, D. R. (1986). *Descriptive phonetics*. New York, NY: Thieme Medical Publishers.

Carrell, J., & Tiffany, W. (1960). *Phonetics: Theory and application to speech improvement*. New York, NY: McGraw-Hill.

Edwards, H. T. (1997). *Applied phonetics* (2nd ed.). San Diego, CA: College-Hill Press.

International Phonetic Association. (1999). *Handbook of the International Phonetic Association*. Cambridge, England: Cambridge University Press.

MacKay, I. R. A. (1987). *Phonetics: The science of speech production*. Boston, MA: Allyn & Bacon.

Sander, E. (1972). When are speech sounds learned? *Journal of Speech and Hearing Disorders*, 7, 55–63.

Shriberg, L., & Kent, R. (2003). *Clinical phonetics* (3rd ed.). Boston, MA: Allyn & Bacon.

Small, L. H. (1999). *Fundamentals of phonetics: A practical guide for students* (3rd ed.). Boston, MA: Allyn & Bacon.

Tiffany, W. R., & Carrell, J. (1977). *Phonetics: Theory and application*. New York, NY: McGraw-Hill.

U.S. Census Bureau. (1990). *Table 5. Detailed list of languages spoken at home for the population 5 years and over by state: 1990*. Retrieved from http://www.census.gov/prod/2010pubs/acs-12.pdf

VanRiper, C. (1979). *An introduction to general American phonetics*. New York, NY: Harper.

Chapter 17

Nasal and Oral Resonant Consonants Analysis and Transcription

PURPOSE

To introduce you to the nasal and oral resonant consonants of United States English.

OBJECTIVES

This chapter will provide you with information regarding:

1. The identification and description of how the United States English stop consonants are produced

2. Different spellings for each stop sound and different sounds for each of the corresponding orthographic letters

3. Rules for spelling and pronunciation of each sound

4. Various contexts in which each sound occurs

5. Examples of cognates and other minimal pairs for auditory discrimination

6. Examples of allophonic variations, dialect differences, and nonnative speaker difficulties

7. Normal development and disordered production of each sound

8. Phonetic transcription exercises throughout the chapter and self-quiz

CHARACTERISTICS OF THE THREE NASAL RESONANT CONSONANTS

The three nasal resonant consonants of United States English are the [m], [n], and [ŋ].

- [m] Bilabial, nasal resonant
- [n] Lingua-alveolar, nasal resonant
- [ŋ] Lingua-velar, nasal resonant

The placement of the articulators for these sounds progresses from front to back: [m] labial (lips); [n] lingua-alveolar (upper gum ridge); [ŋ] lingua-velar (back of tongue in contact with the soft palate).

Nasal sounds have a lower intensity than oral sounds do (Ball & Lowry, 2001). This is likely because of the airflow being directed through the nasal tract. They are produced by alteration of the resonating cavities of the vocal tract (Calvert, 1986). The velopharyngeal port is open to permit open resonation in the nasal cavity. The oral cavity is completely closed off at some point, forcing the flow of air through the nasal cavity. Calvert indicates that for the production of the [m], the resonating "tube" includes the oral cavity occluded at the lips as well as the open nasal cavity. For [n], resonation occurs in the oral cavity behind and in front of the lingua-alveolar closure and between the open lips. The resonance quality in front of the lingua-alveolar area and open lips assists in the differentiation of the [m] and [n]. The oral cavity with open lips in front of the lingua-velar closure contributes resonance to distinguish [ŋ] from the other two nasal consonants. The nasals have some vowel-like qualities because they result from vocal tract resonance.

There is a syllabic function to the [m] and [n]. As discussed earlier, the nucleus of a syllable is a vowel, with a few exceptions to this rule. One of these exceptions is the replacement of a vowel in certain contexts with [m] or [n] when either occurs at the end of a word or in conversational speaking. There are some logical reasons for this. For example, the word *sudden* has two syllables: *sudd-en*. Notice that the *d* and *n* are homorganic (same placement) and there is minimal, if any, movement of the articulators from the one sound to the other to permit a "slot" for a vowel insertion in the second syllable. Consequently, the transcription of *sudden* is [sʌdn̩] with the dot under the [n] to indicate the syllabic function. Other words that contain homorganic placements share this

characteristic, for example, *fountain* [faʊtn̩] and *mountain* [maʊtn̩]. Of course, these and other words can be pronounced more precisely as [faʊtɪn] and [maʊtɪn], but that is not usually the case.

In conversational speaking, a syllabic [m] or [n] may occur in such contexts as *bread and butter* [brɛd n̩ bʌʔɚ] (remember the "flap *t*"); *not until* [nɑt n̩ tɪl]; and *cup and saucer* [kʌp n̩ sɔsɚ].

The nasal [ŋ] differs from the other nasals in a number of ways (Ladefoged, 1993). In United States English, the [ŋ] does not appear in the initial position in words, only in the medial and final positions, as in *singing* [sɪŋɪŋ]. Unlike the other two nasals, the [ŋ] does not function as a syllabic. It is also restricted in context with the preceding vowels of [ɪ], [ɛ], [æ], [ʌ], [ə], [ɑ], and [ɔ]. When the combination of *nk* or *ng* occurs, the *n* becomes an [ŋ], as in *sank* and *song*. One of the peculiarities in pronunciation is demonstrated by the suffix form. For example, the *g* in *sting-er* [sɪŋɚ] is dropped whereas the same *ng* context is maintained in *finger* [fɪŋgɚ]!

The nasal resonant consonants [m], [n], and [ŋ] are discussed individually in this chapter.

PHONETIC SYMBOL [m]

EXHIBIT 17-1	Phonetic Symbol [m]	
Phonetic Symbol	[m]	**[m]**
Grapheme Symbol	m	
Diacritic Symbol	m	
Phonic Symbol	m	
Homorganic Cognate	Bilabial [p] [b] [m] [ʍ]	
Sound Class	Consonant	
Basic Phonetic Features	Placement: Bilabial Manner: Nasal Resonant Voicing: Plus Voice	
International Phonetic Alphabet (IPA) (International Phonetic Association [IPA], 1999)	[m] #114 Voiced, Bilabial, Nasal	

How the Sound Is Produced

The airflow from the lungs activates the vocal folds (voice), and the sound is directed through the open velopharyngeal port into the nasal cavity (nasal resonant) and out the nostrils. The airflow is also directed into the oral cavity. The lips (bilabial) are together, and the position of the tongue may be at a neutral level or beginning to move toward the position of the vowel that follows. The nasal quality of the [m] sound is imparted to the tone because the soft palate is relaxed to permit the cavity above the soft palate (nasopharynx) and the nasal passages to serve as resonators. The teeth may be slightly open during the production of the [m] sound. See **Figure 17-1**.

Different Spellings for the [m] Sound

Transcribe the following words. Refer to the Key at the right upon completion.

Different Spellings   *Key*

m   mother ____   family ____   mʌðɚ, fæmɪli

       team ____   tim

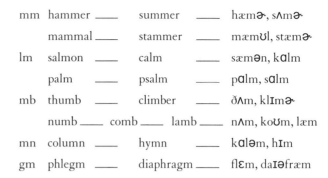

mm	hammer ___	summer	hæmɚ, sʌmɚ
	mammal ___	stammer	mæmʊl, stæmɚ
lm	salmon ___	calm	sæmən, kɑlm
	palm ___	psalm	pɑlm, sɑlm
mb	thumb ___	climber	ðʌm, klaɪmɚ
	numb ___ comb ___ lamb ___		nʌm, koʊm, læm
mn	column ___	hymn	kɑləm, hɪm
gm	phlegm ___	diaphragm ___	flɛm, daɪəfræm

Different Sounds for the Letter *m*

[None]

Rules for Spelling and Pronunciation of the [m] Sound

1. The letter *m* consistently represents the [m] sound, as in *machine, chimney, name*.

2. When two adjacent *m* letters (*mm*) occur, only one [m] sound is pronounced, as in *swimmer, summer, hammock, trimmer*.

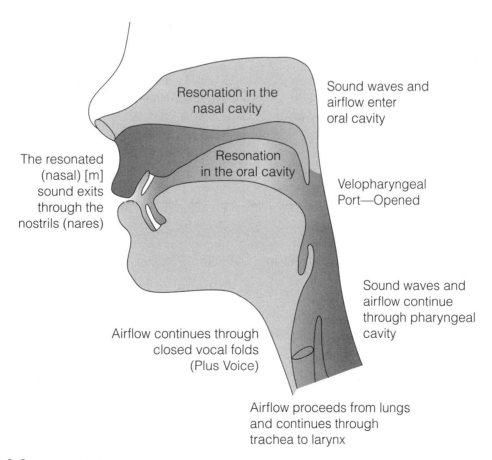

Figure 17-1 [m] pronunciation.

3. In the *lm* context, the *l* is silent when it occurs after *a* or *o*, as in *salmon*.

4. In the *mb* context, the *b* is silent and the [m] becomes the final sound in words such as *numb*, *comb*, *dumb*, *climb*.

5. The *n* is silent in the *mn* context when the [m] is the final sound in the word, as in *column*, *hymn*, *condemn*.

6. The *g* is silent in the *gm* context, as in *phlegm* and *diaphragm*.

Words That Include the [m] Sound

The [m] sound occurs in all three positions, initial, medial, and final. Transcribe the following words. Refer to the Key at the right upon completion.

Initial Consonant		*Key*
marsh ——	mountain ——	mɑrʃ, maʊtən
musician ——	metropolitan ——	mjuzɪʃən, mɛtropɑlɪtən

Medial Consonant

Unstressed Syllable

fireman ——	argument ——	faɪrmæn, arɡumɛnt
hamburger ——	reimburse ——	hæmbɝɡɚ, riɛmbɚs

Stressed Syllable

amuse ——	major ——		əmjuz, meɪdʒɚ
medal ——	movie ——	mattress ——	mɛdḷ, muvi, mætrəs

Final Consonant

flame ——	scream ——	fleɪm, skrim
lame ——	blossom ——	læm, blɔsəm

Initial and Final Consonants

mom ——	maim ——	mɑm, meɪm
maximum ——	monogram ——	mækəməm, mɔnəɡræm

Initial Blend

sm smolder ——	smog ——	smʌðɚ, smɔɡ
smooth ——	smorgasbord ——	smuθ, smɔrɡəsboʊrd

Medial Blends

sm basement ——	classmate ——	beɪsment, klæsmeɪt
dismay ——	transmit ——	dismeɪ, trænsmɪt
rm normal ——	thermos ——	nɔrmʊl, ðɝməs,
farmer ——		fɑrmɚ
airmail ——	foremost ——	ɛrmel, foʊrmoʊst

garment ——			ɡɑrmɛnt
mp computer ——	composition ——		kəmpjutɚ, kɑmpozɪʃən
temporary ——	empower ——		tɛmpɚɛri, ɛmpaʊɚ
attempt ——	lm helmet ——		ətɛmpt, hɛlmɛt,
filmstrip ——			fɪlmstrɪp
hallmark ——	ailment ——		hɑlmɑrk, eɪlmɛnt
installment ——			ɪnstɑlmənt

Final Blends

lm elm ——	film ——	realm ——		ɛlm, fɪlm, rɛlm
helm ——	mp pump ——	champ ——		hɛlm, pʌmp, tʃæmp
bump ——	stamp ——	lamp ——		bʌmp, stæmp, læmp
rm storm ——	worm ——	germ ——		stɔrm, wɝm, ɡɝm
affirm ——	uniform ——			əfɝm, junəfɔrm
mz tombs ——	comes ——	hums ——		tʌmz, kʌmz, hʌmz

Clusters

mpt stumped ——	pumped ——		stʌmpt, pʌmpt
bumped ——	mps shrimps ——		bʌmpt, ʃrɪmps
stamps ——	amps ——		stæmps, æmps

Auditory Discrimination

Transcribe the following words. Refer to the Key at the right upon completion.

Minimal Pairs

[m]	*[n]*	*[m]*	*[ŋ]*	*Key*
me ——	knee ——	dim ——	ding ——	mi, ni, dɪm, dɪŋ
meat ——	neat ——	hum ——	hung ——	mit, nit, hʌm, hʌŋ
meal ——	kneel ——	some ——	sung ——	mɪl, nɪl, sʌm, sʌŋ
foamy ——	phony ——	ram ——	ran ——	foʊmi, foʊni, ræm, ræn

Allophonic and Dialect Variations

The normal nasal resonance may in some cases be assimilated by surrounding vowels, making it difficult to produce and to hear the distinctive nasal quality assigned to the [m] sound as spoken in isolation (Carrell & Tiffany, 1960). Weakening or shortening of the [m] sound may deprive it of a certain sonority but does not interfere with intelligibility. As with all sounds, the context in which it occurs influences the subtle changes in its features, such as in *mom* where in the two [m] sounds are recognized as the same sounds; however, upon closer analysis, there are allophonic differences between the production of the sound in the initial and final positions.

Edwards (1997) indicates that when there is a lengthening of an arresting [m] sound followed by a releasing [m], the second [m] may disappear. The words *Come, Mike* sound like [kʌm: aɪk] combined in a sense as one word, and *Come here* could sound more like "Come mirror" for the same reason. The [m] may also have a different placement of articulation as in *comfort* where the production of the [m] sound shifts from a bilabial to a labiodental position with the upper teeth making contact with the lower lip.

Vowel nasalization replaces the final nasal consonant in African American pronunciation, and the final [m] sound is omitted, as in *come* [kʌ] (Edwards, 1997). There is little variation of the [m] sound (Carrell & Tiffany, 1960). One of the variations is in its function, as explained by Small (1999): In some instances, [m] may become syllabic in conversational speech, depending on the phonetic environment, as in the phrase *wrap them up* [ræpməp]. No doubt the preceding [p] as a bilabial (same as [m]) also plays a role in facilitating the movement to the [m] sound. The [m] and the [b] are produced in the same place of articulation (House, 1998), and if a person's voice quality is denasal because of a blockage in the nasal cavity, the [b] may be substituted for the [m] in conversational speech.

Normal and Deviant Development of the [m] Sound

Children master the [m] sound, as well as the other bilabial sounds [p] and [b], between the ages of 1 and 3 years (Sander, 1972). It is one of the most frequently occurring consonants in United States English speech (Calvert, 1986) and is the easiest to produce of all the consonant phonemes (House, 1998). The [m] sound is one of the first sounds mastered by children (by age 3 years) and is seldom misarticulated (Calvert, 1986).

If any pathologic condition blocks the opening into the nasal pharynx, **denasality**, or the lack of adequate nasal resonance, may be the consequence (Carrell & Tiffany, 1960). Even a severe head cold can produce the same results. Denasality is ordinarily an articulation defect rather than a change in voice quality. Radical changes of all nasals from sonorant to stop consonants may result in changing each nasal to its homorganic stop: [m] becomes [b], [n] becomes [d], and [ŋ] becomes [g].

Nonnative Speaker Pronunciation

Generally, the [m] sound is not a problem for nonnative speakers (Carrell & Tiffany, 1960; Edwards, 1997).

They might have some difficulty distinguishing between the three nasal sounds [n], [m], and [ŋ]. The [m] sound occurs in all of the other 15 prominent languages spoken in the United States, including Spanish, French, German, Italian, Chinese, Tagalog, Polish, Korean, Vietnamese, Portuguese, Japanese, Greek, Arabic, Hindi, and Russian.

Summary

The [m] sound is one of the three nasal consonant sounds. It is consistent in its spelling and sound correspondence and is pronounced as the [m] sound when the letter *m* appears. It is one of the earliest sounds to be mastered and is seldom misarticulated. Nonnative English speakers have little or no difficulty with the sound, particularly because it or its allophonic variations appear in many of the sound systems of languages worldwide.

[m] +

Complete the following word puzzles to increase your phonetic sound/symbol recognition and transcription skills.

Brain Teaser

Provide the orthographic and phonetic spellings of the word that fits the clues given. The first one is completed as an example.

	Orthographic	Phonetic
1. [m] + 7 sounds: often served with cheese	*macaroni*	[_ æ _ ɑ _ oʊ _ i]
2. [m] + 10 sounds: very tiny; not seen with the naked eye	_____	[_ aɪ _ _ o _ _ ɑ _ ɪ _]
3. [m] + 7 sounds: the properties of a magnet	_____	[_ æ _ _ ɛ _ ɪ _]
4. [m] + 10 sounds: something splendid	_____	[_ æ _ _ ɪ _ ɪ _ ɛ _ _]
5. [m] + 8 sounds: uncontrolled growth of tumor	_____	[_ ə _ ɪ _ _ ə _ _]
6. [m] + 6 sounds: human being	_____	[_ æ _ _ aɪ _ _]
7. [m] + 6 sounds: something one reads	_____	[_ æ _ ʌ _ ɪ _]
8. [m] + 5 sounds: tone of a song	_____	[_ ɛ _ oʊ _ i]

9. [m] + 6 sounds: _____ [_ ə _ æ _ I _]
   one who repairs cars

10. [m] + 7 sounds: _____ [_ I _ ə _ I _ i]
    famous river

Key: 1. macaroni [mækərouni]; 2. microscopic [maɪkroskɑpɪk]; 3. magnetic [mægnɛtɪk]; 4. magnificent [mægnɪfɪsɛnt]; 5. malignant [məlɪgnənt]; 6. mankind [mænkaɪnd]; 7. magazine [mægʌzɪn]; 8. melody [mɛloʊdi]; 9. mechanic [məkænɪk]; 10. Mississippi [mɪsəsɪpi]

PHONETIC SYMBOL [n]

EXHIBIT 17-2	Phonetic Symbol [n]	
Phonetic Symbol	[n]	**[n]**
Grapheme Symbol	n	
Diacritic Symbol	n	
Phonic Symbol	n	
Cognate	None	
Homorganic Cognate	Lingua-Alveolar [t], [d], [s], [z], [l], [ʧ], [ʤ]	
Sound Class	Consonant	
Basic Phonetic Features	Placement: Lingua-Alveolar Manner: Nasal Resonant Voicing: Plus Voicing	
IPA (1999)	[n] #116 Voiced, Dental or Alveolar Nasal	

How the Sound Is Produced

The airflow from the lungs makes contact with the closed vocal folds (voiced), and the sound continues through the opened velopharyngeal port and is directed into the nasal cavity where the [n] sound is produced as a nasal resonant as a result of the influence of the resonating characteristics of the sound waves that continue and exit through the nostrils, or **nares**. During this process, the sound waves are also directed through the open oropharynx for resonation of voice in the oral cavity as the sound waves make contact behind the lingua-alveolar closure. This barrier is created as the tip of the tongue closes against the alveolar ridge and the sides of the tongue are pressed against the upper molars. A resonating quality also occurs in front of the lingua-alveolar cavity in the area of the front teeth and lips, which are in an open position. Tongue pressure against the alveolar ridge is less than for two of the [n] sound's homorganic sounds, the [t] and [d]. See **Figure 17-2**.

According to Edwards (1997), some phoneticians consider the [n] sound a **continuant** because of the opened vocal tract through the nasopharynx; that is, the airflow and sound proceed unobstructed above the vocal folds and continue as they exit through the nostrils. VanRiper (1979) shares this viewpoint and considers the [n] sound a lingua-alveolar nasal continuant phoneme. On the other hand, Chomsky and Halle (1968) consider the [n] sound a nasal stop because the airflow and sound are interrupted by the oral cavity blockage. This is consistent with Shriberg and Kent (1994), who indicate that by definition, a nasal consonant (such as [n]) is produced with a complete oral closure (like a stop) but with an open velopharynx so that voicing energy travels out through the nose.

Different Spellings for the [n] Sound

Transcribe the following words. Refer to the Key at the right upon completion.

Different Spellings				*Key*
n	name ___	manual ___	dawn ___	næm, mænul, dɔn
nn	cannot ___	dinner ___	funny ___	kænɔt, dɪnɚ, fʌni

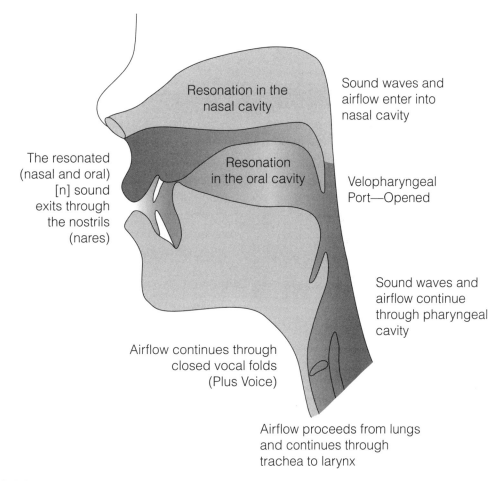

Figure 17-2 [n] pronunciation.

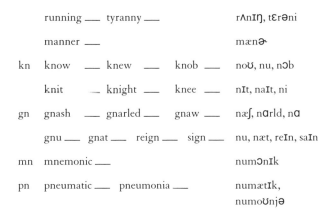

running ___ tyranny ___   rʌnɪŋ, tɛrəni

manner ___   mænɚ

kn   know ___ knew ___ knob ___   noʊ, nu, nɔb

     knit ___ knight ___ knee ___   nɪt, naɪt, ni

gn   gnash ___ gnarled ___ gnaw ___   næʃ, nɑrld, nɑ

     gnu ___ gnat ___ reign ___ sign ___   nu, næt, reɪn, saɪn

mn   mnemonic ___   numɔnɪk

pn   pneumatic ___ pneumonia ___   numætɪk, numoʊnjə

Different Sounds for the Letter *n*

mn   column, solemn (the *n* is silent)

ng [ŋ]   single, sung, tongue

Rules for Spelling and Pronunciation of the [n] Sound

1. The *n* is pronounced as the [n] sound, as in *nun, peanut, can.*

2. The *mn* in the final position is pronounced as [m], as in *solemn, column.*

3. The *mn* in the initial position is pronounced as [n], as in *mnemonic.*

4. Two adjacent *n* letters (*nn*) are pronounced as a single [n] sound, as in *cunning, inning*, and *running*. The [n] is the final sound of the first syllable, although some of its influence may be present in the first part of the second syllable.

5. The *n* is the initial sound in the following contexts: <u>kn</u>ee, <u>gn</u>aw, <u>pn</u>eumonia, and <u>mn</u>emonic. The first phoneme in the [n] blends became silent during MiddleEnglish.

6. The *ng* becomes the [ŋ] sound, as in *sing* [sɪŋ] and *ringing* [rɪŋɪŋ].

The Syllabic [n] Sound

The [n] sound is another of the consonants that can become **syllabic** (function as a vowel), and it does so more often than the [m] or [l] does (Small, 1999; Tiffany &

Carrell, 1977). The syllabic [n] is transcribed as [ņ] with a dot under the [n], as in *fasten* [fæsņ] and *written* [rɪtņ]. The [ņ] represents the "vowel nucleus" rule, thereby functioning as a syllable. This also occurs in conversational speaking; for example, *pants and shirts* is transcribed as [pænts ņ ʃɝts]. The syllabic form of the [n] ([ņ]), such as in *ribbon* [rɪbņ] and *happen* [hæpņ], is used in transcription because the vowel between the two consonants is almost nonexistent. Because of its function as a syllabic, some phoneticians consider the [n] sound a **semivowel**.

Words That Include the [n] Sound

The [n] sound occurs in all three positions, initial, medial, and final. Transcribe the following words. Refer to the Key at the right upon completion.

Initial Consonant			*Key*
note _____	gnat	_____	noʊt, næt
gnarl _____	pneumonia	_____	nɑrl, numoʊnjə

Unstressed Syllable

Medial Consonant

lemonade _____	opener _____	lɛmɔneɪd, oʊpɛnɚ

Stressed Syllable

Medial Consonant

cinnamon _____	mineral _____	sɪnəmən, mɪnɚəl
general _____	manipulate _____	dʒɛnɚəl, mənɪpulet

Final Consonant

green _____	convene _____	grin, kənvin
wagon _____	collection _____	wægən, kəlɛtʃən

Initial and Final Consonants

nun _____	none _____	nine _____	nʌn, nʌn, naɪn

Syllabic Consonant

cotton _____	button _____	fasten _____	kɔtņ, bʌtņ, fæsən

Initial Blend

sn snow _____	sneak _____	snoʊ, snik
snore _____	snail _____	snɔr, sneɪl

Medial Blends

nd handbag _____	Monday _____	hændbæg, mʌndeɪ
thunder _____	condition _____	Ɵʌndɚ, kəndɪʃən

rn furnish _____	warning _____		fɝnɪʃ, wɔrnɪŋ
external _____	tornado _____		ɛkstɝnļ, tɔrneɪdo
ns unseal _____	offensive _____		ənsɪl, ɔfɪnsɪv
uncertain _____	sincere _____		ənsɝtən, sɪnsɪr
nt dental _____	syntax _____		dɛntļ, sɪntæks
contented _____			kɑntɛntɪd
nƟ monthly _____	enthusiast _____		mʌnƟli, ɛnƟuzɪst
anthem _____			ænƟəm

Final Blends

nd tend _____	Ireland _____		tɛnd, aɪɚlənd
commend _____	dividend _____		kɑmɛnd, dɪvədɛnd
nl channel _____	tunnel _____		tʃænəl, tʌnəl
panel _____	national _____		pænəl, næʃənəl
rn corn _____	cavern _____		kɔrn, kævɚn
thorn _____	newborn _____		Ɵɔrn, njubɔrn
ns once _____	rinse _____		wʌns, rɪns
commence _____	fence _____		kʌmɛns, fɛns
nt ant _____	hydrant _____	spent _____	ænt, haɪdrənt, spɛnt
appoint _____	nƟ month _____	tenth _____	əpɔɪnt, mʌnƟ, tɛnƟ
ninth _____	nz tones _____	opens _____	naɪnƟ, toʊnz, oʊpənz
depends _____	rtʃ porch _____	branch _____	dipɛndz, pɔrtʃ, bræntʃ
punch _____	wrench _____		pʌntʃ, rɛntʃ
ndʒ orange _____	manger _____		ɔrɛndʒ, meɪndʒɚ

Clusters

nts or ns tents _____	rents _____		tɛns, rɛns
nʃt benched _____	wrenched _____		bɛnʃt, rɛnʃt
nʒd or nʒ arranged _____	hinged _____		əreɪnʒd, hɪnʒd
nst fenced _____	bounced _____		fɛnst, baʊnst

Auditory Discrimination

Transcribe the following words. Refer to the Key at the right upon completion.

Contrast Minimal Pairs

[n]	[ŋ]	[n]	[m]	*Key*
run ___	rung ___	run ___	rum ___	rʌn, rʌŋ, rʌn, rʌm
thin ___	thing ___	net ___	met ___	Ɵɪn, Ɵɪŋ, nɛt, mɛt
ton ___	tongue ___	no ___	mow ___	tʌn, tʌŋ, noʊ, moʊ

sun ___ sung ___ turns___ terms ___ sʌn, sʌŋ, tɝnz, tɝmz

keen___ king ___ sun ___ sum ___ kin, kiŋ, sʌn, sʌm

Allophonic and Dialect Variations

In addition to the variation as a result of the syllabic [n] discussed earlier, there are considerable allophonic variations in other contexts. For example, the [n] in *knee* may be more forward and even dentalized because of the influence of the front vowel sound that follows [ni] in contrast to the [n] in *new* [nu] or [nju] that is adjacent to a back vowel. It may also become dentalized when it occurs before the labiodental sounds [f] and [v], as in *infinite* and *invade*.

Another assimilative or allophonic change merits attention (Tiffany & Carrell, 1977). When followed by a velar [k] or [g], the [n] may be replaced by [ŋ] (*ng*) and is permissible in some contexts; for example, *conquer* [kɑŋkɚ] and *ink* [iŋk] or [ɪŋk]. It is only in rapid informal speech that pronunciations such as [ɪŋkʌm] for *income* and [ɪŋkwɛst] for *inquest* are acceptable. Otherwise, it may be considered as a substitution error of another nasal resonant consonant.

A different occurrence involves the [n] nasal resonant substitution or allophonic variation in such contexts as when two bilabial sounds, the [m] and [p], are pronounced instead of the [n] and [p], as in *grandpa* [græmpɑ]. This pronunciation appears to be a more natural manner to say such a word.

A lengthening of the [n] sound occurs in such instances, such as *nine nuts* [naɪn:əts], where there is an arrest and release at adjoining syllables. The [n] sound influences other sounds, as in *ridden* (Small, 1999). The "oral" [d] stop is released through the nasal cavity as the velum is lowered in production of the nasal plosive [n].

Edwards (1997) reports that African Americans tend to nasalize the vowel that precedes the [n] sound. For example, the vowel in *run*, which is usually pronounced with only oral resonance, also includes a nasal quality. This is also the same with other speakers who tend to have an increase in nasality in their speech because of regional dialects. If a person's voice is denasal in quality, the [d] may be substituted for the [n] in conversational speech (House, 1998).

Normal and Deviant Development of the [n] Sound

The [n] sound is one of the most frequently occurring sounds (Calvert, 1986) and is second only to the [t] sound in the United States English sound system (Edwards, 1997). It is one of the first sounds that children master by age 3 years (Calvert, 1986; Sander, 1972) and is seldom misarticulated.

The [n] sound is not generally considered a problem (Edwards, 1997). Nasal errors such as with the [n] sound occur only in the very young rather than older children (Shriberg & Kent, 1994). The few errors are (1) deletions and (2) an assortment of variations. It may be difficult to determine whether the [n] sound has been deleted because the assimilative nasality that is normal on the preceding vowel, such as in the word *can* [kæn], may be sufficient to create the impression of the final [n] sound without it being articulated. Compare the [n] sound in the words *no* and *on* and notice the "fading" of the vowel sound into a much weaker [n] sound in *on* as compared with *no*.

Nasal blockage resulting from structural deviations, infections, and other causes may result in a substitution of a denasal sound such as [d], as in *pad* for *pan*, or an intrusion following the [n], as when *pan* becomes *pand*. Devoicing occurs as a result of voiceless emission of the [n] sound, as in *snow*: The [s] is deleted and the [n] becomes devoiced; it is somewhat influenced also by the vowel that follows the [n]. With some practice, you can probably almost pronounce the word *snow* with a devoiced [n], as in [noʊ]. This is also an example of a **cluster reduction** because the [s] sound is deleted. A speaker with a cleft palate may exhibit a voiceless or fricative nasal [n] sound. Such a speaker and others may produce a "glottalized" [n] substitution, as in *enough* [iʔəf] for [inəf] or [ənʌf]. Neurological deficits that result in decreased mobility, endurance, and strength may also affect the production of the [n] sound, particularly during conversational speaking.

Nonnative Speaker Pronunciation

Foreign speakers may need to learn to make the United States English [n] with tongue placement on the alveolar ridge rather than in a more anterior (dental) position involving the upper front teeth (Calvert, 1986). The [n] sound may also be produced in a retroflexed position, adding a different allophonic sound. There may also be a tendency for the [ŋ] sound to be substituted for the [n], as in [sɪŋ] for *sing* [sɪn].

Summary

The [n] sound is one of the three nasal resonant sounds. It is homorganic (lingua-alveolar) with the [t], [d], [s], [z], and [l] and with the first sounds in the affricatives [tʃ] and [dʒ]. The letter *n* represents the [n] sound with the exception of when it is silent, as in *column, solemn*, and in the *ng* context where the two symbols become one sound, the [ŋ] as in *sing*. The [n] sound may function as a semivowel by replacing a vowel, such as in the two-syllable word *fasten* [fæsn̩] or when a phrase such as *shoes and socks* becomes "shoes n̩ socks." The [n] sound is among the first to be acquired, and it occurs in many foreign sound systems with some allophonic variations. Also, nonnative speakers may substitute the [ŋ] sound for the [n]. The peculiar spelling combinations (*knot, gnat*, and *pneumonia*) may present some confusion to nonnative speakers. There is a tendency for the [n] sound to become denasalized among native speakers, including African Americans. The common sound errors among children occur as deletions, denasalization, devoicing, and substitutions.

[n] +

Brain Teaser

Complete the following word game to increase your sound/symbol recognition and transcription skills. Provide the orthographic and phonetic spellings for each of the words.

	Orthographic	Phonetic
1. [n] + 3 sounds: musical scale	_____	[_ oʊ _ _]
2. [n] + 4 sounds: to do something bad	_____	[_ ɑ _ i]
3. [n] + 6 sounds: opposite of positive	_____	[_ e _ ʌ _ ɪ _]
4. [n] + 7 sounds: famous ballet	_____	[_ ə _ _ _ æ _ ɚ]
5. [n] + 6 sounds: Thanksgiving month	_____	[_ o _ ɛ _ _ ɚ]
6. [n] + 5 sounds: western state	_____	[_ ə _ æ _ ə]
7. [n] + 2 sounds: opposite of nephew	_____	[_ i _]
8. [n] + 4 sounds: a fighter's victory	_____	[_ ɑ _ oʊ _]
9. [n] + 2 sounds: a small insect	_____	[_ æ _]
10. [n] + 2 sounds: a figure in royalty	_____	[_ aɪ _]

Key: 1. notes [noʊts]; 2. naughty [aɑti]; 3. negative [neɡʌtɪv]; 4. *Nutcracker* [nətkrækɚ]; 5. November [novɛmbɚ]; 6. Nevada [nəvædə]; 7. niece [nis]; 8. knockout [nɑkaʊt]; 9. gnat [næt]; 10. knight [naɪt].

PHONETIC SYMBOL [ŋ]

EXHIBIT 17-3	**Phonetic Symbol [ŋ]**	
Phonetic Symbol	[ŋ]	**[ŋ]**
Grapheme Symbol	ng	
Diacritic Symbols	ŋ, ŋg, ng	
Phonic Symbol	ŋ	
Homorganic Cognate	Lingua-Alveolar [k], [g], [h], [ʍ]	
Sound Class	Consonant	
Basic Phonetic Features	Placement: Lingua-Alveolar Manner: Nasal Resonant [n] Stop/Plosive [g] Voicing: Plus Voice	
IPA (1999)	[ŋ] #119 Voiced, Alveolar Nasal	

How the Sound Is Produced

The airflow from the lungs activates the vocal folds (voice), and the sound is directed through the open velopharyngeal port. Before the sound enters the nasal cavity and exits out of the nostrils, the back of the tongue (lingua) is in contact with the front portion of the velum (velar). The tongue is held briefly in this position and then released in a motion that resembles the motion for the plosives [k] and [g]. Tongue contact pressure with the velum is less than that for the [g] or [k]. During the production of the [ŋ] sound, the lips and teeth are apart and the tip of the tongue rests behind the lower front teeth. See **Figure 17-3**.

Different Spellings for the [ŋ] Sound

Transcribe the following words. Refer to the Key at the right upon completion.

Different Spellings					*Key*
nk	think	___	thank	___	θɪŋk, θæŋk
	twinkle	___	spunky	___	twɪŋkl̩, spʌŋki

nc	bronco	___	bunko	___		brɑŋkoʊ, bʌŋkoʊ
ng	single	___	angle	___	jungle ___	sɪŋgl̩, æŋgl̩, dʒʌŋgl̩
nd	handkerchief	___				heŋkɝtʃɪf
nx	anxious	___	lynx	___	pharynx ___	æŋksəs, lɪŋks, fɛrɪŋks
ngue	meringue	___	tongue	___		mɝeŋ, tʌŋ
ngs	swings	___	things	___	savings ___	swɪŋz, θɪŋz, seɪvɪŋz

Different Sounds for the Letters *ng*

Transcribe the following words. Refer to the Key at the right upon completion.

			Key
[ŋg]	finger	_____	fɪŋgɚ
[ŋg]	vanguard	_____	væŋgɑrd

Rules for Spelling and Pronunciation of the [ŋ] Sound

I. The [ŋ] sound or spelling never occurs in the initial position of United States English words.

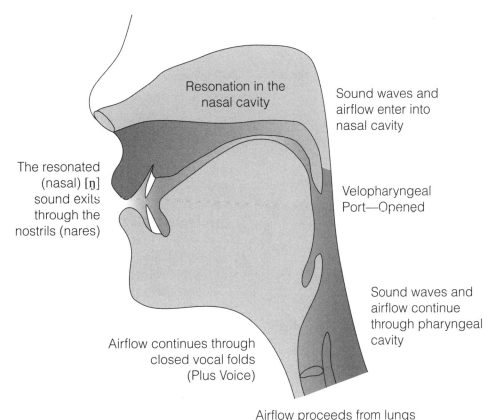

Resonation in the nasal cavity

Sound waves and airflow enter into nasal cavity

The resonated (nasal) [ŋ] sound exits through the nostrils (nares)

Velopharyngeal Port—Opened

Sound waves and airflow continue through pharyngeal cavity

Airflow continues through closed vocal folds (Plus Voice)

Airflow proceeds from lungs and continues through trachea to larynx

Figure 17-3 [ŋ] pronunciation.

2. In the *nc* context, the *n* becomes the [ŋ] sound and the *c* the [k] sound, as in *bronco, bunko* but not as in *pancake* and *encode* where the [n] is pronounced.

3. In the *nk* context, the [ŋ] sound is followed by the voiceless [k] sound, as in *blinker, donkey, twinkle, banking, chipmunk.*

4. In the *ng* context, the [n] sound is followed by the voiced [g] sound, as in *anger, anguish, swing, hanger.* It may not be as obvious in words such as *singer* and *stronger.*

5. An unusual combination is *nd*, as in *handkerchief.*

6. The *n* is pronounced as [ŋ] in the *nx* spelling context, as in *anxiety, anxious, pharynx, larynx.*

7. In words spelled with the *ngue* ending, the *gue* letters are silent and [ŋ] is the final sound, as in *tongue, meringue.*

8. In the letter combination of *ngs*, the *ng* becomes the [ŋ] sound and the *s* is the [z] sound, as in *brings, wrongs, things, paintings.*

Words That Include the [ŋ] Sound

The [ŋ] sound does not occur in the initial or prevocalic sound position but occurs in the medial and final positions. Transcribe the following words. Refer to the Key at the right upon completion.

Initial Consonant   *Key*

[None]

Unstressed Syllable

Medial Consonant

[None]

Stressed Syllable

Medial Consonant

anger	_____	angel	_____	eɪŋɚ, eɪŋʒəl
triangle	_____	stronger	_____	traɪeŋgl, strɑŋgɚ

Final Consonant

cling	_____	collapsing	_____	klɪŋ, kɔlæpsɪŋ
wrong	_____	awarding	_____	rɔŋ, əwɔrdɪŋ

Consonant Blends

<u>ng</u> finger	_____	longer	_____	fɪŋgɚ, lɑŋgɚ

language	_____	<u>nk</u> blanket	_____	læŋkwɪdʒ, bleɪŋkɪt
sink	_____			sɪŋk
<u>nks</u> honks	_____	thinks	_____	hɔŋks, θɪŋks
<u>nkt</u> junked	_____	banked	_____	dʒʌŋkt, beɪŋkt
spanked	_____			speɪŋkt
<u>nd</u> banged	_____	belonged	_____	beɪŋd, bilɑŋd

Auditory Discrimination

Transcribe the following words. Refer to the Key at the right upon completion.

Contrast Minimal Pairs

[ŋ]	[g]	[ŋ]	[n]	*Key*
hung ___	hug ___	king ___	kin ___	hʌŋ, hʌg, kɪŋ, kɪn
ping ___	pig ___	sung ___	sun ___	pɪŋ, pɪg, sʌŋ, sʌn
long ___	log ___	gong ___	gone ___	lɑŋ, lɑg, gɔŋ, gɔn

[ŋ]	[ŋk]	[ŋ]	[ŋg]	*Key*
ring ___	rink ___	finger ___	linger ___	rɪŋ, rɪŋk, fɪŋgɚ, lɪŋgɚ
sung ___	sunk ___			sʌŋ, sʌŋk
clang ___	clank ___			kleɪŋ, kleɪŋk

Allophonic and Dialect Variations

Allophonic variations occur as a result of the context in which the [ŋ] sound is positioned. Three factors that determine these variations are syllable stress, whether the sound occurs in the medial or final position, and the features of the surrounding sounds. Such variations are usually acoustically acceptable to the listener and may hardly be perceived as different. For example, the [ŋ] in *song* and *sing* is different because the vowels are in different positions (back, low, lax vs. front, high, tense). Primary and secondary stress of the two-syllable word *singing* demonstrates the influence of allophonic differences in which the [ŋ] in the first syllable has more strength than the final [ŋ], which often is changed to a nonallophonic [n] sound as in *singin'.*

The physiologic explanation for the tendency of [n] to become [ŋ] before velar sounds is a simple one (Carrell & Tiffany, 1960). The [ŋ] sound is a "tongue-body" consonant. It uses the same part of the tongue that is used to form [k] and [g] and the vowels. Therefore, it is expected that considerable coarticulation among these sounds occurs with the assimilation of features of one to the others.

In informal speech, the [ŋ] (*ing*) ending is frequently pronounced as [ɪn], as in *singing* [sɪŋɪn] and *walking* [wɔkɪn] or [wɑkɪn] (Calvert, 1986). Edwards (1997) indicates that a nasalization of the vowel preceding the [ŋ] occurs in African American speech. In General American speech, the [ŋ] becomes an [n] in such words as *strength* [strɛŋθ], which becomes [strɛnθ], and there may be a stop or hard release in such words as *king* [kɪŋ], which becomes [kɪŋg] and [sɪŋgɚ] for *singer* [sɪŋɚ].

Although the [ŋ] sound is always followed by the voiced, velar stop [g] in such words as *English* and *finger* (Small, 1999), the [ŋ] and [g] combination may be variable as in *hanger* [hæŋgɚ] or [hæŋɚ] (or [heɪŋɚ]) and *singer* [sɪŋgɚ] or [sɪŋɚ], depending on the individual speaker differences and/or dialect. The [ŋ] is produced as a nasal release of the voiced air stream (House, 1998). If a person's voice is denasal in quality (the nasal cavity is blocked), the [g] may be substituted for the [ŋ] in conversational speech.

Normal and Deviant Development of the [ŋ] Sound

The [ŋ] sound is one of the first sounds children master (Calvert, 1986), and Sander (1972) indicates that it is acquired between the ages of 2 and 6 years. A very common error made by beginners is to substitute [n] and [k] as in *thank* [θeɪnk] for [θeɪŋk] and *ink* [ɪnk] for [ɪŋk] (VanRiper, 1979).

The [ŋ] sound may not be developed until as late as 6 years of age, and according to Calvert (1986), it is seldom misarticulated. He states that in informal pronunciation, the *–ing* ending is frequently pronounced as [ɪn] as in *singing* [sɪŋɪn] with the substitution of the [n] for the [ŋ] sound.

As with the other two nasals [n] and [m], one of the difficulties is to determine whether the sound is deleted or not as a result of the assimilation of the preceding vowel influence (Shriberg & Kent, 1994). The word *sang* may sound to the listener as [seɪ] with little or no final [ŋ] influence. Denasalization may occur when the [g] sound is substituted for the [ŋ] sound, as in *thing* [θɪg] for [θɪŋ].

Nonnative Speaker Pronunciation

Foreign dialect errors are not frequent, although a few examples include Yiddish in which the final [ŋ] may have an added stop, as in [goɪŋk] for *going* (Carrell & Tiffany, 1960). Nasals resembling [n] are sometimes present because of the influence of another language. A fronted or palatized [ŋ] or a uvular production is not standard in English but may be heard as variants.

Summary

The [ŋ] is one of the three nasal sounds. It is classified as a lingua-velar, nasal resonant [n] followed by a stop/plosive [g], resulting in the single [ŋ] sound. In United States English, the [ŋ] sound does not appear in the initial position in words, and it is rather consistent in its pronunciation. It is normally acquired between the ages of 2 and 6 years, and in informal speech, the final [ŋ] sound may be substituted with an [n] as in *runnin'*. Nonnative speakers tend to add a [k] sound after the [ŋ] sound, as in *going* [goʊɪŋk]. The [ŋ] sound occurs in approximately 50% of the predominant languages other than English spoken in the United States. Typical speech sound errors include the omission of the [ŋ] and/or the denasalization of the sound. It is not generally considered to be a difficult sound to produce unless there are some pathological deficiencies related to the auditory or neuromuscular mechanisms.

[ŋ] +

Brain Teaser

Complete the following word game to increase your sound/symbol recognition and transcription skills. Provide the orthographic and phonetic spellings for each of the words.

	Orthographic	*Phonetic*
1. 2 sounds + [ŋ]: we sing it	_____	[_ ɑ _]
2. 2 sounds + [ŋ]: the noise of a telephone	_____	[_ ɪ _]
3. 4 sounds + [ŋ]: a season of the year	_____	[_ _ _ ɪ _]
4. 2 sounds + [ŋ]: an object is a	_____	[_ ɪ _]
5. 2 sounds + [ŋ]: a body part	_____	[_ ʌ _]
6. 3 sounds + [ŋ]: informal speech	_____	[_ _ eɪ _]

7. 5 sounds + [ŋ]: _____ [ɛ _ ə _ ɪ _]
   night time

8. 4 sounds + [ŋ]: _____ [_ ɛ _ ɪ _]
   marriage

9. 3 sounds + [ŋ]: _____ [_ _ ɪ _]
   bee "sore"

10. 4 sounds + [ŋ]: _____ [_ eɪ _ ɪ _]
    to do in the oven

Key: 1. song [sɑŋ]; 2. ring [rɪŋ]; 3. spring [sprɪŋ]; 4. thing [Θɪŋ]; 5. tongue [tʌŋ]; 6. slang [slcɪŋ]; 7. evening [ɛvənɪŋ]; 8. wedding [wɛdɪŋ]; 9. sting [stɪŋ]; 10. baking [beɪkɪŋ]

NASAL RESONANT CONSONANTS: CONCLUSION

English has three nasal stop consonants, one bilabial [m], one alveolar [n], and one velar [ŋ] (Edwards, 1997). They have the same placement as oral stops. They involve complete closure between two articulators, but there is no velopharyngeal closure during their production, and the airflow enters into the nasal cavity. Unlike oral stops that include cognate pairs, [p], [b], [t], [d], [k], and [g], all nasal stops are voiced.

CHARACTERISTICS OF THE FOUR ORAL RESONANT CONSONANTS

United States English contains four oral resonant consonants:

- [w] Bilabial, lingua-velar, oral resonant, glide
- [j] Linguapalatal, oral resonant, glide
- [l] Lingua-alveolar, oral resonant, lateral
- [r] Linguapalatal, oral resonant, liquid

The oral resonant consonant [r], the contemporary symbol [ɹ], is discussed previously in this text and is included in this chapter as it relates to the other oral resonant consonants.

The semantic terms phoneticians use to describe the oral resonant sounds vary, and such labels are often abstract, difficult to explain, and difficult to understand conceptually. The terms used in the preceding list are commonly used among phoneticians, but these four sounds are also classified as voiced approximants (Ladefoged, 1993). Ladefoged (1993) considers the [w], [ɹ], and [j] as central approximants and the [l] as a lateral approximant. In United States English, the [w] and [j] do not appear in the final position in words, and when [w] or [l] appear in a consonant blend, they almost become voiceless, as in *twin* and *claim*. Intentionally pronounce the *tw* in *twin* and contrast it with *win* to demonstrate how the voiceless characteristic becomes more apparent. In some dialects, the [j] may also appear as a consonant blend, as in *few* [fju] and *tune* [tjun].

The term *on-glide* is used in conjunction with [w] and [j] in that they glide rapidly into the next sound. The [l] is sometimes referred to as a glide, but more often it is considered a lateral because the tip of the tongue elevates to touch the alveolar ridge and the back of the tongue touches the soft palate, and thus the air flows around the sides of the tongue laterally.

The [r] and [l] are frequently grouped as *liquids*. Unfortunately, this term is difficult to define (Edwards, 1997) and often is confusing. There is nothing particularly "gurgly" or "liquid-like" regarding the production of the [r] and [l] (Edwards, 1997). The term *retroflex* also is used to describe the [r] in that it is produced in a position where the tongue tip flexes toward the back of the oral cavity. To add to the semantic confusion, the oral resonants are also referred to as semivowels or vowelized consonants because of their similarity to vowels.

The quality of resonance of both the oral and nasal consonants may be explained in contrast to how the airflow is modified for stops and fricative consonants. The airflow for stops is interrupted and then released. For fricatives, the airflow is constricted but continues to flow. For oral resonant consonants, the changes in the oral cavity, mainly resulting from lowering or raising the mandible, elevating or lowering the tongue, and varying the opening and rounding of the lips while the velopharyngeal port is closed, shape the oral cavity, which influences the amplification of certain bands of acoustic energy while reducing others. And so instead of an interruption or constriction, the sound waves are acted on as they make contact with the surfaces of the oral cavity and the channels through which they pass. The oral resonant consonants [w], [j], and [l] are individually discussed.

PHONETIC SYMBOL [w]

EXHIBIT 17-4	Phonetic Symbol [w]	

		[w]
Phonetic Symbol	[w]	
Grapheme Symbols	w, wh	
Diacritic Symbol	w	
Phonic Symbol	w	
Cognate	None	
Homorganic Cognate	Lingua-Alveolar [k], [g], [h], [ʍ], [ŋ]	
Sound Class	Consonant/Glide	
Basic Phonetic Features	Placement: Bilabial, Lingua-Velar Manner: Glide Voicing: Plus Voice, Oral Resonant	
IPA (1999)	[w] #170 Voiced, Labial-Velar, Approximant	

How the Sound Is Produced

The airflow from the lungs activates the vibration of the vocal folds (voiced). The velopharyngeal port is closed, and the sound is directed into the oral cavity and through the rounded lips (bilabial) for the production of the [w] sound. No audible friction is created as the airflow proceeds from the vocal folds and exits through the mouth. The original posture of the lips and tongue is quickly modified (glide) by gliding into the position of the vowel sound that follows. See **Figure 17-4**.

During the production of the [w] sound, the airflow contact with the palate is significant as the tongue moves from a high-back position and then makes adjustments for the vowel that follows. Therefore, in a way, the linguapalatal articulators may be included in the description of the placement of the articulators for the production of the [w] sound. The [w] sound is of short duration and is always released into a vowel sound.

Different Spellings for the [w] Sound

Transcribe the following words. Refer to the Key at the right upon completion.

Different Spellings				Key
w	was ___	wear ___	someway ___	wɔz, wɛr, sʌmweɪ
	reward ___	sandwich ___		riwɑrd, sændwɪdʒ

qu	queen ___	quick ___ require ___	kwɪn, kwɪk, rekwaɪr
	consequent ___	liquid ___	kɑnsikwɛnt, lɪkwʊd
gu	agua ___	jaguar ___	ægwɑ, dʒægwɑr
	distinguish ___	linguist ___	dɪstɪŋkwɪʃ, lɪnkwɪst
o	one ___	once ___	wʌn, wʌns
cho	choir ___		kwaɪr
wh	whooping (cough) ___		hupɪŋ
w	owe ___	how ___ low ___	oʊ, haʊ, loʊ

Different Sounds for the Letter *w*

Transcribe the following words. Refer to the Key at the right upon completion.

Phonetic Symbol	Word	Alphabet Letter	Word	Phonetic Symbol	Key
[w]	went	___ w	when ___	[ʍ]	wɛnt, ʍɛn
[w]	was	___ w	write ___	Silent	wɑz, raɪt
[w]	bilingual	___ u	us ___	[ʌ]	baɪlɪŋgwəl, ʌs
[w]	queen	___ u	use ___	[u]	kwin, jus
[w]	one	___ o	on ___	[ɑ]	wʌn, ɑn
Silent	whooping	___ w	which ___	[ʍ]	hupɪŋ, wɪtʃ
Silent	two	___ w	twin ___	[w]	tu, twɪn

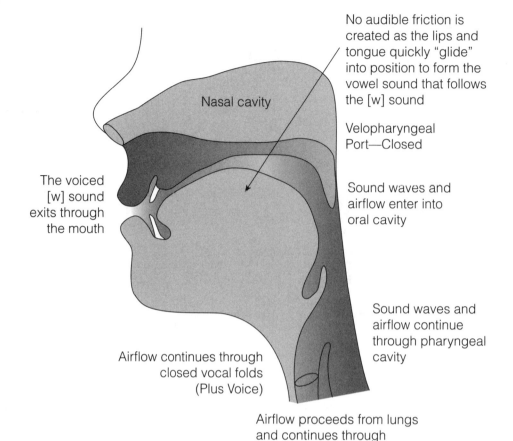

No audible friction is created as the lips and tongue quickly "glide" into position to form the vowel sound that follows the [w] sound

Velopharyngeal Port—Closed

Nasal cavity

Sound waves and airflow enter into oral cavity

The voiced [w] sound exits through the mouth

Sound waves and airflow continue through pharyngeal cavity

Airflow continues through closed vocal folds (Plus Voice)

Airflow proceeds from lungs and continues through trachea to larynx

Figure 17-4 [w] pronunciation.

Rules for Spelling and Pronunciation of the [w] Sound

1. The *w* is pronounced as a [w] sound in the initial and medial positions in words such as *weather, worship, wealthy, hideaway, unaware,* and *sidewalk.*

2. The *u* in the *qu* context is pronounced as [k] [w], as in *quiet, quality, question, frequent, equip,* and *banquet.*

3. In the *gu* context, the *u* functions as a [w] sound, as in *language, iguana, bilingual,* and *penguin.*

4. Words such as *one* and *once* that begin with the *o* letter are begun with a [w] sound, [w] + one.

5. A unique pronunciation occurs with the [w] replacing the *o* letter in the word *choir.* Also, the spelling of *Duane* versus *Dwayne* still has the [w] sound.

6. The word *whooping* (cough) is generally pronounced without any acknowledgment given to the *w,* that is, "hooping cough."

7. Whenever the *w* letter appears at the end of a word, the [w] sound is silent.

8. There is an intrusion of the [w] sound in *memoirs* [mɛmwɑrz].

Words That Include the [w] Sound

Transcribe the following words. Refer to the Key at the right upon completion.

Initial Consonant		Key
warrant _____	worker _____	wɔrənt, wɝkɚ
world _____	"Y" _____	wɝld, waɪ
watch _____	without _____	wɑtʃ, wɪθaʊt

Unstressed Syllable

Medial Consonant

going ____	lower ____	goʊɪŋ, loʊɚ
kiwi ____	homework ____	kiwi, hoʊmwɝk
pathway ____		pæθweɪ

Stressed Syllable

Medial Consonant

away	_____	quickly	_____	əweɪ, kwɪkli
acquiring	_____	anguish	_____	əkwaɪrɪŋ, eɪŋkwɪʃ
bewitch	_____			biwɪtʃ

Initial Blends

sw swing	_____	swift	_____	swɪŋ, swɪft
gw (kw) Gwyn	_____	guava	_____	kwɛn, kwævə
guacamole	_____			kwɔkʌmɑli
tw twine	_____ twin _____ twenty _____			twaɪn, twɪn, twɛnti
dw dwell	_____	Dwayne	_____	dwɛl, dweɪn

Medial Blends

rw doorway	_____	Erwin	_____	dɔrweɪ, ɝwɪn
forward	_____	silverware	_____	fɔrwɝd, sɪlvɚwɛr

Consonant Cluster

skw square	_____			skwɛr
squeaky	_____	squirrel	_____	skwiki, skɚəl̩

Auditory Discrimination

Transcribe the following words. Refer to the Key at the right upon completion.

[w]		[r]		[w]		[v]		Key
wife	__	rife	__	worse	__	verse	__	waɪf, raɪf, wɝs, vɝs
quack	__	crack	__	west	__	vest	__	kwæk, kræk, wɛst, vɛst
wake	__	rake	__	wine	__	vine	__	weɪk, reɪk, waɪn, vaɪn
one	__	run	__	wary	__	very	__	wʌn, rʌn, wɛri, vɛri
wave	__	rave	__	wow	__	vow	__	weɪv, reɪv, waʊ, vaʊ
wed	__	red	__	wail	__	veil	__	wɛd, rɛd, weɪl, veɪl
twill	__	trill	__	waltz	__	vaults	__	twɪl, trɪl, wɔlts, vɔlts
went	__	rent	__	wane	__	vane	__	wɛnt, rɛnt, weɪn, veɪn

[w]		[ʍ] or [hw]		[w]		[f]		Key
way	__	whey	__	wear	__	fair	__	weɪ, ʍeɪ, wɛr, fɛr
weather	__	whether	__	wine	__	fine	__	wɛðɚ, ʍɛðɚ, waɪn, faɪn
wear	__	where	__	wile	__	file	__	wɛr, ʍɛr, waɪl, faɪl
wine	__	whine	__	world	__	furled	__	waɪn, ʍaɪn, wɝld, fɝld
watt	__	what	__	way	__	fey	__	wɔt, ʍʌt, weɪ, feɪ
wile	__	while	__	were	__	fir	__	waɪl, ʍaɪl, wɝs, fɝ
way	__	whey	__	wife	__	fife	__	weɪ, ʍeɪ, waɪf, faɪf
witch	__	which	__	will	__	fill	__	wɪtʃ, ʍɪtʃ, wɪl, fɪl

Allophonic and Dialect Variations

The [w] sound may be produced as a sound that more closely resembles the [ʍ] sound. Although the [w] sound may seem to be a relatively stable sound with little or no variation in speech, this is not the case in a strictly acoustic or physiologic sense (Carrell & Tiffany, 1960). When a vowel and consonant are fairly strongly rounded as in *woo* and *woe*, relatively little unrounding is possible, resulting in extremely close lip rounding that creates a fricative allophonic quality. Similarly, the [w] sound is altered when followed by a front, unrounded vowel, as in *we* [wi]. Carrell and Tiffany (1960) provide a classic example of the change in usage of the [w] sound as presented in the word *toward* [tuwɔrd], which became [twɔrd] and finally [tɔrd]. No significant dialect variation has been reported for [w] (Edwards, 1997).

Normal and Deviant Development of the [w] Sound

The [w] sound is mastered early, by age 3 years (Calvert, 1986), and is seldom misarticulated. The [w] may be omitted as a single sound or in a cluster, as when *queen* [kwin] becomes [kin] (Edwards, 1997).

Nonnative Speaker Pronunciation

In the absence of rounding, a bilabial fricative is produced that may be perceived as a labiodental [v] (Edwards, 1997). Also, tongue position influences the outcome of the sound, resulting in a [g] or a velar fricative allophonic variation.

The U. S. Census Report for 1990 includes a listing of the prominent languages spoken in the United States other than English. According to the *Handbook of the International Phonetic Association* and other sources, the following languages include a [w] sound similar to that of United States English or an allophonic variation of it: Spanish, Chinese, French, Italian, Japanese, Arabic, Polish, Vietnamese, Tagalog, and Russian. Those languages that do not include the [w] in their sound system are German, Greek, Korean, Portuguese, and Hindi.

Summary

The [w] sound is one of the four oral resonant sounds. It does not have a cognate, although there are similarities between the voiceless [ʍ], or as it is sometimes transcribed [hw], particularly because the [w] is quite frequently substituted for the [ʍ]. It is homorganic (lingua-velar) with [k], [g], [h], [ʍ], and [ŋ] and bilabial with [p], [b], [m], and [ʍ]. There are several differences in the use of the letter *w* for the [w] sound as well as other letters that represent the [w] sound such as *u* in *queen*, *o* in *choir*, and silent as in *two*. The [w] sound is mastered early by age 3 years. The [w] appears to be a rather stable sound in its pronunciation except in certain contexts that are influenced by the rounding of the lips.

PHONETIC SYMBOL [J]

EXHIBIT 17-5	Phonetic Symbol [j]	
Phonetic Symbol	[j]	**[j]**
Grapheme Symbols	i, j, y	
Diacritic Symbols	j, y	
Phonic Symbol	j	
Homorganic Cognate	Linguapalatal [ʃ], [ʒ], [r], [h]	
Sound Class	Consonant	
Basic Phonetic Features	Placement: Lingua-Palatal Manner: Glide (Oral Resonant) Voicing: Plus Voice	
IPA (1999)	[j] #153 Voiced, Palatal, Approximant	

How the Sound Is Produced

The [j] sound occurs when the airflow activates the vocal folds (voiced) and the sound is directed upward into the oral cavity. The velopharyngeal port is closed. The tip of the tongue (lingua) is positioned behind the lower front teeth and the front-middle of the tongue is raised high toward the palate (palatal). The [j] sound may also be made with the front of the tongue raised toward, but not touching, the anterior part of the hard palate. The glide is made as the tongue moves to the position from the following vowel sound. See **Figure 17-5**.

Different Spellings for the [j] Sound

Transcribe the following words. Refer to the Key at the right upon completion.

Different Spellings			*Key*
y yellow ___	yet ___	lawyer ___	jɛlo, jɛt, lɔjɚ
yield ___	yoyo ___	coyote ___	jɪld, joʊjo, kaɪjoʊti
j hallelujah ___			haʊləlujə
i union ___	Daniel ___		junjən, dænjʊl
William ___	stallion ___		wɪljəm, stæljən
u blending with [u] for use ___	cute ___		juz, kjut
l bouillon ___			bɔljən
ew blending with [u] as in pew ___	few ___		pju, fju
ue blending with [u] as in Europe ___ fuel ___			jorəp, fjul
[but not in words like *future* and *argue*]			
eu blending with [u] as in feud ___			fjud
e azalea ___			əzeɪljə

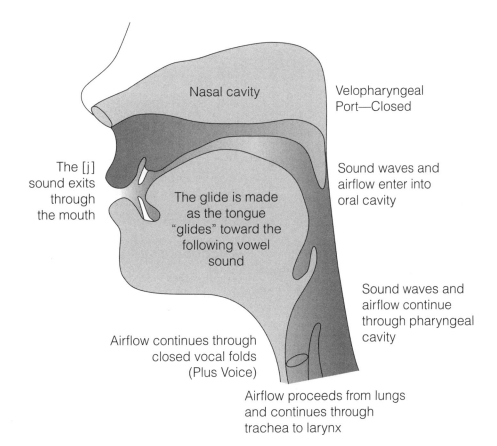

- Nasal cavity
- Velopharyngeal Port—Closed
- The [j] sound exits through the mouth
- The glide is made as the tongue "glides" toward the following vowel sound
- Sound waves and airflow enter into oral cavity
- Sound waves and airflow continue through pharyngeal cavity
- Airflow continues through closed vocal folds (Plus Voice)
- Airflow proceeds from lungs and continues through trachea to larynx

Figure 17-5 [j] pronunciation.

Different Sounds of the Letters That Produce the [j] Sound

Transcribe the following words. Refer to the Key at the right upon completion.

Phonetic Symbol	Word	Alphabet Letter	Word	Phonetic Symbol	Key
[j]	yoyo	___ y	city ___	[i] or [ɪ]	joʊjo, sɪtɪ
[j]	hallelujah ___	j	jam ___	[ʤ]	haʊləlujə, ʤæm
[j]	union ___	i	it ___	[ɪ]	junjən, ɪt

Rules for Spelling and Pronunciation of the [j] Sound

1. The written *y* is pronounced as [j] in the initial position of a word or a syllable, as in *young, yolk, year*, and in the medial position, as in *coyote, lawyer*.

2. With few exceptions, the *j* letter represents the [j] sound, such as *hallelujah*.

3. The [j] sound is represented by the *i* letter, as in *stallion, lion, billiard*.

4. The [j] sound is used in context with [u] (the long *u*), as in *cute*.

5. In the *ew* context, the [j] is pronounced before *ew* ([u]) sound, as in *few, ewe*.

6. In the *ue* ([u]) context, the [j] sound is pronounced, as in *cue, fuel*.

7. In the *eu* ([u]) context, the [j] sound is pronounced, as in *feud, feudal*.

8. With very few exceptions, the [j] has no relation to the *j* letter of the English alphabet.

9. Some words have the [j] sound without a corresponding *y* English alphabet letter.

10. The [j] sound never occurs at the end of a word. The *y* at the end of a word is pronounced as a vowel, as in *city, pretty, tidy*.

Words That Include the [j] Sound

Note: The [j] sound occurs in all three positions, initial, medial, and final. Keep in mind that the [ɑ] and [ɔ] and [j] in the [ju] context is optional depending on dialect.

Also, if the [j] is elongated, there is a tendency for it to glide into a high front vowel such as [ɪ] or [i] such as "A" [eɪjɪ] or [eɪji].

Transcribe the following words. Refer to the Key at the right upon completion.

Initial Consonant   *Key*

yacht ___   yawn ___   jɑt, jɔn

yard ___   your ___ yen ___ youth ___   jɑrd, jɔr, jɛn, juΘ

Unstressed Syllable

Medial Consonant

million ___   kayak ___   mɪljən, kaɪjæk

unused ___   senior ___   amuse ___   ənjuzd, sinjɚ, əmjuz

Stressed Syllable

Medial Consonant

stimulate ___   monument ___   stɪmjulet, mɑnjumɛnt

confusion ___   transfusion ___   kənfjuʃən, trænsfjuʃən

stipulate ___   valiantly ___   stɪpjulet, væljʌntli

Initial Blends

vj view ___ viewed ___ hj hue ___   vju, vjud, hju

human ___ humor ___   hjumən, hjumɚ

humid ___   hjumɪd

fj few ___ fuse ___ kj cue ___cure ___   fju, fjuz, kju, kjur

cute ___ pj puny ___ mj mule ___   kjut, pjuni, mjul

mute ___ mew ___   mjut, mju

Final (dialectal)

A ___   hay ___   I ___   eɪji, heɪji, aɪji

Auditory Discrimination

Transcribe the following words. Refer to the Key at the right upon completion.

[j]	[dʒ]	[j]	[w]	Key
yell ___	jell ___	yield ___	wield ___	jɪl, dʒɛl, jɪld, wɪld
Yale ___	jail ___	Yale ___	wail ___	jeɪl, dʒeɪl, jeɪl, weɪl
yak ___	Jack ___	yet ___	wet ___	jæk, dʒæk, jɛt, wɛt
you'll ___	jewel ___	yell ___	well ___	jul, dʒul, jɛl, wɛl
yo ___	Joe ___	yoke ___	woke ___	joʊ, dʒoʊ, joʊk, woʊk
yolk ___	joke ___	yes ___	Wes ___	joʊk, dʒoʊk, jɛs, wɛs
yaw ___	jaw ___	yacht ___	watt ___	jɑ, dʒɑ, jɑt, wɑt
use ___	juice ___	yaks ___	wax ___	jus, dʒus, jæks, wæks

[j]	[r]	[j]	[l]	Key
you'll ___	rule ___	your ___	lure ___	jul, rul, jɔr, lɔr
yum ___	rum ___	use ___	lose ___	jʌm, rʌm, juz, luz
yen ___	wren ___	year ___	leer ___	jɛn, wrɛn, jɪr, lɪr
yip ___	rip ___	yip ___	lip ___	jɪp, rɪp, jɪp, lɪp
yo ___	row ___	yegg ___	leg ___	joʊ, roʊ, jɛg, lɛg
yak ___	rack ___	yacht ___	lot ___	jæk, ræk, jɑt, lɑt
Yale ___	rail ___	few ___	flew ___	jeɪl, reɪl, fju, flju
you'd ___	rude ___	yo ___	low ___	jud, rud, joʊ, loʊ

Allophonic and Dialect Variations

The [j], when released into [u], is sometimes considered to form a glide–vowel combination or diphthong, [ju] as in *use* [juz] and *few* [fju] (Calvert, 1986). An off-glide is a type of restressing as in *beauty* [beuti] : [bejuti] (Edwards, 1997). The continual motion of the articulators is what characterizes the [j] sound as a glide (Small, 1999). Because the articulators change while gliding from [j] to the following vowel, a corresponding change occurs in relation to the resonance of the vocal tract. Allophonic variations occur as the context varies resulting from the positioning of the prevocalic sound (high, front vs. low, back, etc.). The [j] glide is sometimes called a semivowel because it shares certain features with vowels (Edwards, 1997). For example, the tongue position for the [j] is very similar to that for the vowel [i]. Small (1999) offers this example to demonstrate the similarity in articulation for the glide [j] and the vowel [i]: Prolong the initial [j] phoneme while saying *yam* [jæm] and notice that the [i] vowel will be present before the [j] sound, as in [iiiiijæm].

There are no significant dialect variations (Edwards, 1997) for the [j]. There are some dialectical variations with regard to the use of the [ju] and some speakers sound. They use it distinctly, while others may use it to an allophonic degree or not at all, as in the words *acute, argue, future*.

Normal and Deviant Development of the [j] Sound

Children generally master the [j] sound by age 4 years (Sander, 1972), and satisfactory production does not ordinarily offer much of a problem (Carrell & Tiffany, 1960). Children may learn it readily, although it may be omitted in words such as *yes* [ɛs] and *you* [u], characteristic of "infantile" speech. The [j] sound may be omitted, especially in clusters, and the [w] sound may be substituted for it (Edwards, 1997). Another substitution is the [l] when the [j] assimilates to [l], as in *yellow* [lɛlo].

Nonnative Speaker Pronunciation

For most nonnative speakers, the [j] sound is not a problem, although there may be a tendency for affrication that results in a [ʤ] substitution, as in *yolk* and *joke* both sounding like [ʤoʊk] (Edwards, 1997). The [j] sound is very common among the major modern language sound systems (Carrell & Tiffany, 1960). Nonnative speakers may become confused by misinterpreting the spelling usage of [j] rather than making articulation errors in words such as *jam, jar,* and *judge,* which each begin with the [ʤ] sound. Many words have this sound without there being a corresponding *y* letter, as when *acute* [əkut] may be pronounced [əkjut] (VanRiper, 1979).

According to the U.S. Census Bureau (1990), in addition to English, 15 other languages are spoken in the United States. According to the *Handbook of the International Phonetic Association* (IPA, 1999) and other sources, the languages that have the [j] sound or an allophonic variation of it are Spanish, French, German, Chinese, Korean, Japanese, Arabic, and Hindi. Portuguese does not have the [j] sound.

Summary

The [j] sound is one of the four oral resonant sounds. It does not have a cognate and does not appear in the final positions of United States English words. It is homorganic (linguapalatal) with [ʃ], [ʒ], and [r]. Children master this sound by age 4 years, and it presents some confusion to both native and nonnative speakers because there is not an alphabet letter to represent it. On the contrary, the letter *j* represents the [ʤ] *jam* sound, and the [j] sound is represented by many different letters. One of the major dialect differences is the inclusion of the [j] in words such as *use, few,* and *future.* Phonological deviations include deletion and substitution of the [l] or [w].

PHONETIC SYMBOL [l]

EXHIBIT 17-6 | **Phonetic Symbol [l]**

		[l]
Phonetic Symbol	[l]	
Grapheme Symbol	l	
Diacritic Symbol	l	
Phonic Symbol	l	
Cognate	None	
Homorganic Cognate	Lingua-Alveolar [t], [d], [s], [z], [n]	
Sound Class	Consonant	
Basic Phonetic Features	Placement: Lingua-Alveolar Manner: Lateral Oral Resonant or Glide Voicing: Plus Voice	
IPA (1999)	[l] #155 Voiced, Dental or Alveolar, Lateral, Approximant	

How the Sound Is Produced

The tongue (lingua) is pushed against the back of the upper gum ridge (alveolar), and air is directed laterally (oral resonant) on either or both sides of the tongue.

With the velopharyngeal port closed, the tip of the tongue touches against the alveolar ridge in front and creates openings on both sides. The vocal folds vibrate causing the voiced (voicing) air to escape around the

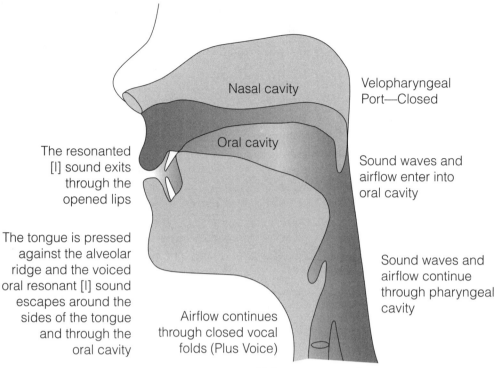

The resonanted [l] sound exits through the opened lips

Nasal cavity

Velopharyngeal Port—Closed

Oral cavity

Sound waves and airflow enter into oral cavity

The tongue is pressed against the alveolar ridge and the voiced oral resonant [l] sound escapes around the sides of the tongue and through the oral cavity

Sound waves and airflow continue through pharyngeal cavity

Airflow continues through closed vocal folds (Plus Voice)

Airflow proceeds from lungs and continues through trachea to larynx

Figure 17-6 [l] pronunciation.

sides of the tongue and through the oral cavity, exiting out the opened lips. See **Figure 17-6**.

Different Spellings for the [l] Sound

Transcribe the following words. Refer to the Key at the right upon completion.

Different Spellings			*Key*
l	like	_____	laɪk
ll	fall	_____	fɑl or fɔl
le	bottle	_____	bɑtl̩ or bɔtl̩
el	funnel	_____	fʌnl̩
sl	island	_____	aɪlænd
ln	kiln	_____	kɪln
cl	muscle	_____	mʌsl̩

Different Sounds of the Letters That Produce the [l] Sound

Transcribe the following words. Refer to the Key at the right upon completion.

		Key
l	silent in palm, talk, calf	pɑm, tɑk, kæf

Rules for Spelling and Pronunciation of the [l] Sound

1. The *l* in spelling contexts is written *l* as in *lamp*, *light*, *let*.

2. The *l* in *half* and in *palm* is silent after the [ɑ] sound in the same syllable.

3. The *l* in *lf* and *l* function as a blend when the letters follow the letters *e*, *o*, or *u* in the same syllable, as in *elf*.

4. Two adjacent *l* letters (*ll*), as in *ball* and *shallow*, are pronounced as one [l] sound.

5. The *l* appears in the *ld* context, as in *told*.

6. The *l* is frequently silent when a final *lk* follows an *a* or *o*, as in *talk* and *folk*, and in such combinations as *ln* in *Lincoln*, *lv* in *halve*, and *lm* in *calm*.

Words That Include the [l] Sound

Transcribe the following words. Refer to the Key at the right upon completion. The [l] sound occurs in all three positions, initial, medial, and final.

Initial Consonant			Key
low ___	lee ___	lay ___	loʊ, li, leɪ
lie ___	lunch ___	lock ___ lamp ___	laɪ, lʌʧ, lɑk, læmp
leg ___			lɛg

Final Consonant

earl ___	ale ___	awl ___	eel ___	ɝ|, eɪl, ɔwl, il

Initial and Final Consonants

Lowell _____	lull _____	loll _____	loʊəl, lɔl, loʊl

Stronger Consonant

hello _____	asleep _____	hɛloʊ, əslip
alarm _____	rely _____	əlɑrm, rilaɪ

Weaker Consonant

careless _____	ability _____	kɛrlɛs, əbɪlɪti
solid _____	pulling _____	sɑləd, pʊlɪŋ

Syllable Consonant

bottle _____	saddle _____	bɔʔl̩, sædl̩
gable _____	battle _____	geɪbl̩, bæʔl̩

Initial Blends

flew ___	glass ___	blue ___	flu, glæs, blu
slick ___	plan ___	glue ___ splash ___	slɪk, plæn, glu, splæʃ

Final Blends

fell _____	hole _____	small _____	fɛl, hoʊl, smɑl
bell _____	mill _____	mail _____	bɛl, mɪl, meɪl

Auditory Discrimination

Transcribe the following words. Refer to the Key at the right upon completion.

[l]	[n]	[l]	[w]	Key
towel ___	town ___	lake ___	wake ___	taʊwəl, taʊn, leɪk, weɪk
let ___	net ___	leak ___	week ___	lɛt, nɛt, lik, wik
line ___	nine ___	slim ___	swim ___	laɪn, naɪn, slɪm, swɪm
tell ___	ten ___	sleep ___	sweep ___	tɛl, tɛn, slip, swip
willing ___	winning ___	later ___	waiter ___	wɪlɪŋ, wɪnɪŋ, leɪtɚ, weɪtɚ
bowl ___	bone ___	lay ___	way ___	boʊl, boʊn, leɪ, weɪ
low ___	no ___	let ___	wet ___	loʊ, noʊ, lɛt, wɛt
slow ___	snow ___	led ___	wed ___	sloʊ, snoʊ, lɛd, wɛd

[l]	[r]	[l]	[j]	Key
blew ___	brew ___	lack ___	yak ___	blu, bru, læk, jæk
lay ___	ray ___	lore ___	yore ___	leɪ, reɪ, lɔr, jɔr
light ___	right ___	clue ___	cue ___	laɪt, raɪt, klu, kju
late ___	rate ___	lung ___	young ___	leɪt, reɪt, lʌŋ, jʌŋ
lies ___	rise ___	local ___	yokel ___	laɪz, raɪz, loʊkɔl, joʊkɔl
cloud ___	crowd ___	lay ___	yea ___	klaʊd, kraʊd, leɪ, jeɪ
pull ___	poor ___	loose ___	use ___	pʊl, pɔr, lus, jus
long ___	wrong ___	let ___	yet ___	lɑŋ, rɑŋ, lɛt, jɛt

Allophonic and Dialect Variations

The phoneme [l] has two separate articulations depending on whether the sound occurs at the initial or final position of a syllable (Small, 1999). When it appears prevocalic as in *log* or *love*, the tongue tip is raised to parallel or to approximate the alveolar ridge while the back of the tongue remains low in the oral cavity. Thus, the airflow is diverted over both sides (lateral) of the tongue. This is the production for the *light* [l]. Almost the reverse occurs when the [l] occurs in the final position of a syllable. The tongue tip, instead of being raised, is lowered and the back of the tongue is raised to approximate the palate as the airflow passes over both sides of the tongue, resulting in a *velarized* allophone of the [l] sound, as in *milk, cruel,* and *careful*. This is the production of the velarized or *dark* [l].

The [l] sound is also velarized as it appears postvocalic and becomes a syllabic consonant, meaning that it functions as a vowel as in *battle*, which is a two-syllable word, *battle*, with no traditional vowel present in the second syllable. The transcribed symbol for such a syllabic [l] is [l̩] with a small dot under the [l]. The [l] sound is devoiced in consonant clusters with voiceless stops, as in *play* and *climb* (Edwards, 1997).

Some United States English speakers substitute a postpalatal or velar [l] in contexts such as *blue* instead of an alveolar or postalveolar [l], which is more common (Edwards, 1997). Edwards also indicates that in both African American and Southern American speech, the [l] is omitted before a consonant, as when *help* [hɛlp] becomes [hɛp], and a substitution of a vowel occurs in the postvocalic position, as when *help* [hɛlp] becomes [hɛəp] and *steel* [stil] becomes [stʊ].

A number of different variants within the class of [l] sounds can be heard in American speech (Carrell & Tiffany, 1960). Preceding and following sounds exert a strong influence on [l], and there is considerable dialectal variation in the pronunciation of this sound. For example, in *million* and *William* the [l] sound becomes the [j] sound, as in [mɪjən] and [wɪjəm].

Normal and Deviant Development of the [l] Sound

Children master the [l] sound late, between the ages of 3 and 6 years, but seldom misarticulate it later in life (Calvert, 1986). The substitution of [w] for [l] is common (Calvert, 1986). The [j] sound and occasionally [d] are also heard, and [l] may be omitted in clusters as in (stop + l) *glass* becomes *gas* (Edwards, 1997). Edwards (1997) indicates that in the final or syllabic position, the [l] may be replaced by [ʊ] or [u] in mild articulation disorders and, in more severe disorders, by [ə], [o], or [ɪ]. In children, the [l] may be missing, as in [ɪto] for *little* and [aɪk] for *like*, and various vowels, principally the [ʊ], [ʌ], [ɛ], [o], and [ə], may be substituted for a final [l] sound, as in [jɪtʌ] for *little* (Carrell & Tiffany, 1960).

Nonnative Speaker Pronunciation

Europeans may articulate the [l] sound forward off the upper teeth rather than farther back off the alveolar ridge, and Asian language speakers produce a sound that resembles the [r] (liquid *r*) sound with the tongue point touching behind the alveolar ridge (Calvert, 1986). The [l] is one of the sounds that is difficult for nonnative speakers to produce and is particularly exhibited in blends such as *pl*, *fl*, and *gl* where the [l] sound may be omitted or produced in an unfamiliar allophonic manner (Edwards, 1997).

The [l] sound is spelled consistently; hence, spelling–pronunciation errors are relatively infrequent, particularly in comparison with some other sounds that have multiple spellings (Carrell & Tiffany, 1960). However, some instances of a silent [l] may occur in United States English, both among nonnative and native speakers who are meticulous in a naïve way, including the [l] sound in *palm* [pɑlm], *salmon* [sælmən], and so forth.

Of the 15 other prominent languages spoken in the United States (U. S. Census Bureau, 1990), the following have the [l] sound, according to the *Handbook of the International Phonetic Association* (IPA, 1999): Spanish, German, Chinese, Korean, Portuguese, Arabic, and Hindi. It is not present in Japanese.

Summary

The [l] sound is one of the four oral resonant sounds. It does not have a cognate and is homorganic (lingua-alveolar) with [t], [d], [s], [z], and [n]. It is consistent in its spelling and pronunciation, although it does occur as a silent "letter" in several instances. Allophonic variations occur as a result of different positions of the tongue, mainly velar or palatal. Children master the [l] sound between ages 3 and 6 years, and later speech sound defects include deletions and substitutions. The [l] sound in the final position may function as a vowel, as in the word *battle*. There are some dialect and nonnative speaker pronunciation differences, and the [l] sound occurs in many of the sound systems of languages worldwide.

It is interesting to note that *l, b, k, m, n,* and *v* have only one sound. The *b, k, l,* and *n* letters may be silent in some words; thus, only *m* and *v* remain constant in sound in all words.

ORAL RESONANT CONSONANTS: CONCLUSION

The three oral resonant consonants are distinguished by their manner of production. The [w] and [j] are classified as glides because the central feature of their articulation is movement toward or away from closure, not the closure itself. The [l] is classified as a lateral because of the lateral emission of the sound over both sides of the tongue.

Children master the [w] sound by age 3 years, and it generally does not present any difficulties to nonnative speakers and is not evident in dialect differences in United States English. The [j] sound is acquired by age 4 and presents some problems to both native and nonnative speakers because of its prominence as a *y* sound, as in *Yolanda*, in many foreign languages, but the *y* is also a vowel sound as in *city*, and the letter *i*, as in *union*, is a [j] sound. In United States English, the usual pronunciation of the *j* is [dʒ], as in *jam* [dʒæm].

The lateral [l] sound is quite consistent in its spelling and pronunciation coordinates, but it does occur as a silent letter or sound in such words as *calf* and *talk*. There are some allophonic variations depending on the sound environment, and it has the function of a vowel in the postvocalic position as in *batt-le*, a two-syllable word with [l] functioning as the vowel nucleus of the final syllable.

REFERENCES

Ball, M. J., & Lowry, O. (2001). *Methods in clinical phonetics*. London, England: Whurr Publishers.

Calvert, D. R. (1986). *Descriptive phonetics*. New York, NY: Thieme Medical Publishers.

Carrell, J., & Tiffany, W. (1960). *Phonetics: Theory and application to speech improvement*. New York, NY: McGraw-Hill.

Chomsky, N., & Halle, M. (1968). *The sound patterns of English*. Cambridge, MA: MIT Press.

Edwards, H. T. (1997). *Applied phonetics* (2nd ed.). San Diego, CA: College-Hill Press.

House, L. (1998). *Introductory phonetics and phonology*. Mahwah, NJ: Lawrence Erlbaum.

International Phonetic Association. (1999). *Handbook of the International Phonetic Association*. Cambridge, England: Cambridge University Press.

Ladefoged, P. (1993). *A course in phonetics* (3rd ed.). Fort Worth, TX: Harcourt Brace College Publishers.

Sander, E. (1972). When are speech sounds learned? *Journal of Speech and Hearing Disorders*, *37*, 55–63.

Shriberg, L. D., & Kent, R. D. (1994). *Clinical phonetics* (2nd ed.). Boston, MA: Allyn & Bacon.

Small, L. H. (1999). *Fundamentals of phonetics (new edition)*. Boston, MA: Allyn & Bacon.

Tiffany, W. R., & Carrell, J. (1977). *Phonetics: Theory and application*. New York, NY: McGraw-Hill.

U.S. Census Bureau. (1990). *Table 5. Detailed list of languages spoken at home for the population 5 years and over by state: 1990.* Retrieved from http://www.census.gov/prod/2010pubs/acs-12.pdf

VanRiper, C. (1979). *An introduction to general American phonetics*. New York, NY: Harper.

Clinical Application: Make Your Own Articulation Test

PURPOSE

To provide you with information concerning the application of phonetic science to basic clinical practice.

OBJECTIVES

This chapter will provide you with information regarding:

1. Basic clinical assessment framework
2. Speech production mechanism
3. Hearing acuity and discrimination
4. Basic model for assessment of speech production
5. Creating your own articulation test

INTRODUCTION

The purpose of this chapter is to provide you with information regarding how you can use the basic principles of phonetic science to acquire information about speech sound defects and take a logical approach to the assessment and treatment of such defects.

BASIC CLINICAL ASSESSMENT FRAMEWORK

Speech Production Mechanism

The basic anatomic structures of speech production discussed in Chapter 6 need to be within the range of normal functioning. A certain level of integrity of the speech production mechanism is needed because all of the structures rely on one another to produce the final results: speech. The lungs, vocal folds, lips, tongue, velum, and so forth need to have muscle tone and neural feedback to produce the sounds. When any of these structures are deformed or absent, compensatory processes may accommodate and result in acceptable sound production. On the other hand, such abnormalities as a cleft palate may limit speech production because, for example, the air pressure needed to produce the plosive sounds [p] and [b] cannot build up.

The hearing mechanism needs to function within normal limits for the reception of speech acuity and discrimination as a listener and for feedback as a speaker. When certain sounds, particularly the high-frequency sounds such as the [f] and voiceless *th* [θ] are difficult to hear, a speaker may be delayed in the acquisition of these sounds. Individuals, in developmental stages as well as nonnative speakers, must become skilled in discriminating one sound from another.

Developmental Acquisition of Speech Sounds

One factor to consider when evaluating the speech sounds of young children is whether the child is within normal range of sounds production and produces the sounds correctly or incorrectly. Knowledge of such information assists you in determining delay or normal development. You need to examine the characteristics of speech sound errors to determine the level of severity. In assessment, you will determine how many different types of speech sound errors there are and at what frequency they occur.

Dialect and Accent Considerations

More often than not, a person's dialect or accent is determined by the production of the vowels and diphthongs and the suprasegmental (prosody) features of rate, rhythm, and intonation. Consonants are usually produced with an allophonic variation that a listener may or may not understand. A main consideration in the assessment of dialect or accent is the need for a change. The traditional definition of a speech defect is "when the speech of the speaker cannot be understood by the listener." Listeners may understand the speech of a person with a dialect or accent but may attend more to the production of the accented speech than to the content. The criteria of what constitutes acceptable speech need to be determined before any recommendation for intervention. In some professional settings, it is almost required that a speaker minimize his or her dialect or accent, and intervention of accent reduction is required. In making such a decision for intervention, the factors of who, what, where need to be considered. The ability to linguistically shift effectively from one speaking style to another should be the overall goal.

PERIMETERS OF ASSESSMENT

Defective Speech Sound Production

Some of the factors to consider in the actual assessment of speech sound production include the following:

1. *Context:* Does the error occur in the production of
   a. A single sound
   b. A single syllable
   c. A short phrase
   d. Conversational speech

2. *Location:* Does the error occur
   a. In the initial position of the word
   b. In the medial position of the word (between the first and last sounds)
   c. In the final position of the word
3. *Type of speech sound error (SODA):*
   a. Substitution of one sound for another
   b. Omission of the sound
   c. Distortion of the sound, such as a lateral lisp
   d. Addition of a sound
4. *Speech feature type:*
   a. Modification of airflow
   b. Placement of articulators
   c. Voicing (plus or minus)

Descriptive Analysis of the Speech Sound Error

Here is an example of a descriptive analysis of a speech sound error:

Transcribed as Spoken	Transcribed as Corrected	Descriptive Analysis	
tæt "cat"	kæt	Position:	Initial sound error
		Type:	Substitution [t] for [k]
		Environment:	CVC
		Placement:	[t] (front) lingua-alveolar
			[k] (back) lingua-velar
		Manner of Airflow Modification:	[t] stop
			[k] stop
		Voicing:	[t] voiceless
			[k] voiceless

Interpretation: Error in placement Compatible manner and voicing. Goal: Target *placement* error. Prove error type in other vowel environment such as the other front vowels:

[t] + [i] [ti]; [t] + [ɪ] /tɪm/
[t] + [e] [teɪk]; [t]+ [ɛ] /tɛn/

to determine if error type /tæ/ is unique to that context only.

Suggested Therapy Goal: Focus on Placement Aspect of Production

Another factor to consider is the phonetic environment of the defective sound. What are the characteristics of the sounds that come before and after the defective sound? What influence do these characteristics have on the production of the defective sound? For example, is there a difference in the production of the defective sound such as the [t] sound, which is a front sound, when it is paired with a front vowel such as [i] in the word *tea* versus when it is paired with a back vowel such as [u] in the word *two*?

YOU ARE ABOUT TO BECOME AN AUTHOR

Thus far, you have been concentrating on the construct of phonetics and its sound/symbol correlates. You should compliment yourself on your achievements in those areas.

Now it is time to apply what you have learned to practice. You are now prepared to create your own articulation test. That's right. You are ready to become an author. What better way to conclude your study of phonetics than to see it in action? So, let's get started.

First, let's briefly review the format of published articulation tests. For example:

1. Pictures of objects that contain the target sound are used (a picture of a house is used to elicit the final [s] sound). These pictures may be in a binder or a set of cards similar to a deck of playing cards.

2. Each of the consonant, vowel, and diphthong sounds are included in the initial, medial (any sound between the first and last sound), and final positions in words.

3. The individual is shown each picture and is asked to say the name of the object.

4. The responses are recorded and a profile of the test results is calculated.

The process is quite straightforward, and administration and scoring are simple. Normative data are used to determine the possible need for speech sound (articulation) intervention.

MY ORIGINAL ARTICULATION TEST

Because this is an initial learning experience, we can simplify it by designing an articulation test that identifies speech production consonant sounds and excludes vowels and diphthongs.

You will be provided with an Articulation Test/Consonants Recording Form and instruction on how to compile your Picture Stimuli Cards. Let's get started!

Step 1. Make a copy of the two-page Articulation Test/Consonants Recording Form, as shown in **Table 18-1**. This will be your master copy.

Step 2. Use card stock and make 35 copies of the following form. This will equal 70 individual cards.

	Circle One
Sound _____ /Word _____	I M F
Modification of Airflow	_____
	_____
Placement of Articulation	_____
	_____
Voice	+ or −

	Circle One
Sound _____ /Word _____	I M F
Modification of Airflow	_____
	_____
Placement of Articulation	_____
	_____
Voice	+ or −

TABLE 18-1   Articulation Test/Consonants Recording Form

Sounds	Words	Correct +	Correct –	Speech Error Type (Write in error sound)				Speech Feature Type			
				S	O	D	A	Modification of Airflow	Placement of Articulation	Plus/Minus Voice	
Plosives											
[b] I											
[b] M											
[b] F											
[p] I											
[p] M											
[p] F											
[d] I											
[d] M											
[d] F											
[t] I											
[t] M											
[t] F											
[g] I											
[g] M											
[g] F											
[k] I											
[k] M											
[k] F											

(continues)

Fricatives										
[v] I										
[v] M										
[v] F										
[f] I										
[f] M										
[f] F										
[ð] I										
[ð] M										
[ð] F										
[θ] I										
[θ] M										
[θ] F										
[z] I										
[z] M										
[z] F										
[s] I										
[s] M										
[s] F										

TABLE 18-1 Articulation Test/Consonants Recording Form (Continued)

Sounds	Words	Correct +	Correct –	Speech Error Type (Write in error sound) S	O	D	A	Speech Feature Type — Modification of Airflow	Placement of Articulation	Plus/Minus Voice
[ʒ] I										
[ʒ] M										
[ʒ] F										
[ʃ] I										
[ʃ] M										
[ʃ] F										
[h] I										
[h] M										
Affricates										
[dʒ] I										
[dʒ] M										
[dʒ] F										
[tʃ] I										
[tʃ] M										
[tʃ] F										
Nasal										
[m] I										
[m] M										
[m] F										

	[n] I	[n] M	[n] F	[ŋ] I	[ŋ] M	[ŋ] F	Oral	[l] I	[l] M	[l] F	[r] I	[r] M	[r] F	[w] I	[w] M	[j] I	[j] M	Summary of Results

Step 3. Place the stack of cards in front of you beside the Articulation Test/Consonants Recording Form.

Step 4. On each card, enter the following, using the symbols on the Recording Form and the information listed in **Table 18-2**.

For example, your first three cards will be as follows:

- [b] I
- [b] M
- [b] F

Manner of modification of airflow: Stop

Place of articulation: Bilabial

Voicing: +

The last two cards will be as follows:

- [j] I
- [j] M

You enter the word later when you have your picture of the target word placed on the opposite side of the card.

TABLE 18-2	Phonetic Symbols and Their Descriptive Features		
	Placement of Articulators	**Manner of Modification of Airflow**	**Voicing**
1. [b]	Bilabial	Stop	Plus
2. [p]	Bilabial	Stop	Minus
3. [t]	Lingua-alveolar	Stop	Minus
4. [d]	Lingua-alveolar	Stop	Plus
5. [k]	Lingua-velar	Stop	Minus
6. [g]	Lingua-velar	Stop	Plus
7. [f]	Labiodental	Fricative	Minus
8. [v]	Labiodental	Fricative	Plus
9. [s]	Lingua-alveolar or Linguadental	Fricative	Minus
10. [z]	Lingua-alveolar or Linguadental	Fricative	Plus
11. [ʃ]	Linguapalatal	Fricative	Minus
12. [ʒ]	Linguapalatal	Fricative	Plus
13. [Θ]	Linguadental	Fricative	Minus
14. [ð]	Linguadental	Fricative	Plus
15. [h]	Linguapalatal *and* Lingua-velar	Fricative	Minus
16. [ʍ]	Lingua-velar *and* Bilabial	Fricative	Minus
17. [tʃ]	Lingua-alveolar *to* Linguapalatal	Affricative	Minus
18. [dʒ]	Lingua-alveolar *to* Linguapalatal	Affricative	Plus
19. [l]	Lingua-alveolar	Oral resonant	Plus
20. [r]	Linguapalatal	Oral resonant	Plus
21. [j]	Linguapalatal	Oral resonant	Plus
22. [w]	Lingua-velar *and* Bilabial	Oral resonant	Plus
23. [m]	Bilabial	Nasal resonant	Plus
24. [n]	Lingua-alveolar	Nasal resonant	Plus
25. [ŋ]	Lingua-velar	Nasal resonant	Plus

Step 5. Number each of your cards in the upper-right corner 1–69.

Step 6. Using the sounds listed on the left-hand side of the Recording Form, find pictures for each of the sounds listed. For example, you need a separate picture for the [b] sound in its three-different positions:

1. Initial: *bird*
2. Medial: *table*
3. Final: *tub*

Step 7. Continue to find the pictures and tape them to the opposite side of the cards. You may find your pictures from a variety of sources, including computer programs, picture dictionaries, and magazines.

Step 8. Enter the name of the picture (object) in the Word column of the Recording Form and next to each sound on the card.

Step 9. You may want to consider laminating your cards.

Step 10. Familiarize yourself with the Instructions for How to Use the Articulation Test/Consonants, which follow. Refer to the Recording Form as you read the instructions.

INSTRUCTIONS FOR HOW TO USE THE ARTICULATION TEST/CONSONANTS

Sounds

Listed are all of the United States English consonant sounds. Note that there are three entries for each sound. This allows for testing for the initial, medial, and final positions.

Words

You need to select the stimulus words for your articulation test. You may want use your computer, magazines, the Internet, or other sources to select pictures/words.

Correct/Incorrect

Enter the response of the person taking the test as correct or incorrect. For example, [tæt] for [kæt] for *cat* would be scored with a minus (–) as incorrect.

Speech Error Type

Enter the type of error:

- S = substitution
- O = omission
- D = distortion
- A = addition

For example, when the test subject speaks a [t] for a [k] in *cat*, you would enter "t" in the S column.

Speech Feature Type

If the error type is the same as the speech feature type, enter *plosive, fricative, affricate, nasal,* or *oral* with a plus sign (+) in the column. If it is different, enter a minus sign (–). For example, for a substitution of a *t* for a *k*, the modification of the airflow is the same (plosive +), but the placement of articulation is different (–), and the voicing is the same. For an example, see **Table 18-3**.

Summary of Results

Identify the articulation errors and write a summary statement using the data recorded on the Articulation Test/Consonants Recording Form. For example:

TABLE 18-3	**Articulation Test/Consonants Recording Form**									

Sounds	Words	Correct +	Correct –	Speech Error Type (Write in error sound) S	O	D	A	Speech Feature Type Modification of Airflow	Placement of Articulation	Plus/Minus Voice
[k] – I	cat		tæt	t				Both plosives	Linguadental	Both voice
[k] – M	nickel	+								
[k] – F	duck	+								

The individual substituted the [t] for the [k] sound in the initial position. Both sounds are plosives and minus voice. The error occurred in the Place of Articulation. The correct [k] sound is a lingua-alveolar, and the [t] sound is a linguadental. The [k] sound in the medial and final positions was correct.

Step 11. Make 10 copies of the two-page Recording Form.

Step 12. Check for completion. You should have the following items:

  1. Sixty-nine cards with pictures on one side and sound/symbol descriptions onthe opposite side.

  2. One master copy of the Recording Form with the words entered in the Word column. (Keep this as the Master Copy for future use.)

  3. Ten copies of the Recording Form.

You are now ready to put your test to the test! Ready. Get set. Go!

PURPOSE OF ADMINISTERING YOUR TEST

Administering this test gives you the opportunity to increase your listening and transcription skills and to have an initial experience in testing. You will participate both as the examiner and the "subject" taking the test. It should also reinforce what you have learned in your study of phonetics.

How to Administer Your Test

Here are some ideas on what to say when you administer your test:

Examiner: (*Present each picture card*) What is this?

Responder: A boat.

Examiner: (*Record the response in the Correct Column using a + sign.*)

                        OR

Responder: A toat.

Examiner: (*Repeat the word, if necessary. Write the incorrect word in the Incorrect Column and put the [t] sound in the S (Substitution) column.*)

You can fill in the Speech Feature Type later by referring to your [t] card.

You would enter a + in the Modification of Airflow column because both the [b] and [t] are plosives, but the errors occur in the Placement of Articulation ([b] bilabial vs. [t] linguadental and Voicing [b]+ vs. [t]–).

Note: Because this is a learning experience, the responder should be encouraged to mispronounce the target words with some frequency. The examiner records only the error of the target sound even though the responder may mispronounce other sounds within the word.

Skill-Building Activities

Continue to seek opportunities to participate both as the examiner and the responder with other class members and friends and family to increase your competency. You may want to consider using a more complex analysis of the testing results by performing the following calculations.

Total number of sounds _____

Total number of errors _____

Percentage of total errors _____

Percentage of errors by position:

_____ Initial position

_____ Medial position

_____ Final position

Percentage of errors by type of error:

_____ Substitution

_____ Omission

_____ Distortion

_____ Addition

Post Script

Congratulations: You Are a Phonetics Scholar!

You are to be commended for your efforts to learn about phonetics. Let's just summarize what you have learned since the time you opened this book. You learned that phonetics is about the sound system of human communication. Each sound has no meaning by itself, and most sounds are maneuverable and can appear anywhere within words. You learned about the International Phonetic Association and the International Phonetic Alphabet that consists of symbols that represent the different sounds of human speech throughout the world.

It's amazing how quickly you learned the phonetic alphabet and began to recognize such symbols as the voiceless *th* [Ө], the voiced *th* [ð], and all of the other unique symbols of consonants, vowels, and diphthongs (remember: difthongs). No doubt you enjoyed the card and dice games and other riddles and exercises as you learned the sounds and their symbols.

Do you recall the discussion on sounds, syllables, and suprasegmentals? You discovered the confusion we have in determining where to divide a word into syllables and the influence of suprasegmental features that indicate whether a word is a noun or verb: **pres**-ent versus pre**sent**. And then there was the ride in the time machine as we ventured through the history of the English language. We found some interesting facts that make us appreciate how much English is really a borrowed composite of many different languages. I hope you enjoyed that ride!

Then, you listened to Shakespeare's prophecy in *Julius Caesar*:

How many ages hence
Shall this our lofty scene be acted o'er
In states unborn and accents yet unknown.

It was interesting to listen to your conversations during the dialect portion of our trip and how when you return to your roots you begin speaking your original dialect automatically even though you may not have spoken it for several years.

You learned to appreciate the method of spelling words phonetically when we analyzed the orthographic method of spelling. It's a wonder that anyone learns how to spell, as illustrated by the poem I wrote for you: *through, hiccough, though,* and *laugh*.

You learned the basic anatomy and physiology of the speech and hearing mechanisms used in the processes of speaking and listening to human speech. You learned such terms as *lingua-alveolar* that describe the placement of the articulators for different speech sounds.

You learned that vowels and diphthongs can be identified by the position of the tongue in the mouth (high, mid, low and front, mid, back), whether or not the tongue is tense or lax, and whether the lips are round or unround. You also studied the characteristics of the consonant sounds in the context of placement of the articulators, modification of the airflow, and voicing. For example, you demonstrated your knowledge by identifying that the descriptors of *stop-bilabial-voiced* describe the [b] sound.

Throughout your study of the United States English sounds, you acquired information concerning the following items:

1. The different spellings and rules of pronunciation for each sound

2. The various contexts in which each sound occurs

3. Examples of allophonic variations, dialect differences, and nonnative speaker difficulties

4. Normal acquisition and disordered production of the sounds

After reading all of the theory and practicing the drillwork to learn about phonetic science and the sound/symbols of the phonetic alphabet, you developed your own articulation test and became an author. By administering your test, you no doubt increased your transcription and listening skills.

Good luck to you, Phonetic Scholar, as you continue to apply what you have learned to the benefit of research and clinical practice in phonetics.

fʌn wɪθ fənɛtɪks

The following pages are provided to increase your sight recognition of sounds/symbols and words and your phonetic transcription skills. *rɪmɛmbɚ tu hæv fʌn!* Please be aware that there may be some dialect difference in some of the transcription.

IDENTIFY THE WORDS

Spell the words that are written in phonetics. Cover the Key until you have written your answers.

One day we went to the **zu** and **watʃd** different **ænəml̩z** and **ɛkzɑtɪk** birds. **wi** saw a bunch of **mʌnkiz** climbing **triz** and a hippo **səbmɚdʒd** in water.

The **ɛləfənts** put on a **ʃo** for us that was **tɚɪfɪk**. There were two **raɪnoz** that were **ɑsʌm**. One of them had a **beibi** following her.

We were getting **hʌngri**, so we stopped to **it**. We had a **hɑtdɑg** and a **drɪnk**. After that, we **sɑ** an **ɛkzɪbɪʃən** of different animals from **æfrɪkə**.

We were tired, so we **lɛft** and **drov** home. It was a **greit** day!

1. _____	9. _____	17. _____
2. _____	10. _____	18. _____
3. _____	11. _____	19. _____
4. _____	12. _____	20. _____
5. _____	13. _____	21. _____
6. _____	14. _____	22. _____
7. _____	15. _____	23. _____
8. _____	16. _____	24. _____

Key: 1. zoo; 2. watched; 3. animals; 4. exotic; 5. We; 6. monkeys; 7. trees; 8. submerged; 9. elephants; 10. show; 11. terrific; 12. rhinos; 13. awesome; 14. baby; 15. hungry; 16. eat; 17. hotdog; 18. drink; 19. saw; 20. exhibition; 21. Africa; 22. left; 23. drove; 24. great

FILL-IN STORY

Using the Words list that follows, identify the phonetic words and fill in the blanks using regular (orthographic) spelling. The phonetic words are written in random order. Happy hunting. Refer to the Key upon completion.

Last _____ we went on a _____ to some _____ parks. We _____ in tents and

_____ our own _____. Some of them were really _____ and others got _____ or were not _____ well _____.

While we were there, we saw some _____ and a _____ deer. We went _____ and caught _____ _____. We _____ them for dinner and they were _____ good.

After dark, we looked up at the _____. They were so _____. We sat around the _____ and _____ _____. They were really _____.

After a _____, we were ready to come home.

Words:

sʌmɚ	kʊkt	maɪti	skɜ˞lz
fraɪd	næʃənəl	kæmpt	bɜ˞nt
fju	traʊt	inəf	teisti
braɪt	stɑrz	kæmpfaɪr	mɪlz
veikeiʃən	twɛlv	mɑrʃmɛloz	jʌmi
wik	dʌn	fɪʃɪŋ	rostd̩

Key:

Last **summer** we went on a **vacation** to some **national** parks. We **camped** in tents and **cooked** our own **meals**. Some of them were really **tasty** and others got **burnt** or were not cooked well **enough**.

While we were there, we saw some **squirrels** and a **few** deer. We went **fishing** and caught **twelve trout**. We **fried** them for dinner and they were **mighty** good.

After dark, we looked up at the **stars**. They were so **bright**. We sat around the **campfire** and **roasted marsh-mallows**. They were really **yummy**.

After a **week**, we were ready to come home.

RIDDLES

Match the phonetic words to the riddles. Cover the Key until you have written your answers.

_____ 1. It is the part of the finger that you can bend.

_____ 2. I am less than seven and more than five.

_____ 3. I am not a duck. I lay eggs and say *cluck-cluck*.

_____ 4. In this room, the cooking is done. Good food is eaten by everyone.

_____ 5. Play in the waves and get wet. Watch the sun as it will set.

_____ 6. I hold liquids and have a spout. Watch the water as it pours out.

_____ 7. When you strike it, it is bright. You will get burnt, so hold it right.

_____ 8. It can be yellow, green, or red. Keeps the doctor away, so it is said.

_____ 9. I am made of wood and have lead. I write the words that are said.

_____ 10. When it is dark at night, turn me on and it is bright.

_____ 11. Email has almost replaced me. It is much faster, I agree.

_____ 12. There are lots of me on a tree. In the fall, I am colorful to see.

a. ʧɪkən	b. sɪks	c. bɪʧ
d. mɛl	e. æpl̩	f. livz
g. pɛnsl̩	h. kɪʧən	i. nək̩l
j. pɪtʒɚ	k. læmp	l. mæʧ

Key: 1. i; 2. b; 3. a; 4. h; 5. c; 6. j; 7. l; 8. e; 9. g; 10. k; 11. d; 12. f

RIDDLES

Phonetically transcribe the answer. Cover the Key until you have written your answers.

1. It is orange and rhymes with *parrot*.
   It grows in the ground. It's a _____.
2. It is not the floor.
   You open it when someone knocks. It's the _____.
3. It hops around and it's hard to grab it.
   You know, it must be a _____.
4. It takes you to a different place.
   Some drivers like to race. It's a _____.
5. We live in it and it rhymes with *mouse*.
   It's a _____.
6. It goes on your wrist and could be gold.
   It could be new or old. It's a _____.
7. It swims and barks like a dog.
   It's surely not a frog. It's a _____.
8. It brings us music and the news.
   Commentators give their views. It's a _____.
9. I am not your eyes or nose.
   I'm part of your face that can open or close.
   I'm your _____.
10. You can blow me up and I float in the air.
    I will explode if you don't handle me with care.
    I'm a _____.
11. It is where you place books and maybe a vase.
    Everything is in its place. It's a _____.

12. Mice like it. It is a real treat.
    We even like it to eat. It is _____.

Key: 1. carrot—kɛrit; 2. door—dor; 3. rabbit—ræbɪt;
4. car—kɑr; 5. house—haʊs; 6. bracelet—breɪslɛt;
7. seal—sɪl; 8. radio—reɪdɪo; 9. mouth—mɑʊθ;
10. balloon—bəlun; 11. shelf—ʃɛlf; 12. cheese—ʧiz

WORD CHAIN

Separate the words from the chain and write them orthographically on the line below each sentence. Refer to the Key upon completion.

1. wʊdjulaɪktugoʊtuðʌbæskɪtbɑlgeɪmwɪθmi?
   _____

2. tudeiwɪlbiɑgreɪtdeituplæntðʌgɑrdən.
   _____

3. junidtugoʊθruðʌɛgzittugɛtaʊtsɑɪd.
   _____

4. ðʌtreinlivəzættuoklokfrʌmðʌsteɪʃən.
   _____

5. ðʌlɪstɪnklʊdədæpləs, eiprɪkɑts, ændgreips.
   _____

6. ðʌskaɪskreipɚwɑzsɪkshəndrɪdfithaɪ.
   _____

7. ðʌkəmputɚkræsʤændðʌdaɪdəwɝlɑst.
   _____

8. ðʌævələnsændhaɪdrɪftswɝdeinʤɚəs.
   _____

9. ðɛɚwɝjəiənsændkɛtsəpɑnðʌhæmbɚgɚz.
   _____

10. ðʌæksədɛntɑnðʌfriweikɑzʤkənʤɛstjən.
    _____

11. ðʌmjuzɪkætðʌrɛstɝɑntwɑztulaʊd.
    _____

12. ðʌɛkzæmɪneɪʃənwɑzisibikəzɑɪhædstʌdid.
    _____

13. ðʌmunlaɪtriflɛkədɑnðʌleik.
    _____

14. ðʌkeibḷkɑrwɑzfʌnturaɪdɪnsænfrænsɪko.
    _____

15. wisætɪnðʌʤəkuziwaɪlɑnðʌkruzʃɪp.
    _____

Key:

1. Would you like to go to the basketball game with me?
2. Today will be a great day to plant the garden.
3. You need to go through the exit to get outside.
4. The train leaves at two o'clock from the station.
5. The list included apples, apricots, and grapes.
6. The skyscraper was six hundred feet high.
7. The computer crashed and the data were lost.
8. The avalanche and high drifts were dangerous.
9. There were onions and ketchup on the hamburgers.
10. The accident on the freeway caused congestion.
11. The music at the restaurant was too loud.
12. The examination was easy because I had studied.
13. The moonlight reflected on the lake.
14. The cable car was fun to ride in San Francisco.
15. We sat in the jacuzzi while on the cruise ship.

WORD CHAINS

Separate the words from the chain and write them orthographically on the line below each sentence. Refer to the Key upon completion.

1. wisɑdəmɛstɪkændforɪnkɑrzætðʌʃo.
   _____

2. ðʌgaɪzɚzwɝriliæktɪvwɪθstim.
   _____

3. ðʌɪkəsændðʌænvḷɑrpɑrtʌvðʌɛɚ.
   _____

4. ðʌsɚfʌsʌvðʌroʊdwɑzbʌmpi.
   _____

5. ðʌdolfɪnswɝvɛriæktɪvɪnðʌoʃən.
   _____

6. maɪsɛlfonnidədtubiʧɑrʤḍ.
   _____

7. skaɪdaɪvɪŋkænbivɛrideiʒɚəsændfʌn.
   _____

8. arɪθmatɪkwɑzizikəmpɛirdtugiɑmɪtri.
   _____

9. trævəlɪŋtuɪndiətukələŋtaɪm.
   _____

10. ðʌdɪkʃənɛrikənteinzmɛnidɪfɝɛntwɝdʒ.

_____

11. ðʌsɑkɚgeimwɑzvɛriɛksaɪtɪŋændwiwʌn.

_____

12. renkɪŋðʌætrəbutsʌvðʌpɚsənwɑzdɪfɪkɑlt.

_____

13. ðʌkjukəmbɚændegplæntwɝdilɪʃəs.

_____

14. sikwɛnsɪŋðʌstɛpsɪnətæskmeɪksðʌjɑbizi.

_____

15. ðʌmɛriɵənwɑzlɑŋændtidiəs.

_____

Key:

1. We saw domestic and foreign cars at the show.
2. The geysers were really active with steam.
3. The incus and the anvil are part of the ear.
4. The surface of the road was bumpy.
5. The dolphins were very active in the ocean.
6. My cell phone needed to be charged.
7. Skydiving can be very dangerous and fun.
8. Arithmetic was easy compared to geometry.
9. Traveling to India took a long time.
10. The dictionary contains many different words.
11. The soccer game was very exciting and we won.
12. Ranking the attributes of the person was difficult.
13. The cucumber and eggplant were delicious.
14. Sequencing the steps in a task makes the job easy.
15. The marathon was long and tedious.

ANAGRAMS

Rearrange the letters phonetically to spell a different word.

1. each _____ 2. odor _____ 3. ape _____
4. who _____ 5. march _____ 6. male _____
7. dust _____ 8. read _____ 9. plug _____
10. mile _____ 11. two _____ 12. robe _____
13. none _____ 14. rock _____ 15. dial _____

Key: 1. ache; 2. door; 3. pea; 4. how; 5. charm; 6. lame;
7. stud; 8. dear; 9. gulp; 10. lime; 11. tow; 12. bore;
13. neon; 14. cork; 15. laid

CREATE A DIFFERENT WORD

Phonetically transcribe a different word by rearranging the letters.

Example: odor   odɚ   door   dor

1. state   _____ _____ _____ _____
2. neon   _____ _____ _____ _____
3. charm   _____ _____ _____ _____
4. gulp   _____ _____ _____ _____
5. each   _____ _____ _____ _____
6. laid   _____ _____ _____ _____
7. race   _____ _____ _____ _____
8. era   _____ _____ _____ _____
9. earn   _____ _____ _____ _____
10. seal   _____ _____ _____ _____
11. rear   _____ _____ _____ _____
12. lame   _____ _____ _____ _____
13. state   _____ _____ _____ _____
14. stud   _____ _____ _____ _____
15. lame   _____ _____ _____ _____
16. felt   _____ _____ _____ _____
17. den   _____ _____ _____ _____
18. mile   _____ _____ _____ _____
19. pea   _____ _____ _____ _____
20. arm   _____ _____ _____ _____

TRANSCRIBE VERBAL ANALOGIES

Phonetically transcribe the words in bold type and complete the analogy.

Example: **March** is to **month** as **Tuesday** is
to _____.

mɑrtʃ is to mʌnɵ as tuzdɑi is to wik.

1. **Man** is to **woman** as **husband** is to _____.
   _____ is to _____ as _____ is to _____.

2. **Hands** are to **fingers** as **feet** are to _____.
   _____ are to _____ as _____ are to _____.

3. **Tennis** is to **racket** as **baseball** is to _____.
   _____ is to _____ as _____ is to _____.

4. **Sit** is to **chair** as **sleep** is to _____.
   _____ is to _____ as _____ is to _____.

5. **Ant** is to **insect** as **robin** is to _____.
   _____ is to _____ as _____ is to _____.

6. **Red** is to **color** as **Ford** is to _____.

_____ is to _____ as _____ is to _____.

7. **Eat** is to **food** as **book** is to _____.

_____ is to _____ as _____ is to _____.

8. **Bread** is to **flour** as **candy** is to _____.

_____ is to _____ as _____ is to _____.

9. **Leg** is to **knee** as **arm** is to _____.

_____ is to _____ as _____ is to _____.

10. **Sink** is to **bathroom** as **bed** is to _____.

_____ is to _____ as _____ is to _____.

Key: 1. waɪf, mæn, wumən, hʌzbɪnd, waɪf; 2. toʊz, hændz, fɪŋgɚz, fit, toʊz; 3. bæt, tɛnis, rækɪt, beisbɔl, bæt; 4. bɛd, sɪt, ʃɛr, slip, bɛd; 5. bɝd, ænt, ɪnsɛkt, rɑbɪn, bɝd; 6. kɑr, rɛd, kʌlɚ, Fɔrd, kɑr; 7. rid, it, fʊd, bʊk, rid; 8. ʃɪgɚ, brɛd, flaʊr, kændi, ʃɪgɚ; 9. ɛlboʊ, lɛg, ni, arm, ɛlboʊ; 10. bɛdrum, siŋk, bæθrum, bɛd, bɛdrum

FILL IN THE BLANKS

Category is Ethnic Foods.

1. ____ aʊ m ____ ____

2. t ____ ____ ɑ l ____

3. ____ u ____ ____ ____ s

Key: ʧaʊmeɪn (chow mein), təmɑli (tamale), kus kus (cous cous)

NONSENSE WORDS

Underline the nonsense word. Refer to the Key upon completion.

Example:	waɪn sʍit	ɑniʍɛr	ʃʍɔ
a	*b*	*c*	*d*
1. baɪdd	briðz	θin	smuðz
2. ʃoʊ	meʃɪn	ʃik	neɪʃən
3. tɪʃu	əʃoʊr	spɛʃʊl	oʊʃen
4. lʌkɚi	səmpl̩	kænʃɛns	ʃaw
5. ʧɪn	sʌn	sɪsɚz	ɛkstrə
6. omɪʃen	ʃɛf	pæʃən	ʃɪgɚ
7. fuʃə	oʃən	səti	naɪs
8. ʃoʊldɚ	rɑʃʊl	məʃɪn	moʊʃən
9. riʒim	fænteɪʒə	rɑʒɚ	gərɑʒ
10. meɪʒɚmɛnt	ɑsɔr	pɪdʒən	prɛsɚ
11. əluʒən	liʒən	rus	beɪz
12. mɛʃɚ	æʒɚ	kɑnfuʃən	mʌsɔʒ
13. viʒən	siʒɚ	gleɪʃɚ	supɚvɪʒən

14. kæʒjuli   ʍɪl   sʍeɪd   wɝθʍaɪl

15. wɪʧ   hɛlmʌt   wɛðɚ   tʍɪŋkl̩

Key: 1. c; 2. b; 3. d; 4. b; 5. c; 6. a; 7. c; 8. b; 9. a; 10. b; 11. c; 12. a; 13. a; 14. c; 15. b

VERBAL ANALOGIES

Phonetically transcribe the words in each set.

Example: water : liquid :: rock : solid <u>wɑtɚ</u> : <u>lɪkwʊd</u> :: <u>rɑk</u> : <u>sɑləd</u>

glove : hand ::	boot : foot	___ : ___ :: ___ : ___
car : driver ::	plane : pilot	___ : ___ :: ___ : ___
paw : dog ::	fin : fish	___ : ___ :: ___ : ___
story : read ::	song : sing	___ : ___ :: ___ : ___
one : three ::	single : triple	___ : ___ :: ___ : ___
wrist : hand ::	ankle : foot	___ : ___ :: ___ : ___
penny : dollar ::	foot : yard	___ : ___ :: ___ : ___
left : right ::	top : bottom	___ : ___ :: ___ : ___
easy : simple ::	hard : difficult	___ : ___ :: ___ : ___

MATCHING

Baseball Level I

Match the city name with the team name.

City		*Team Name*
1. ætlæntə		A. mɛts
2. sæn frænsɪsko		B. rɛdz
3. nu jork		C. breɪvz
4. ʃəkɑgo		D. dɑʤɚz
5. bɑstɪn		E. eɪnʤəlz
6. lɑs ænʤəlɛs		F. rɛd sɑks
7. sɪnsənæti		G. ɪndiɪnz
8. klivlɪn		H. ʤeɪ ɪnts
9. ænəhaɪm		I. pɑdreɪz
10. sæn dieɪgo		J. ʍaɪt sɑks

Baseball Level II

Match the city name with the team name.

Team		*Team Name*
1. m ___ əso ___		A. k ___ b ___
2. æn ___ h ___ m		B. dɑ ___ z
3. s ___ ɑgo		C. ___ ɛt ___
4. h ___ us ___ n		D. ɪn ___ nz

5. l＿＿＿ndʒəl＿＿   E. t＿ɪ＿z

6. kl＿＿lɪ＿   F. br＿＿＿＿

7. ＿ju jo＿＿   G. ＿ndʒə＿＿

8. ＿tl＿n＿＿＿   H. æst＿＿＿＿

NFL Level I

Match the city name with the team name.

City		Team Name	
1.	sæn dieɪgo	A.	fortinaɪnɚz
2.	ʃəkɑgo	B.	dʒaɪənts
3.	dɛnvɚ	C.	kaʊboɪz
4.	sæn frænsɪsko	D.	dɑlfɪnz
5.	nu jork	E.	tʃɑrdʒɚz
6.	bʌfəlo	F.	brɑnkoz
7.	maɪæmi	G.	bɪlz
8.	dæləs	H.	ræmz
9.	seɪnt luɪs	I.	bɛrz

NFL Level II

Match the city name with the team name.

City		Team Name	
1.	maɪ＿m＿	A.	＿eɪd＿z
2.	oʊkl＿＿＿	B.	b＿r＿
3.	d＿＿v＿	C.	r＿m＿
4.	n＿＿＿or＿	D.	d＿＿fɪn＿
5.	bʌf＿＿＿＿	E.	k＿boɪ＿
6.	seɪ＿＿＿＿u＿s	F.	＿aɪ＿nt＿
7.	＿ək＿＿o	G.	b＿＿＿nk＿＿＿
8.	d＿l＿s	H.	b＿＿＿z

NBA Level I

Match the city name with the team name.

City		Team Name	
1.	indiænə	A.	dʒæz
2.	jutɑ	B.	supɚsɑnɪks
3.	finɪks	C.	leɪkɚz
4.	nu jork	D.	hit
5.	lɑs ænd ʒəlɛs	E.	peɪsɚz
6.	sæn æntonio	F.	bəlz
7.	siætəl	G.	spɚz
8.	ʃəkɑgo	H.	sʌnz
9.	maɪæmi	I.	nɪks

NBA Level II

Match the city name with the team name.

City		Team Name	
1.	＿ju dʒ＿zi	A.	t＿eɪ＿lbl＿z＿z
2.	gold＿＿s＿eɪ	B.	＿əl＿
3.	ʃə＿a＿o	C.	s＿p＿sɑn＿k＿
4.	p＿r＿lɪ＿	D.	wor＿＿z
5.	＿ɑrl＿t	E.	k＿＿z
6.	s＿＿təl	F.	＿ɛt＿
7.	＿æk＿＿m＿nt＿	G.	＿æ＿
8.	＿＿tɑ	H.	h＿rn＿ts

NHL Level I

Match the city name with the team name.

City		Team Name	
1.	nu dʒɚzi	A.	reɪndʒɚz
2.	sæn hozeɪ	B.	maɪti dʌks
3.	lɑs ænd ʒəlɛs	C.	oɪlɚz
4.	nu jork	D.	dɛvəlz
5.	ænəhaɪm	E.	flaɪɚz
6.	fɪlədælfiə	F.	fleɪmz
7.	ɛdməntɪn	G.	ʃɑrks
8.	kælgəri	H.	kɪŋz

NHL Level II

Match the city name with the team name.

City		Team Name	
1.	dit＿＿t	A.	k＿＿＿z
2.	n＿＿dʒ＿z＿	B.	fl＿＿z
3.	lɑ＿æ＿＿lɛ＿	C.	＿＿dwi＿＿
4.	＿æn ho＿＿	D.	m＿t＿d＿k＿
5.	＿j＿＿or＿	E.	dɛv＿＿＿
6.	t＿＿ɑnt＿	F.	reɪn＿＿＿＿
7.	f＿＿ə＿ælf＿＿	G.	ʃ＿＿ks
8.	æn＿h＿m	H.	meɪ＿ə＿＿if＿

IPA Distinctive Feature Level I

Match the International Phonetic Alphabet (IPA) symbol in the left column with its distinctive feature in the right column.

IPA Symbol		Distinctive Feature	
1.	tʃ	A.	liŋwɑ-dɛntəl
2.	θ	B.	baɪleɪɪbiəl

3. aʊ   C. ʌnraʊnd
4. b   D. mɪdfrənt
5. i   E. æfrɪkət
6. ɛ   F. dɪfəɑŋ

IPA Distinctive Feature Level II

Match the IPA symbol in the left column with its distinctive feature in the right column.

IPA Symbol   *Distinctive Feature*

1. f   A. æ __ __ kə __
2. ŋ   B. leɪ __ __ __ l-d __ __ __ əl
3. ʤ   C. __ t __ p
4. t   D. ʌn __ __ n __
5. æ   E. l __ __ s
6. ʌ   F. li __ __ w __ - __ __ lə˞

HALF AND HALF

Connect two segments that form a word. Put a line through the segments identified.

səl	təl	sɪv	sɛp
dor	fri	fan	dɛn
tən	fon	təs	glɑ
səm	brɑ	nəm	ælʌ
plo	glɑ	ɪks	ŋkɪ

1. _____
2. _____
3. _____
4. _____
5. _____
6. _____
7. _____
8. _____
9. _____
10. _____

PRESENT–PAST

Transcribe the following words in their present and past tense.

Example: freeze friz   froze froʊz

Ortho   *Phonetic*   *Ortho*   *Phonetic*

1. forget   _____   _____
2. fight   _____   _____
3. fly   _____   _____

4. feed   _____   _____   _____
5. eat   _____   _____   _____
6. drive   _____   _____   _____
7. draw   _____   _____   _____
8. do   _____   _____   _____
9. sleep   _____   _____   _____
10. make   _____   _____   _____
11. leave   _____   _____   _____
12. keep   _____   _____   _____
13. weep   _____   _____   _____
14. spend   _____   _____   _____
15. go   _____   _____   _____

FORWARD AND BACKWARD

Transcribe words phonetically both forward and backward.

Example: but bʌt tʌb

	Forward	*Backward*		*Forward*	*Backward*
1. no	____	____	13. tar	____	____
2. not	____	____	14. won	____	____
3. saw	____	____	15. stop	____	____
4. yam	____	____	16. stab	____	____
5. mood	____	____	17. star	____	____
6. live	____	____	18. span	____	____
7. noel	____	____	19 pot	____	____
8. tub	____	____	20. cod	____	____
9. draw	____	____	21. emit	____	____
10. reed	____	____	22. slap	____	____
11. leg	____	____	23. peek	____	____
12. strap	____	____			

Key: 1. noʊ, ɑn; 2. nɑt, tʌn; 3. sɑ, wʌs; 4. jæm, mei; 5. mʊd, dum; 6. laɪv, ivɪļ; 7. noʊ3l, liɑn; 8. tʌb, bʌt; 9. dɪɑ, wɑrd; 10. reid, dɛr; 11. leig, ʤɛl; 12. stræp, pærts; 13. tɑr, ræt; 14. wʌn, naʊ; 15. stɑp, pæts; 16. stæb, bæts; 17. stɑr, ræts; 18. spæn, næps; 19. pɑt, tæp; 20. kɑd, dɑk; 21. emɛt, təɪm; 22. slæp, paɪlz; 23. pik, kip

SECRET CODE

Identify the number that goes with the phonetic symbol to form your message. Enter the numbers on the broken lines, and write your answer after the message. Inform the receiver of the message to translate the numbers into the words before they look at the answer. You may want to make extra copies of this form.

__ __ __ __ __ __ __ __ __ __

__ __ __ __ __ __ __ __ __

— — — — — — — — — — —

— — — — — — — — — — —

— — — — — — — — — — —

— — — — — — — — — — —

— — — — — — — — — — —

— — — — — — — — — — —

Message: _____

_____

_____

b	d	f	g	h	j	k	l	m	n	ŋ
1	2	3	4	5	6	7	8	9	10	11
p	r	s	t	v	w	ʍ	Θ	ð	ʃ	ʒ
12	13	14	15	16	17	18	19	20	21	22
ʧ	ʤ	i	ɪ	ɛ	e	æ	ɑ	ɔ	o	ʊ
23	24	25	26	27	28	29	30	31	32	33
u	eɪ	oɪ	aɪ	ʌ	ə	ɝ	ɚ			
34	35	36	37	38	39	40	41			

HALF IN HALF OPPOSITES

Following are 20 sets of opposites, such as *in–out*. Put a line through the words in a set when you have identified each opposite.

1.	pænɪk	2.	pæs	3.	gɪv	4.	oʊld
5.	wɝk	6.	glæd	7.	fɝst	8.	hɑt
9.	lʌv	10.	ɪn	11.	laʊd	12.	kɑlm
13.	kʌm	14.	priti	15.	luz	16.	sæd
17.	hɛvi	18.	kip	19.	hɑrd	20.	heɪt
21.	ʌgli	22.	ɑn	23.	laɪt	24.	kwaɪɛt
25.	læf	26.	sæd	27.	nu	28.	hɛd
29.	læst	30.	sɑft	31.	hæpi	32.	fʊt
33.	aʊt	34.	pleɪ	35.	ɔf	36.	risɪv
37.	kraɪ	38.	goʊ	39.	wɪn	40.	koʊld

List the 20 sets of opposites here.

1. _____ 11. _____
2. _____ 12. _____
3. _____ 13. _____
4. _____ 14. _____
5. _____ 15. _____
6. _____ 16. _____
7. _____ 17. _____
8. _____ 18. _____
9. _____ 19. _____
10. _____ 20. _____

Key: panic (1)/calm (12); pass (2)/receive (36); give (3)/keep (18); old (4)/new (27); work (5)/play (34); glad (6)/sad (16 or 26); first (7)/last (29); hot (8)/cold (40); love (9)/hate (20); in (10)/out (33); loud (11)/quiet (24); head (28)/foot (32); come (13)/go (38); pretty (14)/ugly (21); lose (15)/win (39); heavy (17)/light (23); laugh (25)/cry (37); hard (19)/soft (30); on (22)/off (35); happy (31)/sad (26 or 16)

WORDS THAT RHYME

Identify two other words that rhyme with the following words and transcribe them phonetically on the lines provided.

1. dinner ___ ___
2. plow ___ ___
3. shower ___ ___
4. learn ___ ___
5. myrrh ___ ___
6. grab ___ ___
7. boys ___ ___
8. trunk ___ ___
9. pickle ___ ___
10. hello ___ ___

WORD SEARCH

Look for the following words in their transcribed form in the word search grid.

1. deaf   4. septum
2. hertz   5. stop
3. pidgin 6. stress

ɑ	t	s	t	ɑ	p
h	ɝ	t	s	i	ɪ
ɚ	d	r	ɛ	f	ʤ
r	d	ɛ	f	ʌ	ɪ
t	ʌ	s	æ	d	n
s	ɛ	p	t	ə	m

Look for the following words in their transcribed form in the word search grid.

1. dorsum
2. frenum
3. lax
4. liquid
5. rhythm
6. tongue

l	ɪ	k	w	ɪ	d
æ	m	t	ə	s	o
k	ɪ	ʌ	θ	k	r
s	r	ŋ	ɪ	d	s
r	ɪ	ð	ə	m	ə
f	r	i	n	ə	m

Look for the following words in their transcribed form in the word search grid.

1. accent
2. deaf
3. glottis
4. lingual
5. lips
6. prosody
7. tongue

p	g	l	ɑ	t	ə	s
r	s	i	w	ʌ	ʃ	æ
ɑ	o	ŋ	ɚ	ŋ	tʃ	k
s	ɑ	g	j	ɑ	ɛ	s
ə	t	w	d	ɛ	f	ɛ
d	θ	ə	s	r	k	n
i	ŋ	l	ɪ	p	s	t

1. æksɛnt
2. dɛf
3. glɑtɪs
4. lɪŋɡəl
5. lɪps
6. prɑsɪdi
7. ɪʌŋ

Look for the following words in their transcribed form in the word search grid.

1. affricates
2. cartilage
3. intensity
4. intrinsic
5. mandible
6. pharynx
7. phoneme
8. quality
9. stop

f	m	æ	n	d	ɪ	b	ə	l	k
o	v	f	ɛ	r	i	l	s	o	ɑ
f	ɛ	r	ɪ	ŋ	k	s	t	ɚ	r
o	ɚ	ɪ	s	o	tʃ	v	s	u	t

n	ə	k	ʍ	ɑ	l	ə	t	i	ɪ
i	t	ə	s	p	ɪ	dʒ	ɑ	ʌ	l
m	u	t	ʒ	r	ɑ	o	p	ɑ	ə
æ	n	s	ʌ	t	i	ʃ	f	o	dʒ
n	ɪ	n	t	ɛ	n	s	ə	t	i
d	ɪ	n	t	r	ɪ	n	s	ɪ	k

SAME SPELLING, DIFFERENT WORDS

Phonetically transcribe the underlined words in the blanks provided.

Example: To wind waɪnd the windmill the wind wɪnd has to be very strong.

1. The couple decided to desert _____ their tour guide in the desert _____.
2. The wound _____ required a bandage to be wound _____ around it.
3. I will polish _____ the Polish _____ metal.
4. The dove _____ dove _____ back to its nest.
5. He did not object _____ to the object _____ being sold.
6. The drummer had a bass _____ drum at the bass _____ fish bake.
7. He will present _____ the present _____ to the mayor.
8. The lead _____ singer was lead _____ onto the stage.
9. The produce _____ of the field will produce _____ a high yield.
10. The invalid _____ discovered that the ticket was invalid _____.
11. The deadline for the proposal was too close _____ to close _____ it.
12. The buck deer does _____ his thing to attract the does _____.
13. Did I see a tear _____ in the girl's eye when she had a tear _____ in her dress?
14. Before the farmer went to sow _____ the seeds in the field, he fed his sow _____.
15. The authorities had to refuse _____ to allow refuse _____ to be placed outside the bins.

Phonetic Dice Game Score Pad

Name: _____

1. _____
2. _____
3. _____
4. _____
5. _____
6. _____
7. _____
8. _____
9. _____
10. _____

Score: _____

Name: _____

1. _____
2. _____
3. _____
4. _____
5. _____
6. _____
7. _____
8. _____
9. _____
10. _____

Score: _____

Name: _____

1. _____
2. _____
3. _____
4. _____
5. _____
6. _____
7. _____
8. _____
9. _____
10. _____

Score: _____

Name: _____

1. _____
2. _____
3. _____
4. _____
5. _____
6. _____
7. _____
8. _____
9. _____
10. _____

Score: _____

Name: _____

1. _____
2. _____
3. _____
4. _____
5. _____
6. _____
7. _____
8. _____
9. _____
10. _____

Score: _____

Name: _____

1. _____
2. _____
3. _____
4. _____
5. _____
6. _____
7. _____
8. _____
9. _____
10. _____

Score: _____

[l] [p]   [o][ju]
[n][m]   [u]
[k]   [aɪ]
[b][d̠]   [eɪ]
[j] [g]   [e̠] [i]
[h] [f]   [ɾ] [c̠]
[r] [w̠]   [ɔɪ] [l̩]
[v] [t]   [n̩] [ʊ]
[s] [z]   [æ]
[ʧ][ʤ]   [v̄]
[w̄] [ŋ]   [ē]
[Ө] [ʃ]   [ɑ]
[ð] [ʒ]   [ɛ]
[ou]   [ɪ]

Glossary

Abduction   The opening of the vocal folds during the phonation of voiceless sounds. The glottis is open.

Accent   A dialect or native language affected by the manner in which it is pronounced.

Acoustic phonetics   The study of the acoustic aspects of speech sounds that includes the frequency (Hz), duration (length), and intensity (dB).

Adduction   The opposite of abduction; the vocal folds close to create a vibration of voicing phoning.

Affricate   A consonant that begins with a stop and is released as a fricative.

Allophones   Phonemes, such as the initial [p] in *pop* and the final [p] in *pop*, where there is a slight variation in the production of the two sounds.

Allophonic variation   The same sound with slight variation from the other sound. For example, in the word *pop*, the initial *p* is slightly different in production from how the final *p* is produced, but both are recognized as the [p] sound.

Alveolar   The placement of the tongue tip or blade on the gum ridge behind the upper teeth. This includes the [t] and [z].

Alveolar ridge   The gum ridge behind the upper teeth.

Articulation   The configurations made by speech organs in the vocal tract to modify the airstream, such as the restriction created by the tongue and the upper teeth in the sound [s].

Articulatory phonetics   Phonetics that focuses on the speech sound production including manner in which the airflow is modified, voicing, and placement of the articulators.

Audition   The process of the hearing mechanism receiving speech signals and interpreting them.

Bilabial   Articulation of a speech sound such as [p] or [m] in which both lips come together.

Bilabial stop   Production of sounds that involves the upper and lower lips such as the [b] and [p] sounds.

Broad transcription   A method of transcription of phonemes that does not include diacritic markings and that therefore does not demonstrate differences in production.

Clinical phonetics   Phonetics that focuses on the application of phonetic information in a clinical setting.

Cluster reduction   The deletion of one or more phonemes from a consonant blend or cluster.

Cognates   Consonant sounds that are the same in manner and placement but different in voicing, such as [p] and [b].

Cognate pair   Two sounds that are the same in placement of the articulators and manner in which the airflow is modified but different in voicing, such as the [b] "voiced" and the [t] "unvoiced."

Consonant   A sound that is usually found at the beginning or end of a syllable resulting from a partial or complete constriction of the vocal tract.

Denasality   Speech sounds made when the tongue touches the front teeth.

Dental   Refers to the teeth, such as labiodental (lips and teeth) sounds, such as the [f] sound.

Depth   Front to back; used to describe the position of the tongue blade in the production of vowel sounds.

Diacritic markings   Symbols used to modify alphabet letters to show differences in pronunciation.

Diphthongs   Vowels in which the sound begins with one vowel and moves to another vowel, such as the *oi* in *boil*.

Distinctive features   A set of phonemic traits that describe the sounds of human speech.

Epiglottis   A cartilaginous structure that protects the larynx from food and liquids during swallowing.

Flap or tap   A movement of the tongue in contact with another articulator in returning to its resting position.

Frequency   A measurement of the variation in air pressure of a sound wave and perceived as pitch.

Fricatives   Produced by forcing the airstream through a narrow channel, such as for the [f] and [v] sounds.

Glottal stop   A speech sound that is made by allowing air pressure to build up behind the adducted (closed) vocal folds; when the folds are abducted (opened), the drop in pressure creates the glottal stop.

Grapheme   An alphabet letter.

Historical phonetics   The study of the development of a language sound system and its changes over time.

Homorganic   Two consonants that have the same placement of articulation, such as the [v] and [f].

Implosive   A stop that is made with an ingressive glottal airstream such as *Sindhi*.

Intensity   The loudness or amplitude of a sound measured by instrument or perceived by a listener.

International Phonetic Alphabet   Phonetic symbols that are assigned to human speech sounds such as the voiceless *th* [Θ]. In contrast, the orthographic alphabet includes letters that are not sensitive to sound variations.

Intonation   The pattern of pitch changes that happen during a phrase.

Labiodental   A consonant that is made by the upper front teeth connecting with the lower lip; for example, [f] and [v].

Loudness   The auditory perception of a sound whereby a listener can distinguish the difference in degree of loudness but that does not change the meaning.

Mandible   The lower jaw.

Manner of articulation   The modification of the airstream in the production of stops, fricatives, affricates, and other speech sounds.

Narrow transcription   A transcription method that shows the nonphonemic portions of a pronunciation and is also known as close or phonetic transcription.

Obstruents   A category of sounds that are also known as nonresonant consonants that include stops, fricatives, and affricatives.

Orthography   A system of spelling and writing language.

Perceptual phonetics   Characteristics of speech sounds, such as pitch, loudness, length, and quality of tone, as perceived by the listener.

Phonation   The production of sound by vibration of the vocal folds as the airstream passes through the larynx from the lungs.

Phonetics   The study of human speech sounds.

Phonics   A method of identifying the sounds of the language primarily used in the acquisition of reading skills.

Phonology   The description of the patterns of sounds that take place in a language and the system used, for example, how the phonemes are structured to make syllables, words, and sentences.

Places of articulation   Concerned with the physical anatomy (lips, teeth, etc.) in the production of speech sounds.

Plosive   A burst of air that is produced as a result of a stop and release of the airflow, such as the [p], [b], [k], [g], [t], and [d] sounds.

Pragmatic phonetics   Concerned with who is articulating, what the topic is, and situations that affect speech production styles.

Rate   The time it takes to begin and end an utterance.

Retroflex   When the position of the tongue tip is raised and curved back toward the alveolar ridge causing a velar constriction.

Rhythm   The melody of the utterance.

Semi vowel   A consonant sound that is articulated in the same way as a vowel with similar resonant qualities, but does not form a syllable by itself, as in [w] in "*why*."

Sounds   In phonetics, the production of meaningful human sounds including clicks that convey meaning.

Spectrogram   A graph that prints out on a spectrograph the elements of time and intensity.

Stress   Changes that occur affecting pitch, loudness, and duration of speech within an utterance.

Stridency   This term is applied to the fricatives and affricates that are produced in a high-frequency turbulence resulting from the constriction of the airflow.

Suprasegmentals   Units of speech that include changes in stress, intonation, length, and timing.

Syllables   Units of speech that usually consist of a segment of varying acoustic energy, either stressed or not stressed; units of speech that are made of an onset and a rhyme.

Velar   Sounds such as the [k], [g], and [ŋ] that involve the soft palate.

Voiced   A sound that is made with the vibration of vocal folds.

Index

O

P